# Workbook for

# Mosby's Essentials *for* Nursing Assistants

## THIRD EDITION

**Bernie Gorek, RNC, GNP, MA, NHA**
Gerontology Consultant
Greeley, Colorado

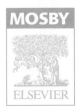

**MOSBY**

ELSEVIER

MOSBY
ELSEVIER

11830 Westline Industrial Drive
St. Louis, Missouri 63146

WORKBOOK FOR MOSBY'S ESSENTIALS FOR NURSING ASSISTANTS      ISBN-13: 978-0-323-03760-0
Third Edition                                                ISBN-10: 0-323-03760-7
**Copyright © 2006, Mosby Inc. All rights reserved.**

---

**Notice**

---

Previous editions copyrighted 2001, 1997 by Mosby, Inc.

**ISBN-13: 978-0-323-03760-0**
**ISBN-10: 0-323-03760-7**

*Executive Editor:* Susan R. Epstein
*Developmental Editor:* Maria Broeker
*Publishing Services Manager:* John Rogers
*Senior Project Manager:* Kathleen L. Teal
*Cover and Text Designer:* Kathi Gosche

Printed in the United States of America

Last digit is the print number:  9  8  7  6  5  4

Working together to grow
libraries in developing countries

www.elsevier.com | www.bookaid.org | www.sabre.org

ELSEVIER    BOOK AID International    Sabre Foundation

In memory of
Cathy Martin
You fought the good fight.
May you find peace.

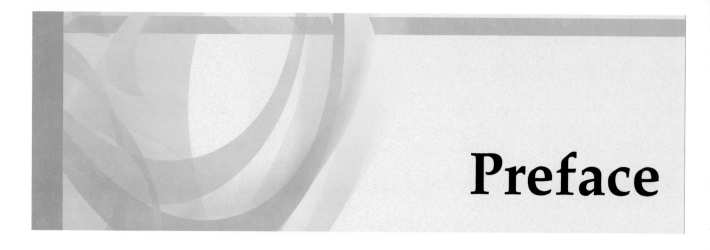

# Preface

This workbook is written to be used with Mosby's *Essentials for Nursing Assistants* textbook, third edition by Sheila A. Sorrentino and Bernie Gorek. Any reference to the "textbook" or to the "book" in this workbook refers to *Mosby's Essentials for Nursing Assistants,* third edition.

This workbook is designed to help you apply what you have learned in each chapter. You are encouraged to use this workbook as a study guide. Various types of questions (Matching, Fill in the Blanks, and Multiple Choice) and **Learning Exercises** are included in each chapter to help you understand and apply the information in the textbook. Questions from *Sorrentino: Mosby's Nursing Assistant Skills Videos* are included in chapters where they apply. The videos are a valuable learning tool. You are encouraged to use them to enhance your learning experience and to reinforce what you read in the textbook.

**Case Studies** are provided for each chapter. They will help you think about what you have learned and apply your knowledge in practical situations. Likewise, the

**Additional Learning Activities** encourage discussion and practical application of the information presented in each chapter. These activities are meant to challenge the student and add to the learning experience.

**Procedure Checklists** are provided that correspond with the procedures in each chapter of Mosby's *Essentials For Nursing Assistants,* third edition. NNAAP™ Skills are identified. These checklists are intended to help you become confident and skilled when performing procedures that affect the quality of care you provide.

Nursing assistants are important members of the health and nursing teams. Completing the exercises in this workbook will increase your knowledge, skills, and confidence. The goal is to prepare you to provide the best possible care and to help you develop pride in the important work you do.

**Bernie Gorek**

# Contents

# 1 Introduction to Health Care Agencies

## OBJECTIVES

The questions and student activities in this chapter will help you meet these objectives.
- Define the key terms listed in this chapter
- Describe hospitals and long-term care centers
- Describe the persons cared for in long-term care centers
- Identify members of the nursing team and the health team
- Describe four nursing care patterns
- Describe programs that pay for health care
- Describe the Omnibus Budget Reconciliation Act of 1987
- Explain resident's rights and patient's rights

## STUDY QUESTIONS

*Crossword*

### Across

1. Fills drug orders written by doctors and monitors and evaluates drug actions and interactions
6. Diagnoses and treats diseases and injuries
7. Assesses and plans for nutritional needs
8. Prevents, diagnoses, and treats foot disorders

### Down

1. Assists persons with musculoskeletal problems; focuses on restoring function and preventing disability
2. Assists with spiritual needs
3. Helps persons and families with social, emotional, and environmental issues affecting illness and recovery
4. Assists nurses in giving nursing care: supervised by a licensed nurse
5. Tests hearing; prescribes hearing aids; works with hearing-impaired persons

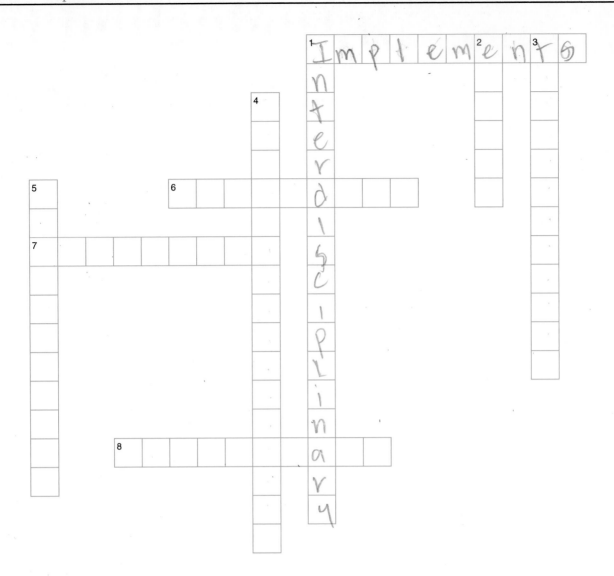

Across:
1. Implements

Down:
1. Interdisciplinary

## Matching

*Match each term with the correct definition.*

1. __A__  Provides a room, meals, laundry, and supervision: residential care facility

2. _____  Staff members who work together to provide health care

3. _____  A nurse who has completed a 1-year nursing program and who has passed a licensing test

4. _____  A person who gives basic nursing care under the supervision of a licensed nurse

5. _____  Provides health care services to persons who need regular or continuous care

6. _____  An agency or program for persons who are dying

7. _____  RNs, LPNs/LVNs, and nursing assistants

8. _____  A law that requires nursing centers to provide care in a manner and in a setting that maintains or improves a person's quality of life, health, and safety

9. _____  Complex medical care or rehabilitation for persons who no longer need hospital care

10. _____  A person who has completed a 2-, 3-, or 4-year nursing program and has passed a licensing test

11. _____  A nursing center that provides complex care for persons with severe health problems

12. __K__  Provides housing, support services, and health care to persons needing help with daily activities

A. Board and care home

B. Health team

C. Omnibus Budget Reconciliation Act of 1987 (OBRA)

D. Licensed practical nurse (LPN)

E. Registered nurse (RN)

F. Nursing center (nursing facility, nursing home)

G. Nursing team

H. Nursing assistant

I. Skilled nursing facility (SNF)

J. Subacute care

K. Assisted living facility

L. Hospice

## Fill in the Blanks

13. Hospitals and long-term care centers provide

    health services. _____

    is the focus of care.

14. Define the following terms:

    A. Acute illness _____

    _____

    B. Chronic illness_____

    _____

    C. Terminal illness_____

    _____

15. _____

    _____

    is a document that explains the person's

    rights and expectations during hospital

    stays.

16. Persons who live in long-term care centers are

    called _____.

17. Long-term care centers are designed to meet the needs of persons who cannot care for themselves at home, but do not need hospital care. Describe the following types of residents cared for in long-term care centers:

    A. Confused and disoriented residents _____

    _____

    _____

    B. Short-term residents_____

    _____

    _____

    C. Mentally ill residents _____

    _____

    _____

18. A disability occurring before 22 years of age is a

    _____.

19. List two other names for nursing center.

    A. _____

    B. _____

20. An Alzheimer's unit is designed for _____.

    _____.

21. A hospital has a governing body called the

    _____.

22. In nursing centers, department heads report to

    _____.

23. Which health team member is responsible for the entire nursing staff and the care given?

    _____

24. Nursing education staff are responsible for:

    A. _____

    B. _____

    C. _____

    D. _____

    E. _____

25. To work in nursing centers, nursing assistants must:

    A. _____

    B. _____

26. Describe primary nursing. _____

    _____

    _____

    _____

27. The goal of the health team is to _____

    _____.

28. _____ is a federal health insurance program for persons 65 years of age and older.

29. Ms. Green is a nursing center resident. She is not able to exercise her rights. Who can do so for her?

    _____

    _____

30. Nursing center must be informed of their rights.

    A. When is this done? _____

    _____

    B. How is this done? _____

    _____

31. Mr. Fink tells you he will not take his walk this

    morning. What should you do? _____

    _____

32. Residents have the right to be free from abuse.

    This includes _____

    _____.

33. Involuntary seclusion involves:

    A. _____

    B. _____

    C. _____

       _____

34. A doctor's order is needed for restraint use. Restraints are not used:

    A. _____

       _____

    B. _____

       _____

35. Nursing center activity programs must promote

    _____

    _____.

36. Write the meanings of the following abbreviations.

    A. LPN _____

    B. NF _____

    C. RN _____

    D. OBRA _____

    E. SNF _____

    F. DON _____

    G. LVN _____

    H. DRG _____

    I. RUG _____

    J. CMG _____

    K. OT _____

    L. PT _____

37. Mr. Martinez is having difficulty swallowing.

    Which health team member evaluates

    swallowing disorders? _____

    _____

38. Mr. Fink cannot hold onto his fork when he tries to eat. Which health team member will evaluate the problem and design eating utensils to help Mr. Fink eat independently?

    _____

*Multiple Choice*

Circle the **BEST** Answer

39. Team nursing:
    A. Focuses on tasks and jobs
    B. Involves a team of nursing staff led by an RN
    C. Involves a primary nurse who is responsible for the person's total care
    D. Is when a case manager coordinates the person's care

40. Which is a health care payment program sponsored by federal and state governments? (Benefits, rules, and eligibility vary from state to state.)
    A. Private insurance
    B. Medicare
    C. Medicaid
    D. Prospective payment

41. Managed care:
    A. Is a health insurance plan sponsored by the federal government
    B. Is a nursing care pattern
    C. Deals with health care delivery and payment
    D. Is required by OBRA

42. This prospective payment system is for SNF payments.
    A. Diagnosis-related groups
    B. Resource utilization groups
    C. Case mix groups
    D. Private insurance

43. Nursing center residents have the right to information. This includes all of the following *except* the right to:
    A. See all of his or her records
    B. Be fully informed of his or her total condition
    C. Information about his or her doctor
    D. Be informed about the condition of his or her roommate

44. If a person does not give consent or refuses treatment, it cannot be given.
    A. True
    B. False

45. Ms. Howard received a letter from her daughter. You know that Ms. Howard cannot read. You can open the letter without her consent.
    A. True
    B. False

46. Which action promotes courteous and dignified care?
    A. Styling the person's hair the way you like it
    B. Rearranging pictures in the person's room
    C. Allowing the person to choose what clothing to wear
    D. Doing everything for the person

47. Which action does *not* promote the person's privacy?
    A. Draping the person properly during care procedures
    B. Knocking on the door before entering the person's room
    C. Closing the bathroom door when the person uses the bathroom
    D. Providing care with the room door open

## MOSBY'S NURSING ASSISTANT SKILLS VIDEOS EXERCISES

## Questions from the "Patient and Resident Rights" Section of the Basic Principles Video

48. Wherever you work, you must be familiar with_____ and _____.

49. List four measures to protect the person's right to privacy.

    A. _____

    B. _____

    C. _____

    D. _____

50. To protect the right to confidentiality, you should

    _____

    _____

51. You protect the right to personal choice by

    _____

    _____

## CASE STUDY

*Mr. George Jansen is a 66-year-old man who had surgery to repair a fractured right hip. His wife died 2 years ago. His son lives in the same town. He is married and has a 16-year-old daughter. Mr. Jansen's son and daughter-in-law work full time. Mr. Jansen lives alone and works part time as a school janitor. This is his third day in the hospital and his second day after surgery. He has Medicare Part A and Part B. His doctor visited Mr. Jansen this morning and told him that he is ready for discharge from the hospital, but that he will need more rehabilitation. The case manager is helping Mr. Hansen with discharge plans.*

*Answer the following questions.*

1. Is Mr. Jansen's condition acute, chronic, or terminal? Explain.

2. Can Mr. Jansen go directly home from the hospital? Explain.

3. What care and services might Mr. Jansen need?

5. What health care agencies might be involved in meeting Mr. Jansen's needs?

4. What health team members might be involved in his care?

6. How might Mr. Jansen pay for his care?

## ADDITIONAL LEARNING ACTIVITIES

1. Look in the yellow pages of the telephone book and list the hospitals, nursing centers, and assisted living facilities in your community. If the services provided are identified, list them.

3. Look at your health insurance policy.
   A. Do you know which services are covered and which are not?

   B. Does your policy limit where you can go for health care? Explain.

2. Collect brochures from the hospitals, nursing centers, and assisted living facilities in your community. Compare the content.
   A. What services are provided?

   B. Are hospice services available?

4. Carefully read the section in this chapter about "resident rights" under OBRA.
   A. Explain why these rights are important to you.

   C. What other information about the hospital, nursing center, and assisted living facility is provided?

   B. Explain how you might react if one or more of your rights were taken away?

# The Nursing Assistant

## OBJECTIVES

The questions and student activities in this chapter will help you meet these objectives.
- Define the key terms listed in this chapter
- Describe the educational requirements for nursing assistants
- Explain what nursing assistants can do and their role limits
- Explain why you need a job description
- Describe the delegation process and how to use the "five rights of delegation"
- Give examples of defamation, assault, battery, false imprisonment, invasion of privacy, and fraud
- Describe how to protect the right to privacy
- Explain the purpose of informed consent
- Describe elder abuse

## STUDY QUESTIONS

*Crossword*

*Across*

2. Negligence by a professional person
4. Intentionally attempting or threatening to touch a person's body without the person's consent
9. Touching a person's body without his or her consent
10. A function, procedure, activity, or work that does not require an RN's professional knowledge or judgement

*Down*

1. A rule of conduct made by a government body
3. A wrong committed against a person or the person's property
5. Making false statements orally
6. Making false statements in print, writing, or through pictures or drawings
7. Knowledge of what is right conduct and wrong conduct
8. An act that violates a criminal law

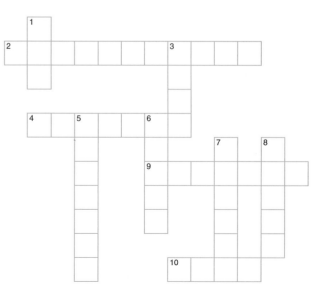

## Matching

*Match each term with the correct definition.*

1. _____ Laws dealing with relationships between people

2. _____ Laws concerned with offenses against the public and society in general

3. _____ Injuring a person's name and reputation by making false statements to a third person

4. _____ To authorize another person to perform a task

5. _____ The intentional mistreatment or harm of another person

6. _____ Saying or doing something to trick, fool, or deceive another person

7. _____ Unlawful restraint or restriction of a person's freedom of movement

8. _____ When a person's name, picture, or private affairs are exposed or made public without consent

9. _____ An unintentional wrong in which a person fails to act in a reasonable and careful manner and causes harm to a person or property

10. _____ A list of responsibilities and functions the agency expects you to perform

A. Delegate

B. Negligence

C. Job description

D. Fraud

E. Civil law

F. False imprisonment

G. Abuse

H. Criminal law

I. Invasion of privacy

J. Defamation

## Fill in the Blanks

11. In order to protect patients and residents from harm, you need to know:

    A. _____

    B. _____

    C. _____

12. OBRA requires each state to have a nursing

    assistant _____

    _____

    It must be completed by nursing assistants

    working in _____.

    _____

13. List the three main content areas included in the National Nurse Aide Assessment Program's (NNAAP) written examination.

    A. _____

    B. _____

    C. _____

14. The _____ is an

    official record of persons who have successfully

    completed a state-approved nursing assistant

    training and competency evaluation

    program.

15. What information about each nursing assistant is contained in the nursing assistant registry?

    A. _____

    _____

    B. _____

    _____

    C. _____

    _____

    D. _____

    _____

    E. _____

    _____

    F. _____

    _____

    G. _____

    _____

16. Nursing agencies must provide educational

    programs for nursing assistants. They must also

    evaluate their work. What is the purpose of

    these requirements? _____

    _____

    _____

    _____

17. To protect persons from harm you must understand:

    A. _____

    B. _____

    C. _____

18. Before you perform a task or procedure, you must make sure that:

    A. _____

    _____

    B. _____

    _____

    C. _____

    _____

    D. _____

    _____

19. The _____

    tells you what the agency expects you to do.

20. Do not take a job that requires you to:

    A. _____

    _____

    B. _____

    _____

    C. _____

    _____

21. List the 8 role limits for nursing assistants. (Things you should never do.)

    A. _____

    _____

    B. _____

    _____

    C. _____

    _____

    D. _____

    _____

    E. _____

    _____

F. _____

_____

G. _____

_____

H. _____

_____

22. RNs can delegate tasks to _____

_____.

23. Before delegating a task to you, the nurse must know:

A. _____

B. _____

C. _____

D. _____

E. _____

24. Delegation decisions must result in

_____.

25. List the five rights of delegation.

A. _____

B. _____

C. _____

D. _____

E. _____

26. An _____

behaves and acts in the right way and does not

harm anyone.

27. Ethical behavior involves not being _____

_____or

_____.

28. False imprisonment involves:

A. _____

B. _____

C. _____

29. The Health Insurance Portability and Accountability Act of 1996 (HIPAA) protects the privacy and security of a person's health information. Protected information refers to:

A. _____

B. _____

30. Failure to comply with HIPAA rules can result

in _____

_____.

31. You are admitting Ms. Hazen to the hospital. You tell her that you are a nurse. This is

_____

32. Consent is informed when _____

_____.

33. Mr. Dunn is unconscious. The doctor orders

intravenous therapy and oxygen. How is legal

consent for these treatments obtained? _____

_____

34. Abuse is a crime. Abuse has one or more of the following elements:

A. _____

B. _____

C. _____

D. _____

E. _____

35. Ms. Reed is left lying in bed all day in the same

position. Her son finds her bed wet with urine

when he visits. This is _____

36. You see Mr. Glen's daughter slap him.

This is _____.

37. Involuntary seclusion is _____.

_____

38. OBRA does not allow nursing centers to employ

persons who _____

_____

_____

_____

## Multiple Choice

Circle the **BEST** Answer

39. OBRA requires each state to have a nursing
assistant training program. How many hours of
instruction does OBRA require?
   A. 16
   B. 40
   C. 50
   D. 75

40. How many attempts does OBRA allow you to
successfully complete the competency
evaluation?
   A. Only one attempt
   B. At least two attempts
   C. At least three attempts
   D. At least four attempts

41. The nursing assistant registry is
   A. A skills evaluation
   B. A list of rules and responsibilities for nursing
   assistants

C. An official record of persons who have
   successfully completed a state
   approved training and competency
   evaluation program
D. A procedure book

42. Retraining and a new competency evaluation
program are required
   A. For nursing assistants who have not worked
   for 2 consecutive years
   B. Whenever a nursing assistant changes jobs
   C. If a nursing assistant has a poor performance
   review
   D. Whenever a nursing assistant is accused
   of abuse

43. Nursing assistants
   A. Function under the supervision nurses
   B. Decide what should or should not be done
   for a person
   C. Supervise other nursing assistants
   D. Take telephone orders from the doctor

44. The nurse asks you to perform a task that is not
in your job description. You should
   A. Perform the task after the nurse shows
   you how
   B. Refuse to perform the task and explain
   why
   C. Ask a co-worker to assist you with
   the task
   D. Report the nurse to the administrator

45. The nurse asks you to apply an ankle brace to
Mr. Grey's right ankle. You do not understand
the directions. What should you do?
   A. Ask Mr. Grey to tell you how to apply
   the brace.
   B. Ask the nursing assistant who cared for
   Mr. Grey yesterday to show you how to
   apply the brace.
   C. Ask another nursing assistant to apply
   the brace.
   D. Explain to the nurse that you do not
   understand the instructions.

46. You agree to perform a task. You must do all
of the following *except*
   A. Complete the task safely.
   B. Ask for help when you are unsure.
   C. Report what you did and your observations
   to the nurse.
   D. Delegate the task to another nursing
   assistant if you are busy.

47. You can refuse to perform a delegated task for all of the following reasons *except*
    A. The task is not in your job description.
    B. You do not know how to use the equipment.
    C. You do not want to perform the task because it is unpleasant.
    D. The nurse's directions are unclear.

48. Nursing assistants *do not* delegate.
    A. True
    B. False

49. Which is not a rule of conduct for nursing assistants?
    A. Respect each person as an individual.
    B. Carry out the directions and instructions of the nurse if you have time.
    C. Be loyal to your employer and co-workers.
    D. Keep the person's information confidential.

50. Which action is *not* a good work ethic?
    A. Completing tasks safely
    B. Providing for privacy when performing care measures
    C. Performing a task that is not in your job description
    D. Asking the nurse to explain instructions if you do not understand

51. Which action protects Mr. Arnold's right to privacy?
    A. Opening his mail without consent
    B. Listening to Mr. Arnold's phone conversation with his daughter
    C. Discussing Mr. Arnold's treatment with his roommate
    D. Asking visitors to leave the room when care is given

52. An RN asks you to perform a task beyond the legal limits of your role. You agree to perform the task. Harm is caused. Who is responsible?
    A. You and the RN
    B. Only the RN
    C. Only you
    D. The entire nursing team

53. Sometimes refusing to follow the nurse's directions is your right and duty.
    A. True
    B. False

54. Two nursing assistants are making fun of the way a resident walks. This is
    A. Sexual abuse
    B. Verbal abuse
    C. Neglect
    D. Physical abuse

55. Ms. Adam's granddaughter takes money from Ms. Adam's purse while Ms. Adams is asleep. This is
    A. Involuntary seclusion
    B. Mental abuse
    C. Financial exploitation
    D. Verbal abuse

56. You suspect a person you are caring for is being abused. You must
    A. Report your observations to the nurse.
    B. Call the police.
    C. Tell a co-worker.
    D. Tell the person's doctor.

57. Threatening a person with punishment is
    A. Physical abuse
    B. Neglect
    C. Emotional abuse
    D. Involuntary seclusion

58. Which is *not* a sign of elder abuse?
    A. Complaints of stiff and painful joints
    B. Weight loss
    C. Bleeding and bruising in the genital area
    D. Frequent injuries

## MOSBY'S NURSING ASSISTANT SKILLS VIDEOS EXERCISES

### Questions from the "Roles and Responsibilities" and "Delegation" Sections of the Basic Principles Video

59. As a nursing assistant, you are a member of

    _____

    that works together for _____

    _____.

60. _____

_____ and

_____

define the roles and functions of each team member.

61. Each member of the nursing team is concerned

with _____

_____

of patients, residents, and their families.

62. _____ function with little

supervision when the person's care is simple

and the person's condition is stable.

63. The tasks you perform and the amount of
supervision you need depend on:

A. _____

B. _____

C. _____

64. Never perform a function or task that _____

_____ or

_____.

65. When deciding what to delegate, the nurse must

protect the person's _____

_____ and can only delegate tasks that are

_____

_____.

66. To ensure that tasks are delegated correctly and

safely, the nurse uses _____

_____.

67. Describe each of "the five rights of delegation"
listed below.

A. "The right task" means _____

_____

_____

B. "The right circumstances means" _____

_____

_____

C. "The right person" means _____

_____

_____

D. "The right directions and communication"

means _____

_____

_____

E. "The right supervision" means _____

_____

_____

68. After you finish a task, you must communicate

with the nurse by reporting _____

_____

_____.

## CASE STUDY

*Miss Mary Adams is a 52-year-old woman. She was admitted to the hospital 2 days ago with nausea and vomiting, and complaints of abdominal pain. The nurse tells you that Miss Adams is very anxious and has some demanding behaviors. Miss Adams has had her signal light on three times in the past 30 minutes. You are walking by her room and you overhear a co-worker talking to Miss Adams in a loud voice. The co-worker tells Miss Adams "I can't keep coming in here to straighten your linens. I am very busy. If you keep putting your signal light on, I will take it away from you. I need to spend my time with patients who really need me."*

*Answer the following questions:*

1. Is your co-worker's behavior toward Miss Adams a form of abuse? Explain.

2. What is your responsibility in this situation?

3. Who should you notify about what you heard?

## ADDITIONAL LEARNING ACTIVITIES

1. Read the rules of conduct for nursing assistants.
   A. Think of and list ways you might apply these rules in a job setting.

2. If you are asked to perform a task that you feel is unsafe, how might you handle it?
   A. What could you say?

   B. Who will you talk to about your concerns?

   B. Discuss the importance of these rules with your classmates.

3. List any job functions that you are opposed to doing for moral or religious reasons.
   A. How will you advise your employer of your concerns?

# 3 Work Ethics

## OBJECTIVES

The questions and student activities in this chapter will help you meet these objectives.
- Define the key terms listed in this chapter
- Describe the practices for good health, hygiene, and professional appearance
- Describe the qualities and traits of a successful nursing assistant
- Explain how to get a job
- Explain how to plan for childcare and transportation
- Describe ethical behavior on the job
- Explain the aspects of harassment
- Explain how to resign from a job
- Identify the common reasons for losing a job

## STUDY QUESTIONS

### Matching

Match each term with the correct definition.

1. _____ Trusting others with personal and private information

2. _____ The most important thing at the time

3. _____ To spread rumors or talk about the private matters of others

4. _____ To trouble, torment, offend, or worry a person by one's behavior or comments

5. _____ Staff members work together as a group; each person does his or her part to provide safe and effective care; staff members help each other as needed

6. _____ Behavior in the workplace

A. Gossip

B. Harassment

C. Confidentiality

D. Teamwork

E. Work ethics

F. Priority

### Fill in the Blanks

7. Ethics deals with _____

_____

8. Work ethics involves:

A. _____

B. _____

C. _____

D. _____

9. You must be _____ and

_____ healthy to function at your best.

10. Good nutrition involves

_____.

11. Regular exercise is needed for _____

_____.

12. If you smoke, you must practice hand washing

and good personal hygiene because _____

_____

_____.

13. You must never report to work under the

influence of alcohol or drugs because _____

_____

_____

_____.

14. Why should you keep your fingernails short

and neatly shaped? _____

_____

15. You should not wear perfume, cologne, or after-

shave lotion to work because _____

_____

_____.

16. List 8 ways to find out about jobs.

A. _____

B. _____

C. _____

D. _____

E. _____

F. _____

G. _____

H. _____

17. Employers want employees who:

A. _____

B. _____

C. _____

D. _____

E. _____

18. Explain why it is important for you to be at

work on time and when scheduled? _____

_____

_____

19. Define the following qualities and traits for
good work ethics:

A. Caring _____

_____

B. Empathetic _____

_____

C. Honest _____

_____

20. You are completing a job application. It is important to follow directions because _____

_____

_____.

21. You are completing a job application. A question on the application does not apply to you. What should you do? _____

_____

22. When completing a job application, you will be asked to supply references. How many references should you be prepared to supply?

_____

What information about each reference should you be prepared to give? _____

_____

_____

23. Lying on a job application is _____.

24. You are reviewing the job description during your job interview. You should advise the interviewer of any functions you cannot perform because of _____

_____.

25. List 3 things you need to do when you accept a job.

A. _____

B. _____

C. _____

26. Some agencies have preceptor programs. A preceptor is _____

_____

_____.

27. _____ and _____ are common reasons for losing a job.

28. List four measures that will help you avoid being part of gossip.

A. _____

_____

B. _____

_____

C. _____

_____

D. _____

_____

29. To eavesdrop means to _____

_____

_____.

30. You are scheduled to return from your meal break at noon. Explain why it is important to return from your meal break on time.

_____

_____.

31. _____,

    _____,

    _____, and

    _____

    help you decide what to do and when to do it.

32. Priorities change as _____

    change.

33. Sexual harassment involves _____

    _____.

34. You are resigning from a job. You should include the following in your written notice:

    A. _____

    B. _____

    C. _____

*Multiple Choice*

Circle the **BEST** Answer

35. To look professional, do all of the following *except*
    A. Wear a clean uniform daily.
    B. Wear a lot of jewelry.
    C. Wear your name badge or photo ID.
    D. Wear a wristwatch with a second hand.

36. You are getting ready for a job interview. You should do all of the following *except*
    A. Bathe, brush your teeth, and wash your hair.
    B. Make sure your hands and fingernails are clean.
    C. Make sure your shoes are clean and in good repair.
    D. Wear clean jeans and a tee-shirt.

37. When you arrive for a job interview, you should
    A. Tell the receptionist your name and why you are there.
    B. Spend time visiting with the receptionist until it is time for your interview.
    C. Ask the receptionist how long you will have to wait.
    D. Ask the receptionist questions about the job.

38. You want to make a good impression for a job interview. You must
    A. Stand until asked to take a seat.
    B. Look down or away from the interviewer when answering questions.
    C. Give short "yes or no" answers.
    D. Give long answers and explanations to all questions.

39. You can ask questions at the end of the interview. Which is *not* a good question?
    A. What is the greatest challenge of this job?
    B. What are the uniform requirements?
    C. Can I have 4 days off next month?
    D. How will my performance be evaluated?

40. How soon after a job interview should you send a thank-you note?
    A. Within 24 hours
    B. Within 3 days
    C. Within 1 week
    D. Whenever you have time

41. You are always willing to help and work with others. You are being
    A. Cheerful
    B. Respectful
    C. Cooperative
    D. Enthusiastic

42. Knowing your feelings, strengths, and weaknesses is the quality of
    A. Cooperation
    B. Self-awareness
    C. Caring
    D. Courtesy

43. You have just completed a 2-week orientation program. You are still not comfortable with some of your job duties. What should you do?
    A. Resign from your job.
    B. Discuss your concerns with the administrator.
    C. Do the best you can.
    D. Ask for more orientation time.

44. Proper speech and language at work involves
   A. Controlling the volume and tone of your voice
   B. Shouting to be heard
   C. Using abusive language when needed
   D. Arguing with the person when you know you are right

45. Which of these statements reflects a negative attitude?
   A. "Can I help you?"
   B. "Please show me how this works."
   C. "I can't, I'm too busy."
   D. "Thank you for your help."

46. You can share information about a resident with
   A. The resident's family
   B. The nurse supervising your work
   C. Your co-worker during lunch
   D. Your family and friends

47. Which action will keep personal matters out of the workplace?
   A. Letting family and friends visit you on the unit
   B. Using an agency copy machine to copy recipes for a co-worker
   C. Taking agency pens and pencils home
   D. Making personal phone calls during meals and breaks

48. Setting priorities involves all of the following *except* deciding
   A. Which person has the greatest needs
   B. What tasks need to be done at a set time
   C. What tasks you enjoy doing most
   D. How much help you need to complete a task

49. Harassment is *not* legal in the workplace.
   A. True
   B. False

50. Harassment involves only sexual behavior.
   A. True
   B. False

51. Victims of sexual harassment are always women.
   A. True
   B. False

52. You feel that you are being harassed at work. You must
   A. Tell your co-worker.
   B. Ignore it. You don't want to cause trouble.
   C. Ask your family and friends for advice.
   D. Report it to the nurse and the human resource officer.

53. Common reasons for losing a job include all of the following *except*
   A. Poor attendance
   B. Falsifying a record
   C. Having, using, or distributing drugs in the work setting
   D. Politely refusing to perform a task you were not trained to do

54. You can lose your job for failing to maintain patient confidentiality.
   A. True
   B. False

## CASE STUDY

*Your co-worker, Linda Evans is often 5 to 10 minutes late for work. She has difficulty completing her assignments. You see her walk by Mr. Daniel's room when his signal light is on. She tells you "He is not my patient and I am too busy to stop and answer his signal light."*

*Answer the following questions.*

1. How might Linda's actions affect the quality of care provided to Mr. Daniel?

2. How might Linda's attitude affect the care of other patients?

3. Is Linda practicing good work ethics? Explain.

4. Can Linda's actions cause her to lose her job? Explain.

5. What are your responsibilities in this situation?

## ADDITIONAL LEARNING ACTIVITIES

1. You are preparing for a job interview. Discuss the following:
   A. How you will make a good impression?

   B. How you will show the employer that you have what he/she is looking for in these areas?
   (1) Hygiene measures

   (2) Professional appearance

   (3) Skills and training

   (4) Values and attitude

2. You want to find the right job. Answer the following questions:
   A. What is important to you?

   B. What questions do you want to ask the employer?

   C. Are there functions you cannot perform because of training, legal, ethical, or religious reasons?

3. You have succeeded in getting the job you want. Now it is important to keep your job. How will you make sure that:
   A. You have dependable transportation?

   B. You have child-care, if needed?

C.  You get to work on time?

4.  Practice writing a thank-you letter following a job interview.

D.  You are available to work at the times you are scheduled?

5.  Practice writing a letter of resignation.

E.  You stay healthy so you can function at your best?

# Communicating With the Health Team

## OBJECTIVES

The questions and student activities in this chapter will help you meet these objectives.
- Define the key terms listed in this chapter
- Describe the rules for good communication
- Explain the purpose, parts, and information found in the medical record
- Describe the legal and ethical aspects of medical records
- Describe the purpose of the Kardex
- Explain your role in the nursing process
- List the information you need to report to the nurse
- List the rules for recording
- Use the 24-hour clock, medical terminology, and abbreviations
- Explain how computers are used in health care
- Explain how to protect the right to privacy when using computers
- Describe the rules for answering phones
- Explain how to deal with conflict

## STUDY QUESTIONS
*Crossword*

### Across

2. Involves measuring if the goals in the planning step of the nursing process were met
5. Data (information) that is seen, heard, felt, or smelled
6. Subjective data
8. Data (things) a person tells you about that you cannot observe through your senses
9. The word element which contains the basic meaning of the word
11. Involves collecting information about the person
14. A clash between opposing interests or ideas
15. The written account of care and observations

### Down

1. Another term for the medical record
3. A shortened form of a word or phrase
4. To perform or carry out
7. Setting priorities and goals
10. Using the senses of sight, hearing, touch, and smell to collect information
12. Objective data
13. The method RNs use to plan and deliver nursing care

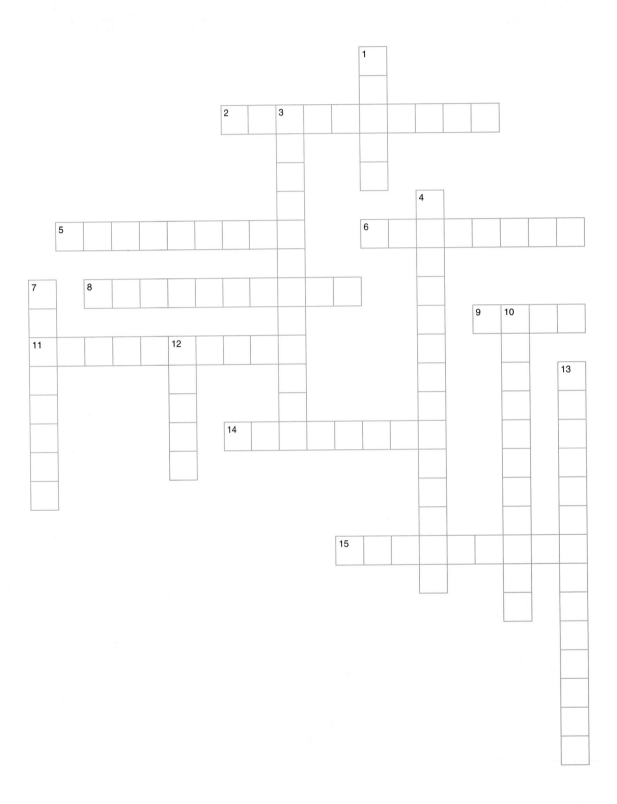

## Matching

*Match each term with the correct definition.*

1. _____ The exchange of information

2. _____ A type of file that summarizes information found in the medical record

3. _____ The identification of a disease or condition by a doctor

4. _____ A written account of a person's condition and response to treatment and care

5. _____ A written guide about the person's care

6. _____ Describes a health problem that can be treated by nursing measures

7. _____ An action or measure taken by the nursing team to help the person reach a goal

8. _____ A written guide giving direction for the resident's care; Required by OBRA.

9. _____ A word element placed before a root; it changes the meaning of a word

10. _____ The oral account of care and observations

11. _____ A word element placed after a root to change the meaning of the word

12. _____ A part of a word

A. Medical diagnosis

B. Prefix

C. Medical record

D. Kardex

E. Communication

F. Nursing intervention

G. Nursing diagnosis

H. Suffix

I. Reporting

J. Word element

K. Comprehensive care plan

L. Nursing care plan

## Fill in the Blanks

13. Health team members share information about:

    A. _____

    B. _____

    C. _____

14. Agency policies about medical records address:

    A. _____

    B. _____

    C. _____

    D. _____

    E. _____

    F. _____

15. If you have access to the medical record

    you must _____

    _____

    _____.

16. What parts of the medical record relate to your work?

    A. _____

    B. _____

    C. _____

    D. _____

    E. _____

17. The _____ is completed

    when the person is admitted to the agency.

    It has the person's identifying information.

18. The graphic sheet is used to record _____

    _____

    _____.

19. In long-term care, summaries of care describe

    _____

    _____.

20. List the five steps of the nursing process in the
    correct order.

    A. _____

    B. _____

    C. _____

    D. _____

    E. _____

21. Indicate whether the observation is subjective or
    objective. (enter "s" or "o")

    A. _____ Pain

    B. _____ Nausea

    C. _____ Vomiting

    D. _____ Dizziness

    E. _____ Clear yellow urine

    F. _____ Warm moist skin

    G. _____ Numbness

    H. _____ Pulse rate of 80 beats per minute

22. _____ are what is

    most important for the person.

23. Goals are aimed at _____

    _____.

24. Describe the purpose of the nursing care plan.

    _____

    _____

    _____

25. The comprehensive care plan identifies:

    A. _____

    B. _____

    C. _____

    D. _____

26. The nurse uses the _____

    to communicate delegated measures and

    tasks to you.

27. You do not understand a task on your
    assignment sheet. What should you do?

    _____

    _____

28. List and define the two types of resident care
    conferences required by OBRA.

    A. _____

    _____

    _____

    B. _____

    _____

    _____

29. Any one who reads your charting should
    know:

    A. _____

    B. _____

    C. _____

30. Convert the following times from standard time to 24-hour clock time.

    A. 6:15 PM _____

    B. 8:00 AM _____

    C. 2:30 PM _____

    D. 5:02 PM _____

    E. 10:55 AM _____

    F. 1:29 PM _____

    G. 1:33 AM _____

    H. 9:00 PM _____

31. Convert the following times from 24-hour clock time to standard time.

    A. 1600 _____

    B. 0945 _____

    C. 1115 _____

    D. 2120 _____

    E. 1705 _____

32. Word elements are:

    A. _____

    B. _____

    C. _____

33. Medical terms are formed by combining word elements. When translating medical terms, begin with the _____.

34. Why is it important to record safety measures (for example: placing the signal light within reach)? _____

    _____

35. Define the following directional terms:

    A. Anterior (ventral) _____

    _____

    B. Distal _____

    _____

    C. Lateral _____

    _____

    D. Medial _____

    _____

    E. Posterior (dorsal) _____

    _____

    F. Proximal _____

36. You are recording care given. You are unsure of an abbreviation. What should you do?

    _____

37. When speaking on the phone, you give much information by:

    A. _____

    B. _____

    C. _____

38. List the information you need to write when taking a phone message.

    A. _____

    B. _____

    C. _____

39. List the steps for transferring a phone call.

    A. _____

    _____

    B. _____

    _____

    C. _____

    _____

40. The problem solving process involves these steps:

    A. _____

    B. _____

    C. _____

    D. _____

    E. _____

    F. _____

41. _____ and

    _____

    help prevent and resolve conflicts.

*Multiple Choice*

Circle the **BEST** Answer

42. For good communication, you should do all of the following *except*
    A. Use familiar words
    B. Be brief and concise
    C. Give unneeded information
    D. Give information in a logical and orderly manner

43. Who has access to a person's medical record?
    A. The person's family members
    B. Staff involved in the person's care
    C. Laundry personnel
    D. Visitors

44. All nursing interventions need a doctor's order.
    A. True
    B. False

45. Care is given during this step of the nursing process.
    A. Assessment
    B. Planning
    C. Implementation
    D. Evaluation

46. Nursing assistants have a key role in the nursing process.
    A. True
    B. False

47. Which statement about resident care conferences is *correct*?
    A. Family members are not allowed to attend.
    B. The resident is required to attend.
    C. Residents may refuse suggestions made by the health team.
    D. Residents attend only if invited by the doctor.

48. You are reporting resident care. Which is *incorrect*?
    A. Report your observations to the nurse.
    B. Report the care that was given by a co-worker.
    C. Reports must be prompt, thorough, and accurate.
    D. Report immediately any changes from normal.

49. When recording, you should do all of the following *except*
    A. Use ink
    B. Use only agency approved abbreviations
    C. Use correct spelling and grammar
    D. Use correcting fluid if you make a mistake

50. When recording you should
    A. Erase errors
    B. Skip lines
    C. Record your judgments
    D. Make sure writing is readable and neat

51. Intake and output is recorded on the
    A. Graphic sheet
    B. Kardex
    C. Admission sheet
    D. Nursing care plan

52. Which is a nursing diagnosis?
    A. Breast cancer
    B. Pneumonia
    C. Bowel incontinence
    D. Diabetes

53. Priorities and goals are set. What step in the nursing process is this?
    A. Assessment
    B. Planning
    C. Implementation
    D. Evaluation

54. Which prefix means "away from"?
    A. ab
    B. anti
    C. dis
    D. epi

55. Which root means "head"?
    A. broncho
    B. cephal (o)
    C. hema
    D. nephr (o)

56. The suffix "algia" means
    A. Cell
    B. Tumor
    C. Disease
    D. Pain

57. What does the medical term "gastritis" mean?
    A. Difficulty urinating
    B. Nerve pain
    C. Inflammation of the stomach
    D. Excision of the ovary

58. Which medical term means study of the skin?
    A. Glossitis
    B. Dermatology
    C. Neuralgia
    D. Bacteriogenic

59. You are using a computer to record care given. Which action will *not* protect the person's privacy?
    A. Preventing others from seeing what is on the screen
    B. Logging off after making an entry
    C. Not leaving printouts where others can read them
    D. Using e-mail to report confidential information

60. Which is *not* a guideline for answering phones?
    A. Give a courteous greeting.
    B. Cover the receiver with your hand when not speaking to the caller.
    C. Return to a caller on hold within 30 seconds.
    D. Do not give confidential information to any caller.

61. Conflict can arise on the job over work schedules, absences, and amount and quality of work. You can do all of the following to help resolve conflicts *except*
    A. Ask your supervisor to meet with you.
    B. Discuss the problem with co-workers during lunch break.
    C. Give facts and specific examples.
    D. Identify ways to solve the problem.

62. Your co-worker frequently does not clean the tub after use. You should
    A. Ask your supervisor for some time to talk privately so you can explain the problem.
    B. Confront your co-worker in the hallway.
    C. Tell the nurse you will not work with the person.
    D. Make sure all team members know how lazy the person is.

## MOSBY'S NURSING ASSISTANT SKILLS VIDEOS EXERCISES

## Questions from the "Nursing Process" Section of the Basic Principles Video

63. The _____ is used to plan and provide nursing care in all health care agencies.

64. You assist with assessment by _____

    _____.

    The nurse uses assessment information to make

    _____.

65. The nursing care plan states _____

    _____

    and identifies _____

    _____

    _____.

66. The nurse involves the entire nursing team in the nursing process.
    A. True
    B. False

## Questions from the "Communication" Section of the Basic Principles Video

67. _____

    is essential for coordinated and effective care.

68. Knowing how to communicate effectively is

    essential for meeting the _____,

    _____, and

    _____ requirements of your work.

69. Communication is oral and written. Information is also conveyed by:

    A. _____

    B. _____

70. For a message to be understood correctly, it

    must be _____,

    _____, and

    _____.

71. What should you do if someone uses a term you

    do not understand? _____

    _____

72. When charting, all entries must include:

    A. _____

    B. _____

## CASE STUDY

*Mr. Juan Gomez is a 75-year-old resident of Valley View Nursing Center. You have been assigned to care for him this morning.*

*Mr. Gomez told you that he had a bowel movement at 0500 (5:00 AM).*

*You helped Mr. Gomez get ready for breakfast by assisting him with mouth care and with washing his face and hands. Mr. Gomez had breakfast sitting in the chair beside his bed. He ate everything on his breakfast tray. After breakfast you took Mr. Gomez for a walk. He walked 20 feet and then complained of being tired, so you assisted him back to his room and helped him into bed.*

*Answer the following questions:*

1. What information would you report and record?

2. Who should you report the information to?

3. What form would you use to record each piece of information?

## ADDITIONAL LEARNING ACTIVITIES

1. Practice answering the phone and taking a written message. You can practice with a classmate or friend.
   A. How would you answer the phone in a professional, courteous manner?

   B. What information should you write down when taking a message?

   C. What steps would you take before putting a person on hold?

2. Practice your observation, recording, and reporting skills. Ask a classmate or member of your family to help. Use Box 4-1 on page 39 in the textbook as a guide for recording your observations.
   A. Talk to the person for about 5 minutes. Use a notepad to write down your observations. Include the following:
      (1) Color and length of hair
      (2) Color of eyes
      (3) Description of any jewelry the person is wearing
      (4) Description of clothing the person is wearing
      (5) Any special features (birth marks, scars, etc.)
      (6) Any information the person gave you about him or herself

   B. Use your notes to give a verbal report.

   C. Discuss the accuracy of your observations.

3. Read the following vignette involving conflict in the workplace. Then answer the questions at the end of the vignette.

   *You are assigned to care for Mrs. Angie Gomez. When you return from your lunch break, Mrs. Gomez's signal light is on. When you answer her signal light, Mrs. Gomez tells you that her light has been on for 25 minutes. Mrs. Gomez also tells you that another nursing assistant walked into her room and told her that she would have to wait until her nursing assistant returned from lunch.*
   A. How would you feel?

   B. What would you say to Mrs. Gomez?

   C. Who would you discuss the situation with?

   D. Where would you discuss the situation?

   E. What steps would you take to solve the problem?

4. Make flash cards of the prefixes, root words, and suffixes in Chapter 4. Write the meaning of each on the back of each flash card. Use the flash cards to help you study and learn medical terms. You can work alone, with a classmate, or with a friend.

# 5 Understanding the Person

## OBJECTIVES

The questions and student activities in this chapter will help you meet these objectives.
- Define the key terms listed in this chapter
- Identify the parts that makeup the whole person and basic needs
- Explain how culture and religion influence health and illness
- Describe the American Hospital Association's *The Patient Care Partnership: Understanding Expectations, Rights, and Responsibilities*
- Describe the feelings and needs of nursing center residents
- Explain how to deal with behavior issues
- Identify the elements needed to communicate
- Describe how to use verbal and nonverbal communication
- Explain the methods for and barriers to good communication
- Explain why family and visitors are important to the person
- Identify the courtesies given to the person and visitors

## STUDY QUESTIONS

*Crossword*

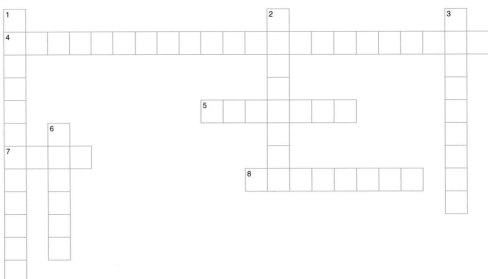

### Across

4. A person's highest potential for mental and physical performance
5. The characteristics of a group of people that are passed from one generation to the next
7. Something necessary or desired for maintaining life and mental well-being
8. Spiritual beliefs, needs, and practices

### Down

1. Messages sent through facial expressions, gestures, posture, hand and body movements, gait, eye contact, and appearance
2. A condition in which the person is unconscious and cannot respond to others
3. Communication that does not use words
6. Communication that uses written or spoken words

## Matching

*Match each term with the correct definition.*

1. _____ Relate to love, closeness, and affection

2. _____ Experiencing one's potential

3. _____ To think well of oneself and to see oneself as useful and having value

4. _____ To focus on verbal and nonverbal communication; using sight, hearing, touch, and smell

A. Self-esteem

B. Love and belonging needs

C. Listening

D. Self-actualization

## Fill in the Blanks

5. The _____ or

_____ is the most

important person in the agency.

6. The whole person has _____,

_____,

_____,

and _____ parts.

7. What is the name of the document that explains the person's rights and expectations during hospital stays?

_____

_____

8. Ms. Mary Martin is a nursing center resident. You

help maintain her optimal level of function by

focusing on her _____, not her

_____.

9. You will be caring for Ms. Martin today. List the courtesies you need to extend before giving care and during care.

A. _____

B. _____

C. _____

D. _____

E. _____

F. _____

10. List the basic needs for life as described by Abraham Maslow (in order of importance).

A. _____

B. _____

C. _____

D. _____

E. _____

11. Persons in hospitals and nursing centers feel safer and more secure if they know what will happen. For every procedure they should know:

    A. _____

    B. _____

    C. _____

    D. _____

12. A person's culture influences health _____

    and _____.

13. List five causes of anger.

    A. _____

    B. _____

    C. _____

    D. _____

    E. _____

14. List six nonverbal signs of anger.

    A. _____

    B. _____

    C. _____

    D. _____

    E. _____

    F. _____

15. Causes of demanding behavior include:

    A. _____

    B. _____

    C. _____

    D. _____

16. Mr. Pete Paulson has difficulty hearing. He also has poor vision. The nurse tells you to write messages to communicate. When writing messages you need to:

    A. _____

    B. _____

    C. _____

17. The meaning of touch depends on _____,

    _____,

    _____, and

    _____.

18. You may use touch to communicate. Touch

    should be _____,

    not _____,

    _____, or

    _____.

19. Listening requires that you care and have interest. You need to follow these guidelines:

    A. _____

    B. _____

    C. _____

    D. _____

    E. _____

20. Giving opinions is a communication barrier.

    Opinions involve _____

    _____.

21. Failure to listen is a communication barrier

    because _____

    _____

    _____.

22. How might illness and disability affect communication?

_____

_____

23. Mr. Pete Paulson has visitors. You need to provide care to Mr. Paulson. What should you do?

_____

_____

_____

*Multiple Choice*

Circle the **BEST** Answer

24. Which needs are the most important for survival?
    A. Self-esteem
    B. Safety and security
    C. Physical
    D. Love and belonging

25. Which needs relate to feeling safe from harm, danger, and fear?
    A. Physical
    B. Safety and security
    C. Love and belonging
    D. Self-esteem

26. Ms. Lois Frank is a nursing center resident. She needs assistance with walking. She wants to attend church services in the center's chapel. You should
    A. Assist her to attend church services.
    B. Tell her family about her request.
    C. Tell her she can attend if she can find a way to get there.
    D. Ask the nurse what to do.

27. Mr. John Reid stays in his room most of the day. He does not attend activities. He does not talk to his family when they visit. This behavior is called
    A. Self-centered behavior
    B. Demanding behavior
    C. Withdrawal
    D. Anger

28. Inappropriate sexual behavior is always on purpose.
    A. True
    B. False

29. A person with aggressive behavior
    A. Is critical of others
    B. May swear, bite, hit, pinch, scratch, or kick
    C. Has little or no contact with others
    D. Has dementia

30. You are giving Ms. Ellen Barr a complete bed bath. She complains about how you are giving the bath. She also tells you that her breakfast was terrible. She says "nobody knows what they are doing and nobody cares about me." You can do all of the following *except*
    A. Explain that you are giving her bath in the right way and you do know what you are doing.
    B. Listen and use silence. Let her express herself.
    C. Stay calm and professional.
    D. Discuss the situation with the nurse.

31. Which action will *not* promote effective communication?
    A. Respecting the person's religion and culture
    B. Giving the person time to process information
    C. Telling the person that you are repeating information
    D. Asking questions to see if the person understood you

32. When using verbal communication, you should
    A. Look away from the person
    B. Speak clearly, slowly, and distinctly
    C. Use slang or vulgar words
    D. Shout to be heard

33. Nonverbal messages more accurately reflect a person's feelings than words do.
    A. True
    B. False

34. Which communication method focuses on certain information?
    A. Listening
    B. Open-ended questions
    C. Clarifying
    D. Direct questions

35. A person's family and visitors
    A. Are treated with courtesy and respect
    B. Often need support and understanding
    C. Are allowed to visit in private
    D. All of the above are correct

36. Using silence shows the person that
    A. You are uncomfortable
    B. You care and respect the person's feelings
    C. You are being rude
    D. You are not listening

37. Which is *not* a communication barrier?
    A. Using touch
    B. Giving opinions
    C. Pat answers
    D. Changing the subject

38. You ask Mr. Adams; "How do you feel about being here?" Which communication method have you used?
    A. A direct question
    B. Clarifying
    C. Silence
    D. An open-ended question

39. Mr. Ben Ortega is comatose. When caring for him, do all of the following *except*
    A. Explain care measures step-by-step as you do them.
    B. Tell him when you are finishing care.
    C. Avoid touching him.
    D. Tell him when you are leaving the room.

40. The presence or absence of family or friends can affect recovery and quality life.
    A. True
    B. False

41. You give visitors support by answering their questions about the person's condition.
    A. True
    B. False

42. You observe that Ms. June Boland's visitor is upsetting her. You must
    A. Ask the visitor to leave.
    B. Report your observation to the nurse.
    C. Ask Ms. Boland if you can help.
    D. Do nothing. It is none of your business.

## CASE STUDY

*Mrs. Sarah Stein was admitted to Pine Crest Nursing Center today. She is an 80-year-old widow of Jewish religion. She came to America from Germany with her parents when she was 12 years old. She speaks German and English fluently. She was a college professor and taught at the local university for 20 years. She was married for 55 years. Her husband died 2 years ago. Mrs. Stein has difficulty hearing and wears eyeglasses. She walks with a cane. Before coming to Pine Crest Nursing Center, she lived with her married daughter for 2 years. Her daughter felt it was no longer safe for her mother to live with her because she was alone most of the day. Mrs. Stein had fallen twice during the past month and has lost 5 pounds.*

*Answer the following questions.*

1. What characteristics make Mrs. Stein unique?

2. How might her culture and religion affect her care plan?

3. How might the RN use the nursing process to help the nursing team meet Mrs. Stein's
   A. Physical needs?

   B. Safety and security needs?

   C. Love and belonging needs?

D. Self-esteem needs?

A.   What measures might help her adjust?

E.  Self-actualization needs?

5. What needs might Mrs. Stein's daughter have?

4. What feelings might Mrs. Stein have about moving to Pine Crest Nursing Center?

A.   What measures might help her adjust?

## ADDITIONAL LEARNING ACTIVITIES

1. Carefully review the Caring about Culture boxes in Chapter 5 in the textbook.
   A. List some ways that knowing about a person's cultural and religious practices might help you give quality care.

   B. Do you have cultural or religious beliefs that are important to you? Explain.

   (1) How do these beliefs influence your health practices?

2. Observe the nonverbal communication during social contacts with family and friends.
   A. Are you aware of your nonverbal communication? Explain.

   B. How do others communicate with you using nonverbal communication?

   C. Do you ever receive mixed messages from a person's verbal and nonverbal communication? Explain.

# 6 Understanding Body Structure and Function

## OBJECTIVES

The questions and student activities in this chapter will help you meet these objectives.
- Define the key terms listed in this chapter
- Identify the basic structures of the cell
- Describe four types of tissue
- Identify the structures of each body system
- Describe the functions of each body system

## STUDY QUESTIONS
*Crossword*

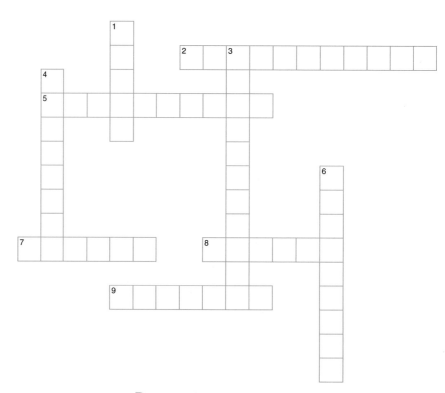

### Across

2. Involuntary muscle contractions in the digestive system that move food through the alimentary canal
5. The burning of food for heat and energy by the cells
7. Organs that work together to perform special functions
8. A groups of cells with similar functions
9. A chemical substance secreted by the glands into the bloodstream

### Down

1. Groups of tissues with the same function
3. The process of supplying the cells with oxygen and removing carbon dioxide from them
4. Protection against a disease or condition; the person will not get or be affected by the disease
6. The process of physically and chemically breaking down food so that it can be absorbed for use by the cells

## Matching

*Match each term with the correct definition.*

1. _____ The basic unit of body structure

2. _____ The skin

3. _____ The point where two or more bones meet

4. _____ Consists of the brain and spinal cord

5. _____ The substance that gives blood its red color

6. _____ The uniting of the sperm and ovum into one cell

A. The integumentary system

B. The central nervous system

C. Cell

D. A joint

E. Fertilization

F. Hemoglobin

## Matching (Immune System)

*The following terms relate to the immune system. Match each term with the correct definition.*

7. _____ The body's reaction to a certain threat

8. _____ Normal body substances that recognize, attack, and destroy abnormal or unwanted substances

9. _____ An abnormal or unwanted substance

10. _____ White blood cells that digest and destroy microorganisms and other unwanted substances

11. _____ White blood cells that produce antibodies

12. _____ The body's reaction to anything that is not a normal body substance

13. _____ React to specific antigens

14. _____ Destroy invading cells

A. B lymphocytes (B cells)

B. Antigens

C. Specific immunity

D. Nonspecific immunity

E. Antibodies

F. T lymphocytes (T cells)

G. Phagocytes

H. Lymphocytes

## Fill in the Blanks

15. Explain why you need to know the body's normal structure and function.

_____

_____

_____

16. List and describe the basic structures of the cell.

A. _____

B. _____

C. _____

D. _____

17. Chromosomes are _____

    _____.

18. Cells reproduce by _____.

    This process is called_____.

19. _____

    tissue covers internal and external body

    surfaces.

20. _____

    tissue stretches and contracts to let the

    body move.

21. What is the function of nerve tissue?

    _____

    _____

22. The largest system is the _____.

23. _____ gives the skin its color.

24. _____,

    _____,

    _____,

    and _____ are skin appendages.

25. List three functions of the musculoskeletal
    system.

    A. _____

    B. _____

    C. _____

26. Name the types of bones and their functions.

    A. _____

    _____

    B. _____

    _____

    C. _____

    _____

    D. _____

    _____

27. A membrane called the _____

    covers bones.

28. _____

    acts a lubricant so the joint can move smoothly.

29. Describe the movement of each type of joint.

    A. Ball-and-socket _____

    _____

    B. Hinge _____

    _____

    C. Pivot _____

    _____

30. _____

    muscles can be consciously controlled.

31. List the three functions of muscles.

    A. _____

    B. _____

    C. _____

32. Strong, tough connective tissues called _____

    _____ connect muscles to bones.

33. The _____

    controls, directs, and coordinates body

    functions.

34. Name and describe the two main divisions of
    the nervous system.

    A. _____

       _____

    B. _____

       _____

35. The three main parts of the brain are:

    A. _____

    B. _____

    C. _____

36. The outside of the cerebrum is called the _____

    _____. It controls

    _____.

37. The brainstem contains the _____,

    _____,

    and _____.

38. The _____

    lies within the spinal column. It contains pathways

    that conduct messages to and from the brain.

39. What is the function of the cerebrospinal fluid?

    _____

    _____

40. The peripheral nervous system has 12 pairs of

    _____ and

    31 pairs of _____.

41. Some peripheral nerves form the _____

    _____.

    This system controls _____

    _____.

42. The autonomic nervous system is divided into

    the _____

    _____ and the

    _____.

43. Name the five senses.

    A. _____

    B. _____

    C. _____

    D. _____

    E. _____

44. Where are touch receptors located?

    _____

45. The _____ gives the eye its color.

46. _____

    varies with the amount of light entering the eye.

47. The ear functions in _____ and

    _____.

48. The circulatory system is made up of the

    _____

    _____, and

    _____.

49. List four functions of the circulatory system.

A. _____

_____

B. _____

_____

C. _____

_____

D. _____

_____

50. The blood consists of _____

_____.

51. _____are needed for blood clotting.

52. The _____ is the

thick, muscular part of the heart.

53. Name and describe the two phases of heart action.

A. _____

_____

B. _____

_____

54. The three groups of blood vessels are:

A. _____

B. _____

C. _____

55. The largest artery is the _____.

56. Arterial blood is rich in _____.

57. The two main veins are:

A. _____

B. _____

58. The respiratory system brings _____

into the lungs and removes _____.

59. Respiration involves _____ and

_____.

60. The _____ is a long

tube that extends from the mouth to the anus.

61. Accessory organs of digestion are the:

A. _____

B. _____

C. _____

D. _____

E. _____

F. _____

62. The waste products of digestion are called

_____.

63. What are the two functions of the urinary system?

A. _____

B. _____

64. Human reproduction results from _____

_____.

65. The male sex glands are called _____.

66. The female sex glands are called _____.

67. The female hormones secreted by the ovaries are

_____ and

_____.

68. The uniting of a sperm and ovum into one cell is

called _____.

69. _____ regulate the

activities of other organs and glands in the body.

70. Where is the pituitary gland located?

_____

_____

71. Thyroid stimulating hormone (TSH) is needed

for _____.

72. Adrenocorticotropic hormone (ACTH)

stimulates the _____.

73. _____ causes

uterine muscles to contract during childbirth.

74. The thyroid gland secretes thyroid hormone.

It regulates _____.

75. List the three groups of hormones secreted by

the adrenal cortex.

A. _____

B. _____

C. _____

76. _____

is needed for sugar to enter the cells.

77. The _____

system protects the body from disease and

infection.

**Multiple Choice**

Circle the **BEST** Answer

78. Which part of the cell controls cell reproduction?
    A. The cell membrane
    B. Protoplasm
    C. The nucleus
    D. Cytoplasm

79. Genes control
    A. Traits parents give to their children
    B. The shape and size of the cell
    C. The function of the cell
    D. Cell division

80. What type of tissue lines the nose and mouth?
    A. Epithelial
    B. Connective
    C. Muscle
    D. Nerve

81. The inner layer of the skin is the
    A. Epithelium
    B. Epidermis
    C. Dermis
    D. Nerve layer

82. Which is *not* a function of the skin?
    A. Preventing bacteria from entering the body
    B. Protecting organs from injury
    C. Regulating body temperature
    D. Maintaining posture

83. Bones and tendons are
    A. Muscle tissue
    B. Nerve tissue
    C. Epithelial tissue
    D. Connective tissue

84. The vertebrae in the spinal column are
    A. Irregular bones
    B. Short bones
    C. Flat bones
    D. Long bones

85. The connective tissue at the end of long bones is
    A. The synovial membrane
    B. Cartilage
    C. Ligaments
    D. Joints

86. Blood cells are made in the
    A. Periosteum
    B. Bone marrow
    C. Synovial membrane
    D. Irregular bone

87. Which is an involuntary muscle?
    A. Arm muscles
    B. Leg muscles
    C. Finger muscles
    D. Stomach muscles

88. Which part of the brain regulates and coordinates body movements?
    A. Cerebellum
    B. Pons
    C. Midbrain
    D. Cerebrum

89. The center of thought and intelligence is the
    A. Spinal column
    B. Brainstem
    C. Cerebrum
    D. Medulla

90. Which part of the brain connects the cerebrum to the spinal cord?
    A. The cerebral cortex
    B. The cerebrum
    C. The myelin sheath
    D. The brainstem

91. The brain and spinal cord are covered by connective tissue called
    A. The medulla
    B. Meninges
    C. The arachnoid
    D. The cortex

92. The sympathetic nervous system
    A. Controls hearing and vision
    B. Causes muscles to relax
    C. Speeds up functions
    D. Slows down functions

93. Which layer of the eye has receptors for vision and the nerve fibers of the optic nerve?
    A. The sclera
    B. The choroid
    C. The pupil
    D. The retina

94. Light enters the eye through the
    A. Cornea
    B. Lens
    C. Optic nerve
    D. Aqueous chamber

95. Which structure separates the external and middle ear?
    A. The pinna
    B. The auditory canal
    C. Cerumen
    D. The tympanic membrane

96. Red blood cells are called
    A. Plasma
    B. Erythrocytes
    C. Hemoglobin
    D. Leukocytes

97. The outer layer of the heart is called the
    A. Pericardium
    B. Heart sac
    C. Myocardium
    D. Endocardium

98. Which chamber of the heart receives blood from the lungs?
    A. The right atrium
    B. The left atrium
    C. The right ventricle
    D. The left ventricle

99. The smallest branch of an artery is
    A. A capillary
    B. A venule
    C. An arteriole
    D. The vena cava

100. The lungs are separated from the abdominal cavity by a muscle called the
    A. Alveoli
    B. Diaphragm
    C. Pleura
    D. Rib cage

101. Where does digestion begin?
    A. In the esophagus
    B. In the stomach
    C. In the large intestine
    D. In the mouth

102. In the stomach, food is mixed and churned with gastric juices to form a semi-liquid substance called
    A. Chyme
    B. Bile
    C. Peristalsis
    D. Saliva

103. The basic working unit of the kidney is the
    A. Glomerulus
    B. Nephron
    C. Renal pelvis
    D. Ureter

104. Urine is stored in the
    A. Bladder
    B. Kidney
    C. Nephron
    D. Urethra

105. Male sex cells are called
    A. Semen
    B. Prostate
    C. Sperm
    D. Testosterone

106. The female sex cell is called
    A. Progesterone
    B. Cervix
    C. Ovum
    D. Vagina

107. The male hormone is
    A. Estrogen
    B. Progesterone
    C. Sperm
    D. Testosterone

108. The tissue lining the uterus is called the
    A. Menstruation
    B. Cervix
    C. Fundus
    D. Endometrium

109. Female external genitalia are called the
    A. Labia
    B. Hymen
    C. Uterus
    D. Vulva

110. Which gland is called the "master gland"?
    A. Pituitary
    B. Thyroid
    C. Adrenal
    D. Parathyroid

111. Insulin is secreted by the
    A. Thyroid
    B. Pancreas
    C. Gonads
    D. Pituitary

112. If there is too little insulin, sugar cannot enter the cells. Excess amounts of sugar build up in the blood. This condition is called
    A. Blood sugar
    B. Glucocorticoid
    C. Diabetes
    D. Epinepherine

*Labeling*

113. Label the three types of joints.

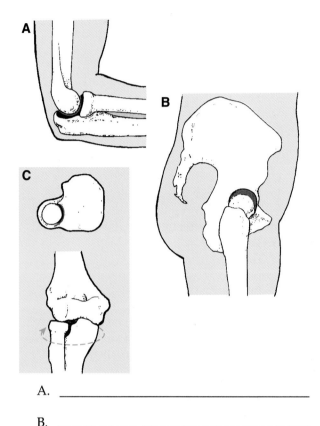

A. _____

B. _____

C. _____

114. Label the major parts of the central nervous system.

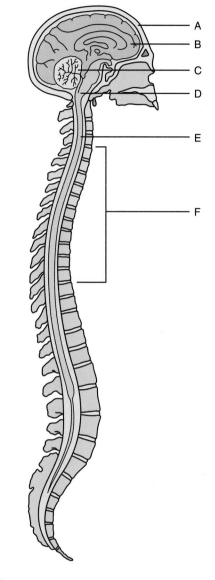

A. _____

B. _____

C. _____

D. _____

E. _____

F. _____

115. Label the structures of the heart.

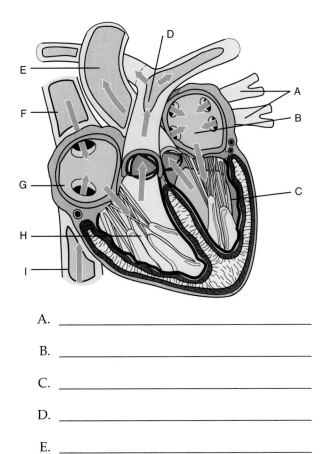

A. _____

B. _____

C. _____

D. _____

E. _____

F. _____

G. _____

H. _____

I. _____

116. Label the structures of the male reproductive system.

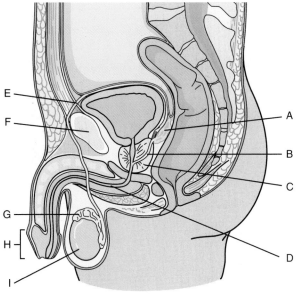

A. _____

B. _____

C. _____

D. _____

E. _____

F. _____

G. _____

H. _____

I. _____

117. Label the structures of the female external genitalia.

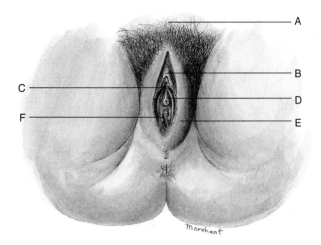

A. _____

B. _____

C. _____

D. _____

E. _____

F. _____

118. Label the glands of the endocrine system.

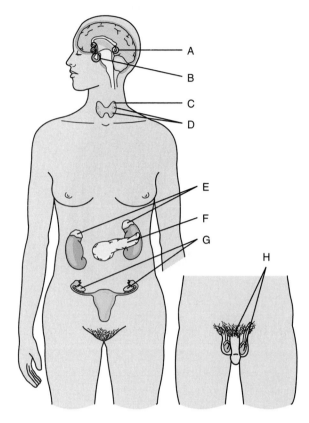

A. _____

B. _____

C. _____

D. _____

E. _____

F. _____

G. _____

H. _____

## CASE STUDY

*This chapter provides the student with a basic knowledge of body structure and function. The body is made up of systems. The systems are related and depend on each other for proper function and survival. Injury or disease of one part affects the whole body.*

*Basic knowledge of the body's structure and function should result in safe and dignified care.*

*Answer the following questions.*

1. How might a basic knowledge of body structure and function help you
   A. Meet the person's physical and safety and security needs?
   B. Understand the reasons for the care you give?
   C. Treat the person and the person's body with dignity and respect?
   D. Make accurate observations about the person?

## ADDITIONAL LEARNING ACTIVITIES

1. List and define the three layers of connective tissue that line the brain and spinal cord. (See page 67 in the textbook.)

2. Describe how the sympathetic nervous system and the parasympathetic nervous system balance each other. (See page 67 in the textbook.)

3. Explain how the eye uses light to see. (See page 68 in the textbook.)

4. Outline how the blood flows through the circulatory system. (See pages 70-71 in the textbook.)

5. Outline the process of respiration. (See pages 71-72 in the textbook.)

6. Outline the process of digestion. (See pages 72-73 in the textbook.)

7. Explain how urine is formed and how it passes through the urinary system. (See page 74 in the textbook.)

8. Outline the process of menstruation. (See pages 76-77 in the textbook.)

9. Outline the process of fertilization. (See page 77 in the textbook.)

10. If available in your school or class site, use anatomical models to practice identifying body structures. You can also practice locating the body structures on your own body.

# 7 Caring For the Older Person

The questions and student activities in this chapter will help you meet these objectives.
- Define the key terms listed in this chapter
- Identify the developmental tasks of each age group
- Identify the social changes common in older adulthood
- Describe the physical changes from aging and the care required
- Describe the gains and losses related to long-term care
- Describe the sexual changes and needs of older persons
- Explain how to deal with sexually aggressive persons

## STUDY QUESTIONS

### Matching

**Match each term with the correct definition.**

1. _____ Difficulty swallowing

2. _____ Difficulty breathing

3. _____ The care of aging people

4. _____ The study of the aging process

5. _____ The time when menstruation stops and menstrual cycles end

6. _____ Between 75 and 84 years of age

7. _____ 85 years of age and older

8. _____ The physical, psychological, social, cultural, and spiritual factors that effect a person's feelings and attitudes about his or her sex

9. _____ Between 65 and 74 years of age

A. Menopause

B. Old-old

C. Young-old

D. Dysphagia

E. Geriatrics

F. Sexuality

G. Dyspnea

H. Old

I. Gerontology

*Fill in the Blanks*

10. With aging, normal changes occur in body

    _____ and

    _____.

    These changes increase the risk for

    _____,

    _____, and

    _____.

11. Growth is _____

    _____.

12. Development relates to _____

    _____

13. Growth and development occur in a

    _____,

    _____,

    and _____.

14. A development task is _____.

15. List five social changes that occur with aging:

    A. _____

    B. _____

    C. _____

    D. _____

    E. _____

16. When a person's partner dies, the person loses

    a _____,

    _____,

    _____,

    and _____.

17. List six age related changes in the musculoskeletal system.

    A. _____

    B. _____

    C. _____

    D. _____

    E. _____

    F. _____

18. List three measures that help prevent bone loss and loss of muscle strength.

    A. _____

    B. _____

    C. _____

19. _____,

    _____, and

    _____

    help prevent respiratory complications from

    bedrest.

20. Persons with _____ or

    _____

    often need foods providing soft bulk, such as

    whole grains, and cooked fruits and vegetables.

21. List four age related changes in the digestive system.

    A. _____

    B. _____

    C. _____

    D. _____

22. As a result of age-related changes in the

    digestive system, _____

    foods are hard to digest and can irritate the

    intestines.

23. List four age related changes in the male
    reproductive system.

    A. _____

    B. _____

    C. _____

    D. _____

24. Nursing centers are designed to meet the needs

    of _____.

25. Nursing center residents may experience some
    or all of the following losses. Loss of:

    A. _____

    B. _____

    C. _____

    D. _____

    E. _____

26. Losses may cause the person to feel

    _____,

    _____,

    and _____.

27. Frequency of sexual activity decreases for many
    men and women. Reasons for this include:

    A. _____

    B. _____

    C. _____

    D. _____

    E. _____

28. You are giving Mr. Peters a bed bath. You notice
    that he is becoming aroused. What actions
    should you take?

    _____

    _____

29. An _____

    is someone who supports or promotes the needs

    and interests of another person.

30. List five functions of a long-term care
    ombudsman.

    A. _____

    B. _____

    C. _____

    D. _____

    E. _____

31. Ombudsman services are useful when:

    A. _____

    _____

    B. _____

    _____

32. Health care agencies must meet certain standards.

    Standards serve to _____

    _____.

33. Surveyors expect the nursing team to work
    together to provide quality care. As a member of
    the nursing team, you must:

    A. _____

    B. _____

    C. _____

    D. _____

    E. _____

F. _____

G. _____

*Multiple Choice*

Circle the **BEST** Answer

34. Which is *not* a developmental task of infancy?
    A. Tolerating separation from parents or primary caregivers
    B. Learning to walk
    C. Learning to eat solid foods
    D. Beginning to have emotional relationships with parents, brothers, and sisters

35. Which is a developmental task of adolescence?
    A. Learning basic reading, writing, and arithmetic skills
    B. Learning how to study
    C. Becoming independent from parents and adults
    D. Selecting a partner

36. Adjusting to decreased strength and loss of health is a developmental task of
    A. Adolescence
    B. Young adulthood
    C. Middle adulthood
    D. Late adulthood

37. Which statement about retirement is *true*?
    A. All people enjoy retirement.
    B. Retirement usually means increased income.
    C. All people retire because they want to.
    D. Some people retire because of poor health or disability.

38. Most older people have regular contact with family and friends.
    A. True
    B. False

39. Some children care for older parents. Which statement is *false*?
    A. This helps some older persons feel secure.
    B. Tensions may occur.
    C. Some older persons lose dignity and self-respect.
    D. This is always a good arrangement for the parent and the child.

40. Changes in the integumentary system include all of the following *except*:
    A. The skin loses its elasticity.
    B. The skin loses its fatty tissue layer.

C. Oil and sweat secretion increases.
D. The skin has fewer nerve endings.

41. Changes in the skin occur with aging. Care measures include all of the following *except*
    A. Using mild soaps or soap substitutes
    B. A daily bath
    C. Using lotions, oils, and creams to prevent drying
    D. Protecting the person from drafts

42. Mr. Jason Samuels complains of cold feet. Which care measure is *correct*?
    A. Soaking his feet in very warm water
    B. Providing him with socks
    C. Giving him a bath
    D. Providing him with a heating pad

43. Age-related changes in the musculoskeletal system cause bones to break easily. Which measure is *not* helpful?
    A. Turning and moving persons gently
    B. Helping persons to get out of bed
    C. Helping persons to walk
    D. Keeping the person in bed as much as possible

44. Which of the following is *not* a result of age-related nervous system changes?
    A. Sensitivity to pain and pressure increase
    B. Blood flow to the brain is decreased
    C. Less sleep is needed
    D. Hearing and vision losses occur

45. Painful injuries or diseases may go unnoticed by an older person because
    A. Older persons are confused
    B. Hearing and vision loss occur
    C. Touch and sensitivity to pain and pressure are reduced
    D. Activity is decreased

46. Changes in the circulatory system results in
    A. Loss of appetite
    B. Poor circulation in many parts of the body
    C. Decreased ability to sleep
    D. Agitation and restlessness

47. Ms. Rose Romero has severe circulatory changes. You know that
    A. Bedrest is needed
    B. Everything must be done for her
    C. Personal care items are kept near by
    D. She is encouraged to walking long distances

48. Which measure does *not* promote normal breathing?
    A. Placing heavy bed linens over the person's chest
    B. Assisting with turning, repositioning, and deep breathing
    C. Positioning the person in semi-Fowler's position
    D. Encouraging the person to be as active as possible

49. Which is *not* a result of age-related changes in the digestive system?
    A. Improved taste and smell
    B. Flatulence and constipation
    C. Indigestion
    D. Swallowing problems

50. Changes in the urinary system result in
    A. Less concentrated urine
    B. Urinary frequency and urgency
    C. Decreased risk for urinary tract infections
    D. Blood in the urine

51. Which measure will help reduce the need to urinate during the night?
    A. Limiting fluid intake to 1000 ml daily
    B. Taking all fluids before 1300 (1:00 PM)
    C. Drinking only water after noon
    D. Taking most fluids before 1700 (5:00 PM)

52. Older persons are at risk for urinary tract infection?
    A. True
    B. False

53. Which is *not* an age-related change in the female reproductive system?
    A. Breasts are less firm and sag.
    B. Vaginal walls become thinner and dryer.
    C. The ovaries and uterus increase in size.
    D. External genitalia shrink and lose elastic tissue.

54. The health team helps nursing center residents cope with loss by
    A. Telling the person not to worry
    B. Ignoring the person's feelings
    C. Feeling sorry for the person
    D. Treating the person with dignity and respect

55. Mr. and Mrs. Adams have been married for 52 years. They no longer have sexual intercourse. You know that
    A. They are too old for sexual intercourse.
    B. They have lost sexual needs and desires.
    C. They can express closeness and intimacy in other ways.
    D. They no longer love one another.

56. A resident makes sexual advances toward you. You should
    A. Refuse to care for the resident
    B. Tell the resident's family
    C. Discuss the problem with the nurse
    D. Ignore it

57. Very few older persons are healthy and live in their own homes.
    A. True
    B. False

58. Love, affection, and intimacy are needed throughout life.
    A. True
    B. False

59. Married couples living in nursing centers are allowed to share the same room?
    A. True
    B. False

60. Ms. Irma Adams and Ms. Lois Moore are nursing center residents. You see them kissing in Ms. Moore's private room. What should you do?
    A. Tell the nurse at once.
    B. Close the door for privacy.
    C. Escort Ms. Adams to her room.
    D. Discuss what you saw with co-workers in the lunch room.

61. Which measure promotes sexuality?
    A. Letting the person practice grooming routines
    B. Choosing clothing for the person
    C. Judging the person's sexual relationships
    D. Entering the person's room without knocking

62. Sexually aggressive behaviors are always intentional.
    A. True
    B. False

63. A person you are caring for touches you in a sexual way. You should do all of the following *except*
    A. Ask the person not to touch you and state the places where you were touched.
    B. Tell the person that the behavior makes you uncomfortable.
    C. Discuss the matter with the nurse.
    D. Tell the person that you will report the behavior to the ombudsman.

64. Mr. Andrews wishes to voice a grievance about his roommate. Which statement is *false*?
    A. Mr. Andrews can share his concerns with anyone outside the center.
    B. Mr. Andrews must discuss his concerns with the nurse.
    C. The center must post the names, addresses, and phone numbers of local and state ombudsmen.
    D. Mr. Andrews has the right to communicate privately with anyone he chooses.

65. You may be involved in a survey process. Which action is *wrong*?
    A. Making sure each person's room is neat and clean
    B. Sharing your complaints about your work schedule with members of the survey team
    C. Protecting each person's rights
    D. Following each person's care plan for how and when to assist him or her

## CASE STUDY

*Mrs. June Chaney and Mr. Warren Anderson live at Green Acres Nursing Center. They have both been widowed for several years. Since moving to Green Acres, they have developed a relationship. They attend the same activities, eat at the same table in the dining room, and sit side by side in the recreation room. They are frequently seen holding hands and kissing. Sometimes they are together in Mrs. Chaney's room with the door closed. Mr. Anderson's son tells you that he is not happy about the relationship and wants you to keep his father and Mrs. Chaney apart.*

*Answer the following questions.*

1. How are Mr. Anderson and Mrs. Chaney expressing their sexuality?

2. Should Mr. Anderson and Mrs. Chaney be allowed to continue their relationship?
   A. If yes, why?

   B. If no, why not?

3. How might you deal with Mr. Anderson's son's concerns?

## ADDITIONAL LEARNING ACTIVITIES

1. Ask an older relative, friend, or neighbor if you can interview him or her. Ask the person:
   A. What physical, social, and psychological changes he or she has experienced over the past 10 to 20 years?

   (1) How has the person adjusted?

   B. What changes have been most difficult to cope with? Explain.

   C. Who provides support for the person?

   D. Does the person have concerns about the future? Explain.

   E. What brings joy and meaning to the person's life?

2. Carefully read about the changes that occur as people age. Think about how these changes might affect you and your life-style as you age.
   A. What are your fears and concerns?

   B. How do you plan to adjust to the changes?

   C. What can you do now to slow or decrease the effects of aging?

   D. Which people and what possessions might you have the most difficulty giving up? Explain.

3. List some ways you can help persons you care for express their sexuality.

4. You may have to deal with persons who are sexually aggressive toward you.
   A. How do you feel about this?

   B. How might you handle these uncomfortable situations?

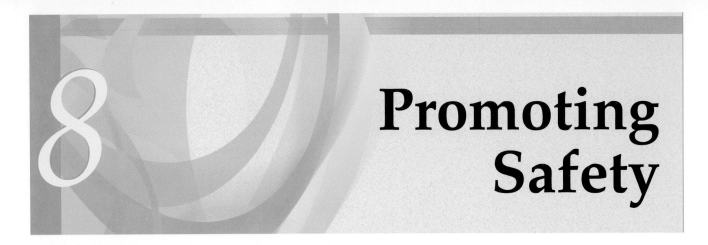

# Promoting Safety

8

## OBJECTIVES

The questions and student activities in this chapter will help you meet these objectives.
- Define the key terms listed in this chapter
- Describe accident risk factors
- Explain why you identify a person before giving care
- Explain how and when to accurately identify a person
- Describe the safety measures to prevent falls, burns, poisoning, and suffocation
- Explain how to safely use bed rails
- Explain how to safely use wheelchairs and stretchers
- Explain how to prevent equipment accidents
- Explain how to handle hazardous substances
- Describe safety measures for fire prevention and oxygen use
- Explain what to do during a fire
- Give examples of natural and human-made disasters
- Describe your role in risk management
- Explain how to protect yourself from workplace violence
- Perform the procedure described in this chapter

## STUDY QUESTIONS

*Matching*

*Match each term with the correct definition.*

1. _____ A sudden catastrophic event in which many people are injured and killed, and property is destroyed

2. _____ A state of being unaware of one's surroundings and being unable to react or respond to people, places, or things

3. _____ The loss of cognitive and social function caused by changes in the brain

4. _____ Any chemical in the workplace that can cause harm

5. _____ Violent acts directed toward persons at work or while on duty

6. _____ When breathing stops from the lack of oxygen

A. Dementia

B. Suffocation

C. Workplace violence

D. Disaster

E. Hazardous substance

F. Coma

*Fill in the Blanks*

7. _____ and

_____

can prevent most accidents.

8. List seven factors which increase the risk of falls and injuries.

A. _____

B. _____

C. _____

D. _____

E. _____

F. _____

G. _____

9. List six drug side effects that increase a person's risk for falls and injuries.

A. _____

B. _____

C. _____

D. _____

E. _____

F. _____

10. Cognitive function involves:

A. _____

B. _____

C. _____

D. _____

E. _____

F. _____

11. You use the _____

to identify the person before giving care.

12. Explain why calling the person by name is not a safe way to identify the person?

_____

_____

13. When checking the ID bracelet with the

assignment sheet, you need to carefully check

the person's full name because _____

_____.

14. Ms. Amelia Kraus is an alert and oriented nursing center resident. She chooses not to wear an ID bracelet. How should you identify her before giving care?

_____

_____

15. You notice that Mr. Lind's ID bracelet is too tight. What should you do?

_____

16. At what time of the day do most falls occur?

_____

17. Explain why falls are more likely to occur during shift changes.

_____

_____

_____

18. List four bathroom safety measures to prevent falls.

    A. _____

    B. _____

    C. _____

    D. _____

19. Explain why wheeled equipment is pulled, not pushed through doorways.

    _____

    _____

    _____

20. Why should you do a safety check of the person's room after visitors leave?

    _____

    _____

    _____

21. Mr. Paul Gomez's care plan states that he needs bed rails. When must his bed rails be up?

    _____

22. Persons at greatest risk of entrapment when bed rails are used are those who:

    A. _____

    B. _____

    C. _____

    D. _____

    E. _____

    F. _____

    G. _____

    H. _____

23. Bed rails are considered restraints. When can they be used?

    A. _____

    B. _____

24. How will you know which patients or residents use bed rails?

    _____

25. Ms. Paula Perkins uses bed rails. You need to:

    A. _____

    B. _____

    C. _____

26. Mr. Mark Masters does not use bed rails. How will you promote his safety when giving care?

    _____

    _____

27. _____

    give support to persons who are weak or

    unsteady when walking.

28. Bed wheels have locks to prevent the bed from moving. You need to lock bed wheels when:

    A. _____

    B. _____

29. List four common causes of burns.

    A. _____

    B. _____

    C. _____

    D. _____

30. List five common causes of suffocation.

    A. _____

    B. _____

    C. _____

    D. _____

    E. _____

31. When is equipment unsafe?

    A. _____

    B. _____

    C. _____

32. Frayed cords and overloaded electrical outlets

    can cause _____ ,

    _____ ,

    and _____ .

33. List seven warning signs of a faulty electrical item.

    A. _____

    B. _____

    C. _____

    D. _____

    E. _____

    F. _____

    G. _____

34. Where should you connect bed power cords?

    _____

35. Explain why you should turn off equipment before unplugging it.

    _____

    _____

36. How many workers are needed to safely transfer a person to a stretcher?

    _____

37. When can you leave a person on a stretcher alone?

    _____

38. Exposure to hazardous substances can occur in the workplace. List seven hazardous substances found in health care agencies.

    A. _____

    B. _____

    C. _____

    D. _____

    E. _____

    F. _____

    G. _____

39. Every hazardous substance has a material safety data sheet (MSDS). You need to check the MSDS before:

    A. _____

    B. _____

    C. _____

40. List the three things needed for a fire.

    A. _____

    B. _____

    C. _____

41. The word RACE will help you remember what to do first if a fire occurs. What do the letters R-A-C-E stand for?

    A. R _____

    B. A _____

    C. C _____

    D. E_____

42. You answer the phone at the nurses' station. The caller tells you there is a bomb in the hospital. What should you do?

_____

43. Explain why nurses and nursing assistants are at risk for workplace violence.

_____

_____

44. _____ involves

identifying and controlling risks and safety

hazards affecting the agency.

45. The intent of risk management is to:

A. _____

B. _____

C. _____

D. _____

46. Errors in care must be reported at once. Errors in care include:

A. _____

B. _____

C. _____

47. _____

occurs when the person or his or her property is

harmed.

*Multiple Choice*

Circle the **BEST** Answer

48. Cognitive relates to:
    A. Dementia
    B. Impaired hearing
    C. Knowledge
    D. Balance and coordination

49. A history of falls increases the risk of falling again.
    A. True
    B. False

50. Which is a factor increasing the risk of falls?
    A. Wearing eye glasses
    B. Wearing hearing aides
    C. Pediculosis capitis
    D. Foot problems

51. Ms. Louise Adams is incontinent of urine. She is at increased risk of falling.
    A. True
    B. False

52. Which is *not* a safety measure to prevent falls?
    A. The bed is kept in the highest horizontal position.
    B. Furniture is placed for easy movement.
    C. Bed wheels are locked for transfers.
    D. Crutches, canes, and walkers have non-skid tips.

53. Which statement about bed rails is *false*?
    A. Bed rails are considered restraints by OBRA.
    B. Bed rails are necessary for all nursing center residents.
    C. A person can get caught or entangled in bed rails.
    D. The person or legal representative must give consent for raised bed rails.

54. Ms. Paula Perkins uses bed rails. You promote her comfort by
    A. Making sure needed items are within reach
    B. Keeping the bed in the highest horizontal position
    C. Raising both bed rails when giving care
    D. Leaving her alone when the bed is raised

55. Bed wheels must be locked at all times except when moving the bed.
    A. True
    B. False

56. Safety measures to prevent burns include all of the following *except*
    A. Do not allow smoking in bed.
    B. Do not allow smoking near oxygen equipment.
    C. Measure bath water temperature before the person gets into the tub.
    D. Turn on hot water first, then cold water.

57. You can help prevent poisoning by
    A. Removing all personal care items from the person's room
    B. Inspecting the person's drawers every shift
    C. Following agency policy for storing personal care items
    D. Reminding patients and residents not to drink shampoo, mouth wash, or lotion

58. Which measure helps prevent suffocation?
    A. Leaving a person alone in the bathtub
    B. Giving small amounts of oral foods and fluids to persons with feeding tubes
    C. Using bed rails for all patients and residents
    D. Reporting loose teeth or dentures to the nurse

59. Which action will *not* help prevent equipment accidents?
    A. Inspecting power cords for damage
    B. Using two pronged plugs on all electrical devices
    C. Keeping electrical items away from water
    D. Turning off equipment before unplugging it

60. Which measure promotes wheelchair safety?
    A. Make sure the casters point toward the back of the chair.
    B. Position the person's feet on the footplates.
    C. Pull the chair backward when transporting the person.
    D. Have the person stand on the footplates when transferring from the wheelchair.

61. Mr. Andy Rice needs to be moved to another room on a stretcher. Which action will *not* promote stretcher safety?
    A. Locking the stretcher wheels before transferring him to the stretcher
    B. Fastening the safety straps when he is properly positioned on the stretcher
    C. Raising the side rails and keeping them up during transport
    D. Moving the stretcher head first

62. You find a bottle of liquid in the tub room without a label. You should
    A. Open the bottle to see what is inside.
    B. Leave the bottle and get the nurse.
    C. Take the bottle to the nurse and explain the problem.
    D. Ask a co-worker what is in the bottle.

63. When must you check material safety data sheets (MSDS)?
    A. Before using a hazardous substance
    B. Before cleaning up a leak or spill
    C. Before disposing of a hazardous substance
    D. All of the above are correct

64. Which is *not* a fire prevention measure?
    A. Following safety measures for oxygen use
    B. Supervising persons who smoke
    C. Emptying ashtrays into metal wastebaskets lined with plastic bags
    D. Storing flammable liquids in their original containers

65. The first thing you must do when a fire occurs is to
    A. Pull the fire alarm
    B. Rescue persons in immediate danger
    C. Get the fire extinguisher
    D. Turn off electrical equipment

66. Do not use elevators if there is a fire.
    A. True
    B. False

67. Mr. Peter Tate is receiving oxygen therapy. Which is *false*?
    A. A "No Smoking" sign is placed on his door and near his bed.
    B. Smoking materials are kept in his bedside stand.
    C. Mr. Tate and his visitors are reminded not to smoke in his room.
    D. Materials that ignite easily are removed from his room.

68. Special safety precautions are practiced where oxygen is used and stored.
    A. True
    B. False

69. When dealing with an agitated or aggressive person you should
    A. Use touch to calm the person.
    B. Keep your hands free.
    C. Tell the person to calm down.
    D. Stand close to the person.

70. To help keep personal belongings safe, you need to
    A. Send all personal belongings home with the family.
    B. Complete a personal belongings list.
    C. Lock all personal belongings in a safe.
    D. Keep all personal belongings in the person's closet.

71. In nursing centers, personal belongings are labeled with the person's name.
    A. True
    B. False

72. Accidents and errors in care are reported only if someone is injured.
    A. True
    B. False

73. You promote safety by doing as much for the person as possible.
    A. True
    B. False

74. You notice that a light bulb has burned out in a resident's bathroom. You need to
    A. Get a new light bulb and change the light bulb.
    B. Do nothing. Assume the nurse already knows about the problem.
    C. Tell the resident to be extra careful when using the bathroom.
    D. Tell the nurse at once.

## MOSBY'S NURSING ASSISTANT SKILLS VIDEOS EXERCISES

## Questions from the "Preventing Falls" Section of the Safety and Restraints Video

75. Being in an unfamiliar environment increases the risk of accidents.
    A. True
    B. False

76. As a member of the nursing team, you are responsible for:

    A. _____

    B. _____

    C. _____

    D. _____

    E. _____

    F. _____

77. List the safety measures practiced when assisting Mr. Rydell to the bathroom.

    A. _____

    _____

    B. _____

    _____

    C. _____

    _____

    D. _____

    _____

    E. _____

    _____

    F. _____

    _____

    G. _____

    _____

    H. _____

    _____

    I. _____

    _____

    J. _____

    _____

    K. _____

    _____

78. What safety measures were practiced after assisting Mr. Rydell back to bed?

A. _____

_____

B. _____

_____

C. _____

_____

## CASE STUDY

*Mr. John Wilson is 80 years old. He is a resident at Pine View Nursing Center. He is recovering from surgery to repair a fractured right leg. He is learning to use a walker. He is receiving oxygen for a chronic lung disease. He wears eyeglasses and has very poor vision without his glasses. Mr. Wilson has smoked a pack of cigarettes a day for the past 60 years. He is alert and oriented and able to make his needs known.*

*Answer the following questions.*

1. What accident risk factors does Mr. Wilson have?

2. What types of accidents or injuries is Mr. Wilson at risk for?

3. What nursing measures might help decrease Mr. Wilson's risks for accidents and injury?

4. What is your role in providing a safe environment for Mr. Wilson?

## ADDITIONAL LEARNING ACTIVITIES

1. Carefully review the safety measures to prevent falls, burns, poisoning, and suffocation.
   A. List the safety measures you practice related to each in your home.

   B. List the safety measures you practice related to falls, burns, poisoning, and suffocation in your workplace?

   C. Is your home safe and free from safety hazards? Explain.

   D. Do you have a fire safety plan in your home? Explain.

E. If you do not already have one, develop an evacuation plan for your home. Make sure that there are at least 2 possible exits from each room. Have regular fire drills with your family.

2. Make a list of emergency phone numbers. (Poison control, police, ambulance, hospital, and doctor). Keep the list by each phone in your home. Make sure all family members know where the list is.

3. Carefully review the procedure for using a fire extinguisher.
   A. Under the supervision of your instructor practice the procedure. Use the procedure checklist on page 206 as a guide.

# Restraint Alternatives and Safe Restraint Use

## OBJECTIVES

The questions and student activities in this chapter will help you meet these objectives.
- Define the key terms listed in this chapter
- Describe the purpose and complications of restraints

- Identify restraint alternatives
- Explain how to use restraints safely
- Perform the procedure described in this chapter

## STUDY QUESTIONS

*Matching*

*Match each term with the correct definition.*

1. _____ Any action that punishes or penalizes a person

2. _____ A restraint attached to the person's body and to a fixed (non-movable) object

3. _____ Any item, object, device, garment, material, or drug that limits or restricts a person's freedom of movement or access to one's body

4. _____ A restraint near but not directly attached to the person's body

A. Restraint

B. Passive physical restraint

C. Active physical restraint

D. Discipline

*Fill in the Blanks*

5. _____

_____

and _____,

have guidelines about restraint use.

So do _____ and

_____.

6. List seven risks of restraint use.

A. _____

B. _____

C. _____

D. _____

E. _____

F. _____

G. _____

7. Restraints cannot be used for staff convenience. Convenience is any action that:

   A. _____

   B. _____

   C. _____

8. The nurse restrains Mr. Gomez in the chair in his room so he can make rounds without being interrupted. This action is _____

   _____.

9. Restraints are used only when necessary to

   _____.

10. According to OBRA and CMS, physical restraints include these points:

    A. _____

    _____

    B. _____

    _____

    C. _____

    _____

    D. _____

    _____

11. Drugs are restraints if they:

    A. _____

    B. _____

12. The doctor may order drugs to help persons who are confused or agitated. What is the goal?

    _____

    _____

13. List six mental effects of restraint use.

    A. _____

    B. _____

    C. _____

    D. _____

    E. _____

    F. _____

14. List six legal aspects of restraint use:

    A. _____

    _____

    B. _____

    _____

    C. _____

    _____

    D. _____

    _____

    E. _____

    _____

    F. _____

    _____

15. Mrs. Monroe's doctor writes an order for a restraint. What information does the doctor's order include?

    A. _____

    B. _____

    C. _____

    D. _____

16. The nurse tells you to apply a wrist restraint to Mr. Clark's right wrist. You do not understand why the restraint is being used. What should you do and why?

    _____

    _____

    _____

17. Explain why you should never secure restraints to the bed rails.

    _____

    _____

    _____

18. You apply a belt restraint to Ms. Monroe when she is in her wheelchair. What information must you report to the nurse?

    A. _____

    B. _____

    C. _____

    D. _____

    E. _____

    F. _____

    G. _____

    H. _____

    I. _____

    J. _____

19. You are applying a belt restraint to Mr. Norris. He is confused and resists your efforts. What should you do?

    _____

    _____

20. Before you apply any restraint, what information do you need from the nurse and the care plan?

    A. _____

    B. _____

    C. _____

    D. _____

    E. _____

    F. _____

    G. _____

    H. _____

    I. _____

    J. _____

    K. _____

    L. _____

21. Mr. Clark has a wrist restraint on his right wrist. You are checking the circulation in his right wrist. What signs and symptoms must you report to the nurse at once?

    A. _____

    B. _____

    C. _____

    D. _____

22. Why are persons restrained in the supine position monitored constantly?

    _____

23. What is the purpose of bed rail covers and gap protectors?

    _____

24. When applying a restraint to a person's chest, you must _____

    _____

    _____.

25. Criss-crossing vest restraints in back can cause

_____ .

26. You must remove Mr. Clark's restraint at least every 2 hours. What care measures do you need to perform before you reapply the restraint?

A. _____

B. _____

C. _____

D. _____

E. _____

F. _____

*Multiple Choice*

Circle the **BEST** Answer

27. Knowing and treating the cause of certain behaviors can prevent restraint use.
A. True
B. False

28. Physical restraints
A. Restrict freedom of movement or access to one's body
B. Must be used to control a person's behavior
C. Are effective in preventing falls
D. Should never be used

29. Which of the following is a physical restraint?
A. The person is moved closer to the nurses' station.
B. The person is taken to a supervised activity.
C. The person wears padded hip protectors under his or her clothing.
D. The person's chair is placed so close to the wall that the person cannot move.

30. The most serious risk from restraints is
A. Loss of dignity
B. Fractured hip
C. Increased agitation
D. Death from strangulation

31. Which is *not* a restraint alternative?
A. An exercise program is provided.
B. A floor cushion is placed next to the person's bed.
C. The person's bed sheets are tucked in so tightly that the person cannot move.
D. Extra time is spent with the person who is restless.

32. Which of the following measures is a restraint alternative?
A. The person is kept in his or her room with the door closed.
B. The person wanders in a safe area.
C. The person's wheelchair is placed tight against a table. The wheelchair wheels are locked.
D. Bed rails are used to keep the person in bed.

33. Restraints cannot be used without consent.
A. True
B. False

34. Mr. Norris is confused. He cannot give informed consent for restraint use. Who does so for him?
A. The doctor
B. The RN
C. The agency's administrator
D. Mr. Norris's legal representative

35. You may need to apply restraints or care for persons who are restrained. Which action is *unsafe*?
A. Using the restraint noted in the person's care plan
B. Using only restraints that have manufacturer instructions and warning labels
C. Using a restraint to position a person on the toilet
D. Padding bony areas and skin

36. For safe use of restraints
A. Keep bed rails down when using vest, jacket, or belt restraints.
B. Position the person in the supine position when using vest, belt, or jacket restraints.
C. Tie restraints according to agency policy.
D. Secure restraints to the bed rail.

37. A belt restraint is used to restrain a person on the toilet.
A. True
B. False

38. Back cushions are used when a person is restrained in a chair.
    A. True
    B. False

39. How often do you need to check the person's circulation if mitt, wrist, or ankle restraints are used?
    A. At least every 15 minutes
    B. At least every 30 minutes
    C. Every hour
    D. Every 2 hours

40. Restraints can increase confusion and agitation.
    A. True
    B. False

41. Which restraints limit arm movements?
    A. Mitt restraints
    B. Wrist restraints
    C. Belt restraints
    D. Vest restraints

42. Which type of restraint is the *most* restrictive?
    A. A mitt restraint
    B. A wrist restraint
    C. A belt restraint
    D. A vest restraint

43. You are applying a wrist restraint. The person is in bed. Where should you tie the straps?
    A. To the headboard
    B. To the bed rail, out of the person's reach
    C. To the foot board
    D. To the movable part of the bed frame, out of the person's reach

## MOSBY'S NURSING SKILLS VIDEO EXERCISES

### Questions from the "Using Restraint Alternatives, Safe Use of Restraints, and Monitoring Restraint Use" Sections of the *Safety and Restraints* Video

44. Restraints are used only as a last resort, when other measures have failed to do one or all of the following:

    A. _____

    B. _____

    C. _____

45. Explain what "the least restrictive device" means.

    _____

    _____

46. For which persons are vest or jacket restraints ordered?

    _____

    _____

47. For which persons are mitt restraints ordered?

    _____

    _____

    _____

48. The person with a _____,

    _____ or

    _____,

    restraint is at great risk for strangulation.

49. If a person with a vest, jacket, or belt restraint is

    having difficulty breathing or is not breathing,

    you must _____.

50. _____,

    _____,

    _____, and

    _____,

    may prevent accidents, injury, and restraint use.

## CASE STUDY

*Mr. Howard Hein is a 76-year-old man in the hospital. He is recovering from abdominal surgery. He has a large abdominal dressing. He is receiving intravenous (IV) therapy (receiving nutrition and medications through a catheter in his vein). The (IV) catheter is in his left arm. He receives pain medication every 4 hours.*

*Mr. Hein is very restless and moves around a lot in bed. He is agitated at times. He has removed his abdominal dressing and has pulled the IV catheter from his arm. The RN has scheduled an emergency care planning conference.*

*Mr. Hein has a daughter, a son, and 2 adult grandchildren who visit daily. The daughter and son will be attending the care planning conference.*

*Answer the following questions.*

1. What safety risk factors does Mr. Hein have?

2. What behaviors does Mr. Hein have that interfere with his treatment?

3. What are some of the possible causes for Mr. Hein's behavior?

4. What restraint alternatives might the health team try?

5. Before the doctor orders the restraint, what must he or she do?

6. If a restraint is ordered:
   A. What are the risk factors?

   B. What safety measures must be followed?

   C. What must be reported and recorded about the restraint?

   D. How will you provide for Mr. Hein's basic needs?

   E. How will you provide for Mr. Hein's quality of life?

## ADDITIONAL LEARNING ACTIVITIES

1. You are caring for a person who is restrained. List some things you can do to protect the person's quality of life. Discuss how you would want to be treated.

2. Under the supervision of your instructor, practice the procedure for applying restraints with a classmate.
   A. Use the procedure checklist on pages 207-210 to evaluate your technique. Remember that restraints can cause serious injury and even death. They must always be applied correctly.

3. Under the supervision of your instructor, allow a classmate to practice applying restraints to you. Discuss how it feels to be restrained. Answer these questions.
   A. Did you feel safe? Explain.

   B. Did you feel comfortable? Explain.

   C. Did you feel in control? Explain.

   D. What fears did you have?

4. Imagine that you are in a nursing center or hospital. You are having a lot pain. You do not know the staff. The medication you are taking makes you drowsy. You are not sure what day it is. You have an IV in your right arm and a tube in your nose. You are frightened.
   A. What behaviors might you have?

   B. What could be some reasons for your behavior?

   C. Might the staff believe that you are confused? Explain.

   D. Would you feel safer and less fearful if you were restrained?

   E. What measures might make you feel safe and less fearful?

# Preventing Infection

## OBJECTIVES

The questions and student activities in this chapter will help you meet these objectives.
- Define the key terms listed in this chapter
- Identify what microbes need to live and grow
- List the signs and symptoms of infection
- Explain the chain of infection
- Describe the practices of medical asepsis
- Describe disinfection and sterilization methods
- Explain how to care for equipment and supplies
- Explain Isolation Precautions
- Describe Standard Precautions and the Bloodborne Pathogen Standard
- Perform the procedures described in this chapter

## STUDY QUESTIONS

*Crossword*

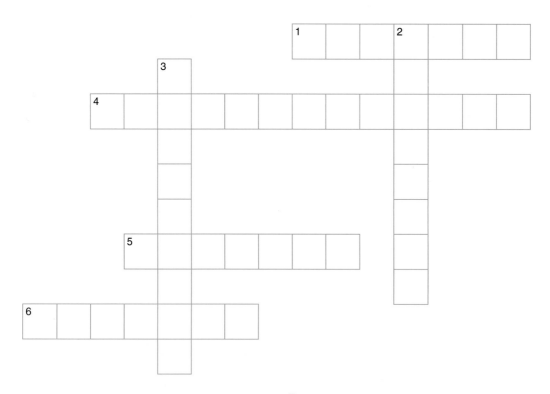

*Across*

1. Being free of disease-producing microbes
4. The process of becoming unclean
5. The absence of all microbes
6. A microorganism

*Down*

2. A microbe that is harmful and can cause an infection
3. A disease resulting from the invasion and growth of microbes in the body

## Matching

*Match each term with the correct definition.*

1. _____ Items contaminated with blood, body fluids, secretions, or excretions

2. _____ A human or animal that is a reservoir for microbes, but does not have signs and symptoms of infection

3. _____ The process of destroying pathogens

4. _____ A disease caused by pathogens that spread easily; a contagious disease

5. _____ Practices used to remove or destroy pathogens and to prevent their spread from one person or place to another person or place; clean technique

6. _____ A small living plant or animal seen only with a microscope; a microbe

7. _____ A microbe that does not usually cause an infection

8. _____ The process of destroying all microbes

A. Carrier

B. Microorganism

C. Sterilization

D. Biohazardous waste

E. Medical asepsis

F. Disinfection

G. Non-pathogen

H. Communicable disease

## Fill in the Blanks

9. Where are microbes found?

_____

10. Microbes need a _____ to live and grow.

11. _____organisms can resist the

effects of antibiotics.

12. A _____

infection is in a body part.

A _____ infection

involves the whole body.

13. The chain of infection is a process. Describe the process.

_____

_____

_____

_____

14. List the portals of exit and the portals of entry used by pathogens to leave and enter the body.

A. _____

B. _____

C. _____

D. _____

E. _____

F. _____

15. The _____

system protects the body against disease and

infection.

16. In medical asepsis, an item or area is _____

_____ when it is free of pathogens.

17. Mr. Pete Peterson has dementia. He does not understand aseptic practices. When do you need to assist him with hand washing?

    A. _____

    B. _____

    C. _____

    D. _____

18. Explain why hand lotion or cream is applied to the hands after practicing hand hygiene.

    _____

    _____

19. Germicides are _____

    _____.

20. List three aseptic measures that help protect the susceptible host.

    A. _____

    B. _____

    C. _____

21. _____

    are used to keep pathogens within a certain area.

22. Isolation Precautions are based on _____

    _____

23. _____ are used

    for all persons.

24. Standard Precautions prevent the spread of infection from:

    A. _____

    B. _____

    C. _____

    D. _____

25. List four measures needed for respiratory hygiene/cough etiquette

    A. _____

    _____

    B. _____

    _____

    C. _____

    _____

    D. _____

    _____

26. List the three types of Transmission-Based Precautions.

    A. _____

    B. _____

    C. _____

27. Mr. Chin Lee is on Droplet Precautions. What information do you need form the nurse and the care plan before providing care?

    A. _____

    B. _____

28. The nurse tells you that you need to wear PPE. List the order in which you should don PPE.

    A. _____

    B. _____

    C. _____

    D. _____

29. Wear gloves whenever contact with _____,

    _____,

    _____,

    _____,

    _____, and

    _____

    is likely.

30. You notice an itchy rash on your hands after you remove your gloves. What should you do?

    _____

31. Some patients and residents are allergic to latex. Where will you find this information?

    _____

32. Masks prevent the spread of microbes from the

    _____.

33. Contact precautions are used for known or unknown infections involving microbes transmitted by:

    A. _____

       _____

    B. _____

       _____

34. A patient is in Isolation Precautions. Explain how contaminated items are removed from the person's room.

    _____

    _____

35. Double bagging of items is not needed unless

    _____.

36. Goggles and face shields can change how you look. Before putting on PPE, you need to:

    A. _____

    B. _____

37. _____

    protects against exposure to the AIDS virus

    (HIV) and the hepatitis B virus (HBV).

38. Bloodborne pathogens are spread to others by

    _____

    and _____.

39. Immunity means _____

    _____.

40. You need to discard contaminated needles

    and sharp instruments in containers that are

    _____,

    _____, and

    _____.

41. List the times you need to decontaminate work surfaces.

    A. _____

    B. _____

    C. _____

    D. _____

42. What should you use to clean up broken glass?

    _____

43. An exposure incident is _____

    _____.

44. Parenteral means _____

_____.

45. The source individual is _____

_____.

46. The Centers for Disease Control and Prevention

(CDC) serves to _____

_____.

*Multiple Choice*

Circle the **BEST** Answer

47. A carrier can pass a pathogen to others.
    A. True
    B. False

48. Microbes are destroyed by
    A. Water
    B. A warm environment
    C. A dark environment
    D. Heat and light

49. Which of the following is *not* a sign or symptom of infection?
    A. Fever
    B. Increased appetite
    C. Pain and tenderness
    D. Redness and swelling

50. The most important measure to prevent the spread of infection is
    A. Sterilization of equipment
    B. Hand hygiene
    C. Surgical asepsis
    D. Isolation Precautions

51. An alcohol-based hand rub can be used to decontaminate your hands
    A. When they are visibly dirty or soiled with blood, body fluids, secretions, or excretions
    B. Before eating
    C. After using the restroom
    D. After removing gloves

52. Which is *not* a rule for hand washing with soap and water?
    A. Wash your hands under warm running water.
    B. Stand away from the sink.
    C. Keep your hands and forearms higher than your elbows.
    D. Rub your palms together to work up a good lather.

53. When cleaning equipment, do all of the following *except*
    A. Wear personal protective equipment.
    B. Rinse the item in hot water first.
    C. Wash the item with soap and hot water.
    D. Scrub thoroughly. Use a brush if necessary.

54. Disposable gloves are worn when using chemical disinfectants.
    A. True
    B. False

55. All non-pathogens and pathogens are destroyed by
    A. Disinfection
    B. Cleaning
    C. Sterilization
    D. Handwashing

56. Which aseptic measure controls reservoirs?
    A. Washing the overbed table with soap and water before placing a meal tray on it.
    B. Wearing personal protective equipment as needed
    C. Holding soiled linens away from your uniform
    D. Providing good skin care

57. Which aseptic measure controls a portal of entry?
    A. Cleaning away from your body
    B. Providing perineal care after bowel elimination
    C. Emptying urinals promptly
    D. Cleaning and disinfecting the shower after use

58. Which of the following is an aseptic measure?
    A. Taking equipment from one person's room to another
    B. Holding equipment and linen close to your uniform
    C. Covering your nose and mouth when coughing or sneezing
    D. Shaking linen to remove wrinkles

59. You help prevent the spread of infection by
    A. Cleaning toward your body
    B. Using leakproof plastic bags for soiled linens
    C. Holding equipment and linens against your uniform
    D. Cleaning from the dirtiest area to the cleanest area

60. Which is *not* a rule for Isolation Precautions?
    A. Collect all needed items before entering the room.
    B. Use paper towels to handle contaminated items.
    C. Do not touch any clean area or object if your hands are contaminated.
    D. Wear gloves to turn faucets on and off.

61. Standard Precautions involve
    A. Washing your hands every hour
    B. Wearing gloves for all patient and resident care
    C. Decontaminating your hands right away after removing gloves
    D. Wearing the same gloves for all tasks and procedures on the same person

62. Persons on Isolation Precautions may feel lonely. You can help the person by doing all of the following *except*:
    A. Encouraging family to stay away to prevent the spread of microbes
    B. Providing hobby materials if possible
    C. Organizing your work so you can stay to visit with the person
    D. Saying "Hello" from the doorway often

63. Remember the following when wearing gloves.
    A. Gloves are easier to put on when hands are wet.
    B. Remove a torn glove when you complete the task.
    C. The same pair of gloves are worn for persons in the same room.
    D. Change gloves when moving from a contaminated body site to a clean body site.

64. Gloves are removed so the inside part is on the outside. The inside is clean.
    A. True
    B. False

65. A wet or moist mask is contaminated.
    A. True
    B. False

66. Protective gowns
    A. Must cover you from your neck to your knees
    B. Open in the front
    C. Are used more than once
    D. Are clean on the outside

67. The Bloodborne Pathogen Standard is a regulation of
    A. OBRA
    B. Medicare
    C. OSHA
    D. Medicaid

68. Hepatitis B is spread by
    A. The fecal-oral route
    B. Blood and sexual contact
    C. Contaminated water
    D. Coughing and sneezing

69. Which statement about the hepatitis B vaccine is *false*?
    A. You can receive it within 10 working days of being hired.
    B. You can refuse the vaccination.
    C. If you refuse the vaccination, you can have it at a later time.
    D. You pay for the vaccination.

70. Which work practice is required by OSHA?
    A. Store food and drinks where blood or OPIM are kept.
    B. Practice hand hygiene before removing gloves.
    C. Wash hands as soon as possible after skin contact with blood or OPIM.
    D. Recap and remove needles by hand.

71. Which is *not* a safety measure for using personal protective equipment (PPE)?
    A. Remove PPE when it becomes contaminated.
    B. Wash and decontaminate disposable gloves for reuse.
    C. Place used PPE in marked containers or areas.
    D. Wear gloves when you expect contact with blood or OPIM.

72. OSHA requires all of these measures for contaminated laundry *except*
    A. Handle it as little as possible.
    B. Wear gloves or other needed OPIM.
    C. Bag contaminated laundry in the dirty utility room.
    D. Place wet, contaminated laundry in leak-proof containers before transport.

73. When do you need to report an exposure
    incident?
    A. At once
    B. At the end of your shift
    C. Only if you request blood testing
    D. When you have time

74. The Centers for Disease Control and Prevention is
    A. A state agency
    B. An OBRA agency
    C. A federal agency
    D. A survey team

75. Ms. Jean Monroe is on Isolation Precautions.
    Your co-worker, Mary, is assigned to care for
    Ms. Monroe. Mary asks you to help answer
    the signal lights of her other patients while she
    is in Ms. Monroe's room. You should
    A. Do so willingly and pleasantly
    B. Tell Mary that you have your own
       work to do
    C. Report Mary's behavior to the nurse
    D. Ignore the request and complete your own
       assignment

## MOSBY'S NURSING ASSISTANT SKILLS VIDEO EXERCISES

### Questions from "Medical Asepsis" Section of the Basic Principles Video

76. Practices to remove or destroy microbes and to

    prevent them from spreading are called _____

    _____.

77. To prevent the spread of microbes, you must
    wash your hands:

    A. _____

    B. _____

    C. _____

    D. _____

78. Besides hand washing, other measures to
    prevent the spread of microbes include:

    A. _____

    _____

    B. _____

    _____

    C. _____

    _____

    D. _____

    _____

    E. _____

    _____

    F. _____

    _____

    G. _____

    _____

    H. _____

    _____

    I. _____

    _____

## CASE STUDY

*Miss Joan McMillan is a 60-year-old patient. She was admitted to the hospital with influenza. She has been placed in a private room and is on Droplet Precautions. Miss McMillan is hearing impaired. She has difficulty seeing without her eyeglasses. She has very few visitors. She lives in her own home in a small rural town about 50 miles from the hospital.*

*Answer the following questions.*

1. What signs and symptoms might Miss McMillan have?

2. What practices are required when providing care for Miss McMillan?

3. What guidelines will you follow if you need to transport Miss McMillan to another area of the hospital for tests?

4. How will you meet Miss McMillan's love, belonging, and self-esteem needs?

## ADDITIONAL LEARNING ACTIVITIES

1. List the measures you practice in your personal life to prevent infection.

2. List the special care needs of persons on Isolation Precautions. Describe how you can help meet their needs?

3. View the CD Companion: Skills to help you learn and practice the Hand Washing Procedure.

4. Carefully review the procedures in Chapter 10. Using the procedure checklists provided on pages 211-214:
   A. Practice the procedures for hand washing, removing gloves, donning and removing a gown, and donning and removing a mask.

   B. Observe a classmate performing the procedures.

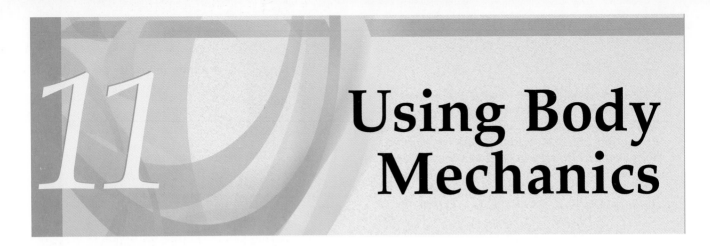

# Using Body Mechanics

## OBJECTIVES

The questions and student activities in this chapter will help you meet these objectives.
- Define the key terms listed in this chapter
- Explain the purpose and rules of body mechanics
- Explain how ergonomics can prevent workplace accidents
- Identify comfort and safety measures for moving and turning persons in bed
- Explain how to safely perform transfers
- Explain why body alignment and position changes are important
- Identify the comfort and safety measures for positioning a person
- Position persons in the basic bed positions and in a chair
- Perform the procedures described in this chapter

## STUDY QUESTIONS

*Matching*

Match each term with the correct definition.

1. _____ The area on which an object rests

2. _____ Using the body in an efficient and careful way

3. _____ The back-lying or supine position

4. _____ The way the head, trunk, arms, and legs are aligned with one another

5. _____ A semi-sitting position; the head of the bed is raised between 45 and 60 degrees

6. _____ The side-lying position

7. _____ The rubbing of one surface against another

8. _____ Turning the person as a unit, in alignment, with one motion

9. _____ Body alignment

10. _____ Lying on the abdomen with the head turned to one side

11. _____ The lateral position

A. Body mechanics

B. Friction

C. Logrolling

D. Shearing

E. Base of support

F. Sims' position

G. Body alignment

H. Dorsal recumbent position

I. Fowler's position

J. Posture

12. _____ A left side-lying position in which the upper leg is sharply flexed so it is not on the lower leg and the lower arm is behind the person

13. _____ A belt used to support persons who are unsteady or disabled: a gait belt

14. _____ When skin sticks to a surface while muscles slide in the direction the body is moving

K. Side-lying position

L. Transfer belt

M. Prone position

N. Lateral position

*Fill in the Blanks*

15. _____

lets the body move and function with strength

and efficiency.

16. The strongest and largest muscles are in the

_____,

_____,

_____, and

_____.

17. For good body mechanics, you need to _____

_____

to lift a heavy object.

18. Ergonomics is _____

_____

19. The goal of ergonomics is to _____

_____.

20. Musculoskeletal disorders (MSDs) are _____

_____

_____.

21. To reduce friction and shearing, you need to

_____.

22. You need to move Mr. Green up in bed. How will you promote his mental comfort?

_____

23. You are getting ready to move Mr. Stevens up in bed. Why should you place the pillow against the headboard?

_____

_____

24. It is best to have help and to use an assist device when moving persons up in bed. You can perform this procedure alone *only if*:

A. _____

B. _____

C. _____

D. _____

E. _____

F. _____

G. _____

25. Explain why an assist device is used to move persons up in bed.

_____

_____

26. Some persons are moved up in bed with an assist device. With a co-worker's help, use an assist device for persons who:

A. _____

B. _____

C. _____

D. _____

27. You are moving Ms. Peters up in bed using a lift sheet. How should you stand?

    _____

    _____

    _____

28. Explain why you need to move Mr. Lewis to the side of the bed before turning him.

    _____

    _____

29. You will move Mr. Lewis in segments. Which part of his body do you need to move first?

    _____

30. What information do you need from the nurse and the care plan before turning a person?

    A. _____

    B. _____

    C. _____

    D. _____

    E. _____

    F. _____

    G. _____

    H. _____

31. Why is it important to position the person in good alignment after turning him or her?

    _____

    _____

32. Logrolling is used to turn the following persons:

    A. _____

    B. _____

    C. _____

33. You are assisting Ms. Young to dangle. She complains of feeling dizzy. What should you do?

    _____

34. You are assisting Mr. Joe Burch to dangle. After he is in the sitting position, you need to check his condition by:

    A. _____

    B. _____

    C. _____

    D. _____

35. To transfer a person means _____

    _____.

36. Explain why you need to know about areas of weakness before you transfer a person?

    _____

    _____

    _____

37. What observations do you need to report and record after transferring a person?

    A. _____

    _____

    B. _____

    _____

    C. _____

    _____

    D. _____

    _____

38. The person wears _____

    footwear for transfers.

39. You are transferring a person from the chair to the bed. The number of staff members needed for a transfer depends on the person's

    _____,

    _____, and

    _____.

40. You are preparing to transfer Ms. Ann Jensen from her wheelchair to bed. Her left side is her weak side. How will you position her wheelchair for the transfer?

    _____

    _____

41. The nurse tells you to transfer Mr. Ben Brown using a mechanical lift. You have not used the lift before. What should you do?

    _____

    _____

    _____

42. How will you promote Mr. Brown's mental comfort when using a mechanical lift to transfer him?

    _____

    _____

43. How is the wheelchair positioned for wheelchair to toilet transfers?

    _____

    _____

    _____

    _____

44. List four reasons that frequent position changes and good alignment are needed.

    A. _____

    B. _____

    C. _____

    D. _____

45. What information do you need from the nurse and the care plan before you position or reposition a person?

    A. _____

    B. _____

    C. _____

    D. _____

    E. _____

    F. _____

    G. _____

    H. _____

46. Pressure ulcers are serious threats from:

    A. _____

    B. _____

47. A contracture is _____

    _____

48. You are positioning Ms. Barnett in Fowler's position. For good alignment, you need to:

    A. _____

    B. _____

    C. _____

49. You have positioned Mr. Carson in the prone position. Where should you place small pillows?

_____

50. You are positioning Mr. Carson in a chair. For good alignment you need to:

A. _____

_____

B. _____

_____

C. _____

_____

*Multiple Choice*

Circle the **BEST** Answer

51. Which is *not* involved in good body mechanics?
    A. Keep objects close to your body when you lift, move, or carry them.
    B. Push, slide, or pull heavy objects.
    C. Work with sudden motions.
    D. Turn your whole body when changing the direction of your movement.

52. To pick up a box using good body mechanics, you
    A. Use the muscles of the lower back.
    B. Bend your hips and knees.
    C. Hold the box away from your body.
    D. Stand with your feet very close together.

53. Before moving a person in bed, you need the following information from the nurse and the care plan *except*:
    A. Any position limits or restrictions
    B. How to use body mechanics
    C. How many workers are needed
    D. If the person uses bed rails

54. A lift sheet is used to move Ms. Lee up in bed. Which is *false*?
    A. Two workers are needed to move Ms. Lee.
    B. Shearing and friction are reduced.
    C. Place the sheet under Ms. Lee from her waist to her knees.
    D. Roll the sides of the lift sheet up close to Ms. Lee.

55. Two or three staff members are needed to logroll a person.
    A. True
    B. False

56. Ms. Vance is 90 years old and has arthritis. Before turning her, you need to move her to the side of bed. You need to move her in segments.
    A. True
    B. False

57. You are helping Ms. Young to dangle. Which is *incorrect*?
    A. Provide support if necessary.
    B. Ask her how she feels.
    C. Check her pulse and respirations.
    D. Leave her alone if she tells you she is OK.

58. Transfer belts are always applied over clothing.
    A. True
    B. False

59. You are applying a transfer belt on Ms. Perez. Which is *incorrect*?
    A. The belt should be snug, but should not cause discomfort or impair breathing.
    B. You should be able to slide your open, flat hand under the belt.
    C. Make sure her breasts are not caught under the belt.
    D. Place the buckle in back over her spine.

60. When preparing to dangle a person, the head of the bed should be
    A. As flat as possible
    B. Slightly raised
    C. Raised to a sitting position
    D. In the position the person prefers

61. When using a transfer belt to transfer a person, you grasp the belt:
    A. Underneath the belt at each side
    B. In the back near the person's spine
    C. In the front close to the midline
    D. Where it is most comfortable for you

62. You are transferring Ms. Bertha Blair from her bed to the chair. Which is *correct*?
    A. Ms. Blair wears non-skid footwear.
    B. Ms. Blair is helped out of bed on her weak side.
    C. The bed is kept in the high position.
    D. Ms. Blair places her arms around your neck.

63. You are assisting Mr. Ben Blake to transfer from his bed to his wheelchair. You must do all of the following *except*:
    A. Lock wheelchair wheels.
    B. Make sure wheelchair footplates are down.
    C. Remove or swing the front rigging out of the way.
    D. Lower the bed to its lowest position.

64. Which statement about mechanical lifts is *false*?
    A. Persons who cannot help themselves are transferred with mechanical lifts.
    B. The slings, straps, hooks, and chains must be in good repair.
    C. The person's weight must not exceed the lift's capacity.
    D. If you know how to use one type of lift, you know how to use all types.

65. You are using a mechanical lift to transfer Mr. Brown. You should instruct him to hold onto the swivel bar.
    A. True
    B. False

66. Before transferring a person to the toilet, you need to:
    A. Practice hand hygiene.
    B. Remove the elevated toilet seat.
    C. Check the towel bar to make sure it is secure.
    D. Have the person wear warm slippers.

67. To safely position a person, you need to do all of the following *except*:
    A. Use good body mechanics.
    B. Explain the procedure to the person.
    C. Position the person as quickly as possible.
    D. Place the signal light within reach after positioning.

68. Which action will *not* help prevent contractures?
    A. Keeping the person in the supine position as much as possible
    B. Repositioning the person according to the care plan
    C. Assisting with exercise as directed
    D. Encouraging activity according to the care plan

69. You are repositioning Mr. Green in the wheelchair. He is able to assist. Which is *correct*?
    A. Stand behind him.
    B. Ask him to place his folded hands in his lap.
    C. Position his feet on the footplates.
    D. Lock the wheelchair wheels.

70. You need to reposition Ms. Howard in her wheelchair. She cannot assist. A mechanical lift is used.
    the wheelchair.
    A. True
    B. False

71. Residents and patients are repositioned at least:
    A. Every hour
    B. Every 2 hours
    C. Every 4 hours
    D. Once each shift

72. Which action promotes the person's independence?
    A. Positioning the person's wheelchair so the person can see outside
    B. Letting the person stay in the same position for up to 4 hours
    C. Letting the person help as much as safely possible
    D. Arranging the person's room for your convenience

73. Moving, turning, transferring, and positioning a person should be done by one worker whenever possible.
    A. True
    B. False

## Labeling

### Label each position

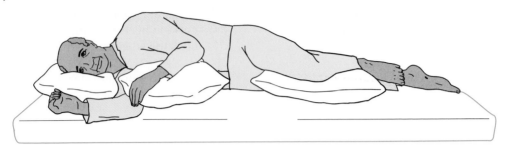

74. _____

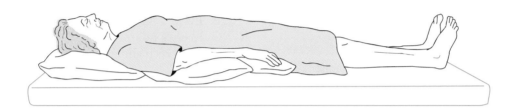

75. _____

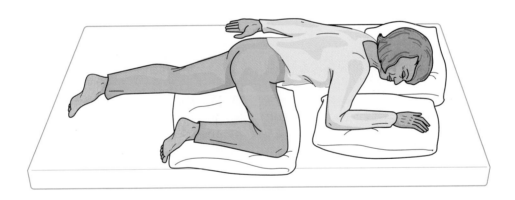

76. _____

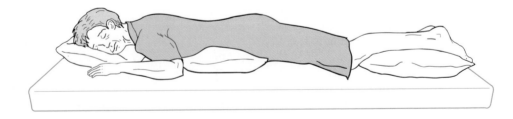

77. _____

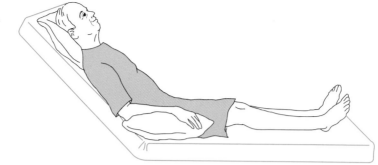

78. _____

## MOSBY'S NURSING ASSISTANT SKILLS VIDEOS EXERCISES

**Questions from the "Principles of Body Mechanics, Moving a Person Up in Bed, Turning and Positioning, Dangling, and Transfer" Sections of the Body Mechanics and Exercise Video**

79. How you perform your tasks as a nursing assistant affects:

   A. _____

   B. _____

80. The principles of body mechanics involve:

   A. _____

   B. _____

   C. _____

81. When you are delegated lifting, moving, positioning, and transferring activities, you need to:

   A. _____

   _____

   B. _____

   _____

   C. _____

   _____

   D. _____

   _____

E. _____

   _____

F. _____

   _____

G. _____

   _____

82. You are preparing to transfer Mr. Anderson. How will you know how much help he needs?

   _____

83. When transferring a person from the bed to the wheelchair, where is the wheelchair back positioned?

   _____

84. The transfer belt was placed just below Mr. Anderson's rib cage with the buckle centered in the front.
   A. True
   B. False

85. Where did the nurse place her hands to transfer Mr. Anderson when not using the transfer belt?

   _____

86. After transferring a person, where should the wheelchair be positioned?

   _____

## CASE STUDY

*Mr. John Lind is a 70-year-old resident living in Pine View Nursing Center. He is 5 feet and 11inches tall and weighs 190 pounds. Mr. Lind cannot walk. He uses a wheelchair. He cannot stand alone. He is able to bear some weight on his legs to assist with transfers from his bed to his wheelchair and from his wheel chair onto the toilet. His right side is his strong side. Mr. Lind has some difficulty breathing when lying flat in bed. He needs help to change positions when in bed.*

*Answer the following questions.*

1. What factors does the nursing team need to consider when planning for Mr. Lind's safety?

2. What skin problems is Mr. Lind at risk for?

3. How can you protect Mr. Lind from friction and shearing during transfers and when turning and moving him in bed?

4. When assisting Mr. Lind with transfers, which side will you move first?

5. How often do you need to help Mr. Lind reposition himself in bed? In the wheelchair?

6. What steps will you take to help Mr. Lind reposition himself in his wheelchair?

7. Which position will Mr. Lind probably prefer when he is in bed? Why?

## ADDITIONAL LEARNING ACTIVITIES

1. Review the rules for body mechanics
   A. Do you practice these rules in your daily activities? Explain.

   B. Do you practice these rules in your work activities? Explain.

   C. How can you change how you move and work to decrease your risk for injury?

2. List the measures needed for good alignment for each of the following positions (See pages 172 and 174 in the textbook.)
   A. Fowler's position

   B. Supine position

   C. Lateral position

   D. Sims' position

   E. Chair position

3. Describe how you would reposition a person in the chair or wheelchair: (See page 176 in the textbook.)
   A. If the person is alert, cooperative, can follow instructions, and has the strength to help

   B. If the person cannot assist with repositioning

4. View the CD Companion: Skills to help you learn and practice the following procedures:
   A. Turning and Positioning the person

   B. Transferring the Person to a Chair or Wheelchair

5. Review the procedures described in Chapter 11.
   A. Under the supervision of your instructor, practice each procedure.
      (1) Use the procedure checklists provided on pages 215-236.

      (2) Take your turn being the patient or resident.

      (3) Discuss the experience with your classmates and instructor. Answer these questions.
         a. Did you feel safe? Explain.

         b. Did you feel comfortable? Explain.

6. Practice proper positioning (Fowler's, supine, prone, lateral, and Sims') with a classmate or family member. Use pillows to promote comfort and body alignment. Assume each position yourself.

# 12 Assisting With Comfort

## OBJECTIVES

The questions and student activities in this chapter will help you meet these objectives.
- Define the key terms listed in this chapter
- Describe how to control temperature, odors, noise, and lighting for the person's comfort
- Describe the basic bed positions
- Describe how to use the furniture and equipment in the person's unit
- Describe four ways to make beds
- Handle linens following the rules of medical asepsis
- Describe the factors that affect sleep and the common sleep disorders
- Identify the nursing measures that promote sleep
- Perform the procedures described in this chapter

## STUDY QUESTIONS

*Matching*

*Match each term with the correct definition.*

1. _____ Having the means to be completely free from public view while in bed

2. _____ A chronic condition in which the person cannot sleep or stay asleep all night

3. _____ The amount and quality of sleep are decreased

4. _____ The head of the bed is raised 30 degrees; or the head of the bed is raised 30 degrees and the knee portion is raised 15 degrees

5. _____ The sleeping person leaves the bed and walks about

6. _____ The head of the bed is lowered and the foot of the bed is raised

7. _____ The head of the bed is raised, and the foot of the bed is lowered

8. _____ A semi-sitting position; the head of the bed is raised between 45 and 60 degrees

A. Reverse-Trendelenburg's position

B. Insomnia

C. Full visual privacy

D. Sleep deprivation

E. Sleepwalking

F. Semi-Fowler's position

G. Fowler's position

H. Trendelenburg's position

*Fill in the Blanks*

9. _____ is a state of well-being.

10. The person's unit is _____

    _____.

    This area is _____.

11. To protect old and ill persons from drafts, you
    need to:

    A. _____

    B. _____

    C. _____

    D. _____

    E. _____

    F. _____

12. Smoking causes odors. If you smoke, you need to:

    A. _____

    B. _____

    C. _____

13. Common health care sounds frighten and
    irritate some people. List four ways to help
    decrease noise.

    A. _____

    B. _____

    C. _____

    D. _____

14. Explain why hospital beds are raised horizontally
    to give care.

    _____

    _____

15. Mr. Harvey has a manual bed. Explain why it is
    important to keep the cranks down when not
    in use.

    _____

    _____

16. List the five basic bed positions.

    A. _____

    B. _____

    C. _____

    D. _____

    E. _____

17. Bed wheels must be locked when you:

    A. _____

    B. _____

18. The overbed table is used for _____

    _____

    _____.

19. Explain the purpose of raised toilet seats.

    _____

    _____

20. A _____

    bed is not in use. Top linens are not folded back.

21. A surgical bed is also called _____

    _____.

22. Place clean linens on a _____.

23. When are wet damp or soiled linens changed?

    _____

24. What is the purpose of a cotton drawsheet?

    _____

25. What information do you need from the nurse
    and the care plan before making a bed?

    A. _____

    B. _____

    C. _____

    D. _____

    E. _____

    F. _____

    G. _____

    H. _____

26. Why is it important to follow Standard
    Precautions and the Bloodborne Pathogen
    Standard when removing linen from the
    person's bed?

    _____

    _____

27. After making a bed, you must _____

    _____

    _____.

28. You are putting the top sheet on a closed bed.

    The hem-stitching should face _____

    _____.

29. Describe how you should place the pillow on
    the person's bed.

    _____

    _____

30. A closed bed becomes an open bed by _____

    _____.

31. List six factors that affect sleep.

    A. _____

    B. _____

    C. _____

    D. _____

    E. _____

    F. _____

32. Sleep disorders involve _____

    _____.

*Multiple Choice*

Circle the **BEST** Answer

33. To maintain the person's unit, you need to:
    A. Adjust the temperature so it is comfortable for you.
    B. Arrange personal items the way you prefer.
    C. Keep the signal light within reach at all times.
    D. Empty the person's wastebasket weekly.

34. You are assisting Mr. John Martin with his bath. You notice many small scraps of paper with notes on them lying on his bedside stand. You can throw them in the trash to keep his unit neat and clean.
    A. True
    B. False

35. Which room temperature range is usually comfortable for most healthy people.
    A. 65° F to 68° F
    B. 68° F to 74° F
    C. 72° F to 82° F
    D. 82° F to 90° F

36. Which action will *not* help reduce odors?
    A. Dispose of incontinence products at the end of your shift.
    B. Check incontinent persons often.
    C. Keep laundry containers closed.
    D. Provide good hygiene.

37. Good lighting is needed for safety and comfort. You need to:
    A. Provide bright light to help the person relax.
    B. Provide dim lighting during the night.
    C. Adjust lighting the way visitors request.
    D. Keep light controls within the person's reach.

38. Which bed positions require a doctor's order?
    A. Flat and Fowler's
    B. Fowler's and semi-Fowler's
    C. Semi-Fowler's and reverse Trendelenburg's
    D. Trendelenburg's and reverse Trendelenburg's

39. Mr. Harvey tells you he does not like his mattress because it is too hard. What should you do?
    A. Tell him it is the only mattress available.
    B. Call maintenance and ask for a new mattress.
    C. Tell the nurse about Mr. Harvey's complaint.
    D. Ask Mr. Harvey's family to bring him a more comfortable mattress.

40. Which item *cannot* be placed on the overbed table?
    A. A bedpan
    B. The water pitcher
    C. A box of tissues
    D. A book

41. Where should you store the person's bedpan and toilet paper?
    A. On the overbed table
    B. On the lower shelf in the bedside stand
    C. Under the bed
    D. In the person's bathroom

42. Each person's unit must have at least one chair. The chair must:
    A. Be a reclining chair
    B. Be a straight back chair
    C. Not tip or move during transfers
    D. Be provided by the person or family

43. The privacy curtain must be pulled completely around the person's bed
    A. Always when giving care
    B. Only when the person's roommate is present
    C. Only when the room door is open
    D. Only if the person requests it to be

44. Ms. Emma Franks is confused. Therefore she does not need a signal light.
    A. True
    B. False

45. For the person's safety, you must:
    A. Keep the signal light within the person's reach.
    B. Place the signal light on the person's weak side.
    C. Remind the person to signal only in emergencies.
    D. Take the signal light away from a person if he or she uses it too often.

46. OBRA requires closet space for each nursing center resident.
    A. True
    B. False

47. To keep beds neat and clean, you need to:
    A. Straighten linens whenever loose or wrinkled.
    B. Check for and remove food and crumbs once each shift.
    C. Straighten linens whenever they become wet, soiled, or damp.
    D. Change all linens daily.

48. What type of bed is made for residents who are out of bed for a short time?
    A. A closed bed
    B. An occupied bed
    C. An open bed
    D. A surgical bed

49. You are making a closed bed for a new resident. Which piece of linen is placed on the bed first?
    A. Bottom sheet
    B. Cotton draw sheet
    C. Mattress pad
    D. Pillow case

50. What type of bed is made after a person is discharged?
    A. An open bed
    B. A closed bed
    C. An occupied bed
    D. A surgical bed

51. You are making an occupied bed. Which is *incorrect*?
    A. Keep the bed in the lowest position.
    B. If the person uses bed rails, the far bed rail is up.
    C. Keep the person in good alignment.
    D. After making the bed, lock the bed wheels.

52. You have finished making a surgical bed for a resident arriving by stretcher. You should leave the bed in its highest position.
    A. True
    B. False

53. Which is a rule for bedmaking?
    A. Shake linens to remove wrinkles.
    B. Hold linens against your uniform.
    C. Place dirty linen on the floor.
    D. Follow the rules of medical asepsis.

54. You brought an extra pillowcase into a patient's room. What should you do?
    A. Take it back to the linen closet.
    B. Put it in the dirty laundry.
    C. Use it for another patient.
    D. Put it in the patient's closet.

55. During sleep
    A. Tissue healing and repair occur.
    B. Stress and tension increase.
    C. The body uses more energy than when awake.
    D. Body functions speed up.

56. Which of these measures will *not* promote sleep?
    A. Giving a back massage
    B. Providing soft music
    C. Keeping the room cool and well lighted
    D. Good body alignment

57. Mrs. Adams asks for a bed time snack. Which does *not* help promote sleep?
    A. Coffee and a brownie
    B. Milk
    C. Toast
    D. Crackers and milk

## MOSBY'S NURSING ASSISTANT SKILLS VIDEOS EXERCISES

### Questions from the Bedmaking Video

58. Linens are always changed when _____

    _____.

59. Follow these procedure guidelines when making a bed:

    A. _____

    B. _____

    C. _____

    D. _____

60. Wash your hands _____

    handling clean linens and _____

    handling dirty linens.

61. Your uniform is considered _____.

    Linens must be held _____.

62. You must never place clean or soiled linens

    _____.

63. Never shake linens because _____

    _____.

64. How should you fold the bedspread and blanket if they will be reused?

   _____

   _____

65. Which piece of linen is used to cover the person before the top sheet is removed?

   _____

66. When fanfolding bottom linens, you need to keep the side that touched the person

   _____ .

67. Before putting on clean linens, you need to

   _____ .

68. Place the clean bottom sheet on the bed with the

   hem stitching _____ .

69. The cotton drawsheet must cover the entire plastic drawsheet.
   A. True
   B. False

70. Top linens must be loose enough to allow

   _____ .

71. All top linens are tucked under the mattress together.
   A. True
   B. False

72. After making the bed you need to:

   A. _____

   B. _____

   C. _____

   D. _____

   E. _____

   F. _____

   G. _____

## CASE STUDY

*Ms. Angela Lopez and Ms. Lois Green share a room at Pine View Nursing Center.*

*Ms. Lopez has the bed by the window. She likes to sleep with the window open. She likes the privacy curtain between her bed and Ms. Green's bed open so she can see out the door. Ms. Lopez has a large family and many friends who visit often. They often bring her ethnic foods. She sometimes hides food in her drawers and closet.*

*Ms. Green is a very private person. She chills easily. She likes to go to bed early. Listening to opera music helps her fall asleep. Ms. Jones has many figurines, which she likes to display in a cabinet she brought from home. She worries about them getting broken. She also brought her own reclining chair from home.*

*Answer the following questions.*

1. What challenges does the interdisciplinary health team have in meeting the needs of each resident?

2. How can the rights of each resident be promoted?

3. How can the interdisciplinary health team promote each person's comfort and quality of life?

## ADDITIONAL LEARNING ACTIVITIES

1. Discuss the importance of personal space in your daily life. Answer the following questions:
   A. How would you feel about sharing a room with another person?

   B. How would you decide what items to take with you and what items to leave behind?

2. Make a list of factors that affect your ability to sleep. Answer the following questions.

   A. What temperatures are most comfortable for you? How do you adapt to changes in temperature?

   B. Are there certain odors that prevent sleep? How do you control the odors in your environment?

   C. How do noises and sounds affect your ability to sleep? What sounds keep you awake? Are there sounds that help you relax?

   D. How do you control the light in your environment to help you sleep?

   E. Do you have certain rituals that help you sleep? Explain.

   F. How might you use what you know about your personal comfort needs to help you provide better care.

3. How much sleep do you need to feel rested?

   A. How does lack of sleep affect your daily activities?

4. Practice gathering linen in the correct order for bedmaking. List the correct order on an index card. Carry the card with you until you have the order memorized.

5. View the CD Companion: Skills to help you learn and practice the Making an Occupied Bed Procedure.

6. Practice the procedures in Chapter 12. Use the procedure checklists provided on pp. 237-245.

7. Observe classmates performing the procedures in Chapter 12. Use the procedure checklists provided on pp. 237-245.

# 13 Assisting With Hygiene

## OBJECTIVES

The questions and student activities in this chapter will help you meet these objectives.
- Define the key terms listed in this chapter
- Describe the care given before and after breakfast, after lunch, and in the evening
- Describe the rules for bathing
- Identify safety measures for tub baths and showers
- Explain the purposes of a back massage
- Explain the purposes of perineal care
- Identify the observations to make while assisting with hygiene
- Perform the procedures described in this chapter

## STUDY QUESTIONS

### Matching

*Match each term with the correct definition.*

1. _____ Routine care before breakfast

2. _____ Routine hygiene done after lunch and the evening meal

3. _____ Breathing fluid or an object into the lungs

4. _____ Care given at bedtime

5. _____ Mouth care

6. _____ Cleaning the genital and anal areas

7. _____ Care given after breakfast

A. Morning care

B. Oral hygiene

C. Evening care (PM care)

D. Early morning care (AM care)

E. Afternoon care

F. Aspiration

G. Perineal care (pericare)

### Fill in the Blanks

8. The _____

   is the body's first line of defense against disease.

9. Intact skin prevents _____

   from entering the body.

10. You will assist patients and residents with

    personal hygiene. You need to protect the right

    to _____ and

    _____.

11. Mr. Gene Jones has his own teeth. You assist him with oral hygiene. What observations do you need to report and record?

    A. _____

    B. _____

    C. _____

    D. _____

    E. _____

12. Explain why a tooth brush with soft bristles is used to brush the person's teeth.

    _____

13. Explain why you need to follow Standard Precautions and the Bloodborne Pathogen Standard when giving oral hygiene.

    _____

    _____

    _____

14. Many people brush their own teeth. You may have to brush the teeth of persons who:

    A. _____

    B. _____

    C. _____

15. Explain why flossing is done.

    _____

    _____

16. Explain the steps in brushing teeth.

    A. _____

    _____

    B. _____

    _____

    C. _____

    _____

    D. _____

    _____

17. You are giving oral care to an unconscious person. To prevent aspiration, you need to:

    A. _____

    B. _____

18. You are using a sponge swab to give oral hygiene to an unconscious person. Explain why you need to make sure the sponge is tight on the stick.

    _____

    _____

19. Ms. Roberta Smith removed her dentures and placed them under her pillow. While you were straightening her pillow, the dentures fell off the bed and broke. What should you do?

    _____

    _____

20. Mr. John Roberts wears an upper denture. You need to remove the denture for him. Explain how you would do so.

    _____

    _____

    _____

    _____

21. List eight benefits of bathing.

   A. _____

   B. _____

   C. _____

   D. _____

   E. _____

   F. _____

   G. _____

   H. _____

22. The bathing method for each person depends on:

   A. _____

   B. _____

   C. _____

23. You are giving Ms. Peters a tub bath. What observations do you need to report and record?

   A. _____

   B. _____

   C. _____

   D. _____

   E. _____

   F. _____

   G. _____

   H. _____

   I. _____

   J. _____

24. Do not use powder near persons with

   respiratory disorders because _____

   _____ .

25. To safely apply powder, you need to:

   A. _____

   B. _____

   C. _____

26. Explain why you should allow the person to use the bathroom, commode, bedpan, or urinal before bathing.

   _____

   _____

27. You are giving Mr. Rust a complete bed bath. Why should you wait to remove his gown until after you wash his face, ears, and neck?

   _____

   _____

28. A partial bath involves bathing the _____ ,

   _____ ,

   _____ ,

   _____ ,

   _____ ,

   and _____ .

29. You protect the persons privacy during a shower by:

   A. _____

   B. _____

30. What information do you need from the nurse and the care plan before giving a shower or tub bath?

   A. _____

   B. _____

   C. _____

   D. _____

   E. _____

   F. _____

31. Mr. Harris uses bar soap for his tub bath. Why is bar soap kept in the soap dish between latherings?

_____

_____

32. Before giving a back massage, you need to observe the skin for:

A. _____

B. _____

C. _____

D. _____

33. List three methods used to warm lotion before applying it.

A. _____

B. _____

C. _____

34. Which position is best for giving a back massage?

_____

35. You need to give a back massage to Mr. Martinez. He is 90 years old and has arthritis in his hips and knees. Which position will likely be most comfortable for him?

_____

36. Perineal care involves _____

_____.

37. Explain why perineal care is given?

_____

_____

38. When is perineal care given?

A. _____

B. _____

39. When giving perineal care, work from

_____ to

_____.

40. You have given perineal care to Ms. Hanson. What observations do you need to report and record?

A. _____

B. _____

C. _____

D. _____

41. You are giving perineal care to Mr. Martinez. Explain how you will clean the tip of his penis.

_____

_____

_____

## Multiple Choice

Circle the **BEST** Answer

42. Before giving oral hygiene, you need the following information from the nurse and the care plan *except*:
    A. The type of oral hygiene to give
    B. The type of toothbrush to use
    C. If flossing is needed
    D. How much help the person needs

43. Which action is *incorrect* when flossing the person's teeth?
    A. Hold the floss between the middle fingers of each hand.
    B. Start at the upper back tooth on the right side.
    C. Move the floss gently up and down between the teeth.
    D. Use a new piece of floss for each tooth.

44. When providing mouth care to the unconscious person, you:
    A. Use your fingers to hold the mouth open.
    B. Position the person on his or her back.
    C. Use a hard bristle toothbrush.
    D. Explain what you are doing step by step.

45. How often is mouth care given to unconscious persons?
    A. At least every 2 hours
    B. Twice a day
    C. Every 4 hours
    D. Every 6 hours

46. You are giving mouth care to an unconscious person. Which action is *incorrect*?
    A. Provide for privacy.
    B. Place a towel under the person's face.
    C. Place a kidney basin under the chin.
    D. With the tongue blade, use force to separate the upper and lower teeth.

47. When cleaning dentures, you need to:
    A. Use hot water
    B. Firmly hold them over a basin of water lined with a towel
    C. Use a sponge swab to clean them
    D. Store them dry in a container with a lid

48. Which is *not* a rule for bathing?
    A. Follow the care plan for bathing method.
    B. Allow personal choice whenever possible.
    C. Cover the person for warmth and privacy.
    D. Briskly rub the person dry with a clean towel.

49. Mr. Albert Martinez has dementia. He becomes agitated when you try to give him a tub bath. Which measure might be helpful?
    A. Trying to hurry Mr. Martinez to get the bath over with as soon as possible
    B. Explaining to Mr. Martinez that there is nothing to be afraid of
    C. Trying the bath later
    D. Getting help to force Mr. Martinez into the tub

50. Water temperature for a complete bed bath is usually between
    A. 95° F and 100° F
    B. 100° F and 110° F
    C. 110° F and 115° F
    D. 115° F and 120° F

51. You give Mr. Jones a complete bed bath. Do all of the following *except*:
    A. Expose only the body part needed.
    B. Change the water if it is soapy or cool.
    C. Provide for privacy.
    D. Place the bed in the lowest horizontal position.

52. To wash around the person's eyes
    A. Use warm soapy water.
    B. Wipe from the outer to the inner aspect of the eye.
    C. Clean around the near eye first.
    D. Use a clean part of the washcloth for each stroke.

53. Risks from tub baths and showers include
    A. Falls, chilling, and burns
    B. Dementia, confusion, and restlessness
    C. Skin breakdown and infection
    D. Hypertension and shortness of breath

54. You are giving Mrs. Smith a tub bath. Which is *true*?
    A. The bath should last 30 minutes.
    B. The tub bath may cause her to feel faint and weak.
    C. Use bath oils in the water.
    D. Drain the tub after Mrs. Smith gets out of the tub.

55. Shower chair wheels are locked during the shower.
    A. True
    B. False

56. Which is *not* a safety measure for tub baths and showers?
    A. Clean the tub or shower before and after use.
    B. Place needed items within the person's reach.
    C. Place the signal light within the person's reach.
    D. Have the person use the towel bars for support.

57. When giving a shower, turn hot water on first, then the cold water.
    A. True
    B. False

58. Fill the tub before the person gets into it.
    A. True
    B. False

59. Mr. Harris can bathe alone in the tub. How often do you need to check on him?
    A. Every 5 minutes
    B. Every 15 minutes
    C. Whenever you have time
    D. Only when Mr. Harris turns on his signal light

60. When giving a back massage, you do all of the following *except*:
    A. Warm the lotion before applying.
    B. Use firm strokes.
    C. Always keep your hands in contact with the person's skin.
    D. Massage bony areas that are reddened.

61. A back massage is safe for all persons.
    A. True
    B. False

62. When giving a back massage, use fast movements to relax the person.
    A. True
    B. False

63. You have given a back massage to Ms. Jean Hansen. What do you need to report and record?
    A. The type of lotion used
    B. How you warmed the lotion
    C. How long the massage lasted
    D. Breaks in the skin and reddened areas

64. You are giving perineal care to Ms. Hansen. Which is *correct*?
    A. Cover her with a draw sheet.
    B. Use hot water.
    C. Rinse thoroughly.
    D. Rub the area dry after rinsing.

65. When giving perineal care, you need to use a clean part of the washcloth for each stroke.
    A. True
    B. False

66. You protect the person's right to privacy by
    A. Exposing the person during bathing procedures
    B. Allowing visitors to stay in the room when giving care
    C. Providing care with the room door open
    D. Covering persons who are taken to and from tub and shower rooms

## MOSBY'S NURSING ASSISTANT SKILLS VIDEOS EXERCISES

### Questions from the "Oral Hygiene" Section of the Personal Hygiene and Grooming Video

67. By giving skillful and considerate care, you:

    A. _____

    B. _____

68. Oral hygiene is important for the following reasons:

    A. _____

    B. _____

69. When delegated oral hygiene, you need to follow these procedure guidelines:
    A. Follow the nurses directions and the care plan for:

    (1) _____

    (2) _____

    (3) _____

    B. Follow Standard Precautions and the

    Bloodborne Pathogen Standard because

    _____

    _____.

    C. Provide for the person's privacy, comfort,

    and safety taking special care to prevent

    _____.

    D. Give explanations of each procedure and

    your actions as you give care. This is

    especially important when caring for the

    unconscious person because _____

    _____.

70. Mrs. Callahan was able to assist with her oral hygiene. List the supplies provided for Mrs. Callahan.

  A. _____

  B. _____

  C. _____

  D. _____

  E. _____

  F. _____

71. Aspiration can cause _____ and

  _____.

72. List the supplies needed when giving oral care to the unconscious person.

  A. _____

  B. _____

  C. _____

  D. _____

  E. _____

  F. _____

  G. _____

  H. _____

73. How was Mr. Harris positioned for oral care?

  _____

  _____

74. To clean dentures, you need these supplies:

  A. _____

  B. _____

  C. _____

  D. _____

  E. _____

  F. _____

  G. _____

  H. _____

  I. _____

75. Explain why the sink is lined with a towel and filled with water when cleaning dentures.

  _____

76. As you clean dentures, you need to note:

  A. _____

  B. _____

  C. _____

77. Dentures are stored in the denture cup filled with cool water because

  _____

  _____.

## Questions from the Bathing Video

78. Bathing is necessary to clean the skin of _____,

  _____,

  _____,

  _____, and

  _____.

79. When you are delegated a person's bath or shower, you must follow procedure guidelines. The nurse's directions and the care plan tell you:

  A. _____

  B. _____

  C. _____

80. When giving a bath or shower, you provide for the person's warmth, privacy, and safety by:

    A. _____

    B. _____

    C. _____

    D. _____

81. You must give explanations about the procedure in the language the person understands.
    A. True
    B. False

82. Explain why you need to use proper positioning and body mechanics.

    _____

    _____

83. Before starting the bed bath you need to ask for

    help if _____

    _____

    _____.

84. Before starting the bed bath, adjust the bed height

    to promote _____.

85. You do not have a bath thermometer. How should you test water temperature for a bed bath?

    _____

86. You need to wear gloves if there is the potential

    for contact with _____

    _____.

87. How did the nursing assistant protect Mr. Bennett's privacy while removing his gown?

    _____

88. Soaking the feet is avoided when the person has

    _____ or

    _____.

89. Before washing the person's back and buttocks,

    you need to _____.

90. You need to provide for _____

    any time you are giving personal care.

91. Report reddened areas to the nurse immediately.
    A. True
    B. False

92. Explain why you should not massage reddened areas.

    _____

    _____

    _____

93. You should always encourage the person to let you do his or her perineal care.
    A. True
    B. False

94. Before beginning perineal care, you need to

    _____.

95. When washing the scrotum, you need to

    observe for _____

    _____.

96. When giving female perineal care, wash from the anus to the vagina.
    A. True
    B. False

## CASE STUDY

*Ms. Mary Chin is a resident of Pine View Nursing Center. She is alert and can make her needs known. She is continent of bowel and bladder. You are assigned to her care today. Your assignment sheet tells you that Ms. Chin:*

- *Uses a wheelchair to get around*
- *Eats all of her meals in the dining room*
- *Has an upper and lower denture*
- *Needs a whirlpool tub bath today*
  - *She likes her bath at 10 AM.*
- *Gets a back massage after her bath*

*Answer the following questions.*

1. What care do you need to give Ms. Chin before breakfast?

2. What care do you need to give Ms. Chin after breakfast?

3. What information do you need from the nurse and the care plan before you give Ms. Chin her bath?

4. What observations do you need to make when giving Ms. Chin a bath?

5. How will you promote Ms. Chin's right to privacy?

6. How will you promote Ms. Chin's right to personal choice?

## ADDITIONAL LEARNING ACTIVITIES

1. Discuss the importance of hygiene and cleanliness in your personal life.
   A. Explain how important it is for you to feel clean and free from unpleasant odors when you are around other people.

   B. List the personal care routines you practice daily to promote cleanliness?

2. Has illness ever prevented you from carrying out your daily hygiene routines? Explain.

   A. Discuss how this affected your personal comfort.

3. View the CD Companion: Skills to help you learn and practice the following procedures:
   A. Brushing the Person's Teeth

   B. Providing Mouth Care For the Unconscious Person

   C. Providing Denture Care

   D. Giving a Complete Bed Bath

   E. Giving a Back Massage

F. Giving Female Perineal Care

G. Giving Male Perineal Care

4. The procedures in this chapter require you to provide personal care to another person. They must be performed in a way that respects the person's privacy and dignity. It will help you to understand how the person feels if you practice the procedures with a classmate. Take your turn being the patient or resident. Under the supervision of your instructor, use the procedure checklist provided on pages 246-269 to practice the procedures in Chapter 13. Use a simulator to practice female and male perineal care.
   A. After practicing each procedure, discuss your experience.

# 14 Assisting With Grooming

## OBJECTIVES

The questions and student activities in this chapter will help you meet these objectives.
- Define the key terms listed in this chapter
- Explain the importance of hair care, shaving, and nail and foot care
- Describe the safety measures for shaving a person
- Describe the rules for changing clothing and gowns
- Perform the procedures described in this chapter

## STUDY QUESTIONS

### Matching

Match each term with the correct definition.

1. _____ Hair loss

2. _____ Excessive amount of dry, white flakes from the scalp

3. _____ Excessive body hair in women and children

4. _____ Infestation with lice

5. _____ Being in or on a host

6. _____ Prevents or slows down blood clotting

A. Hirsutism

B. Alopecia

C. Anticoagulant

D. Pediculosis

E. Dandruff

F. Infestation

### Fill in the Blanks

7. The nursing process reflects the person's:

   A. _____

   B. _____

   C. _____

   D. _____

   E. _____

8. Hirsutism results from _____

   _____.

9. Lice spread to others through:

   A. _____

   B. _____

   C. _____

   D. _____

   E. _____

10. Brushing and combing hair are part of

    _____ ,

    _____ , and

    _____ care.

11. _____

    chooses how to brush, comb, and style hair.

12. You have finished brushing Ms. Reed's hair. What observations do you need to report and record?

    A. _____

    B. _____

    C. _____

    D. _____

    E. _____

    F. _____

    G. _____

13. Ms. Ambrose is dressed for the day. She asks you to brush her hair. Explain why you should place a towel across her shoulders before you begin.

    _____

    _____

14. The nurse tells you which shampooing method to use. The shampooing method depends on:

    A. _____

    B. _____

    C. _____

15. List four shampooing methods.

    A. _____

    B. _____

    C. _____

    D. _____

16. You have finished shampooing Mr. John Baird's hair. What observations do you need to report and record?

    A. _____

    B. _____

    C. _____

    D. _____

17. You used a medicated shampoo for Mr. Baird. What should you do with the shampoo when you are finished shampooing Mr. Baird's hair?

    _____

    _____

18. Mr. James is 80 years old. He cannot tip his head back. You are shampooing his hair in the tub. How would you keep soap out of his eyes while shampooing his hair?

    _____

    _____

    _____

    _____

19. What type of shaver is used for a person taking an anticoagulant drug?

    _____

20. Shave in the direction of hair growth when

    shaving _____

    _____ .

21. Explain why you should not use a safety razor to shave a person with dementia.

    _____

    _____

22. When shaving a person, what observations do you need to report at once?

    A. _____

    B. _____

    C. _____

23. Where are used razor blades and disposable shavers discarded?

    _____

24. Never trim or shave a beard or mustache

    without _____.

25. You are giving foot care to Ms. Martin. What observations do you need to report and record?

    A. _____

    B. _____

    C. _____

    D. _____

    E. _____

26. You do not cut or trim toenails if a person:

    A. _____

    B. _____

    C. _____

    D. _____

27. How are fingernails trimmed?

    _____

    _____

28. List the rules to follow when changing gowns or clothing?

    A. _____

    B. _____

    C. _____

    D. _____

    E. _____

    F. _____

29. What information do you need from the nurse and the care plan before changing clothing?

    A. _____

    B. _____

    C. _____

    D. _____

*Multiple Choice*

Circle the **BEST** Answer

30. Infestation of the scalp with lice is:
    A. Pediculosis capitis
    B. Pediculosis pubis
    C. Pediculosis corporis
    D. Dandruff

31. Brushing and combing hair is
    A. Done whenever needed
    B. Done when you have time
    C. Not your responsibility
    D. Always done by the patient or resident

32. When giving hair care, you
    A. Decide how to style the person's hair.
    B. Start at the scalp and brush and comb to the hair ends.
    C. Cut matted and tangled hair.
    D. Braid long hair to keep it neat.

33. Before shampooing a person's hair, you need the following information from the nurse and the care plan *except*:
    A. When to shampoo the person's hair
    B. What method to use
    C. The person's position restrictions or limits
    D. How long the person's hair is

34. Mr. James has limited range of motion in his neck. He is not shampooed
    A. In bed
    B. In the shower
    C. In the tub
    D. At the sink or on a stretcher

35. If a person receives a cut during shaving, you:
    A. Apply after-shave lotion to the cut.
    B. Apply direct pressure to the cut.
    C. Put a dressing on the cut
    D. Put a piece of tissue on the cut.

36. Mr. White has a beard. You do all of the following *except*:
    A. Wash and comb the beard daily.
    B. Ask Mr. White how to groom his beard.
    C. Trim the beard once a week.
    D. Wash the beard whenever mouth or nose drainage is present.

37. Use nail clippers to cut fingernails. Never use scissors.
    A. True
    B. False

38. Nails are easier to trim and clean
    A. In the morning
    B. Before the bath
    C. After soaking or bathing
    D. At bedtime

39. When trimming fingernails, you:
    A. Let the fingernails soak for 30 minutes before starting.
    B. Clip the fingernails in a curved shape.
    C. Be careful not to damage surrounding tissue.
    D. Use a scissors.

40. Feet are soaked for
    A. 5 to 10 minutes
    B. 15 to 20 minutes
    C. 25 to 30 minutes
    D. 30 minutes

41. If there is injury or paralysis, the gown is removed from
    A. The strong side first
    B. The weak side first
    C. The right side first
    D. The left side first

42. Mr. Adam Green has an IV in his right arm. He has an IV pump and a standard gown. You are changing his gown. You know that
    A. His right arm is put through the sleeve first.
    B. His left arm is put through the sleeve first.
    C. His gown is not changed until he no longer has the IV.
    D. His right arm is not put through the sleeve.

43. Encourage the person to do as much for him or herself as safely possible.
    A. True
    B. False

44. You promote courteous and dignified care by
    A. Combing the person's hair the way you like it
    B. Making sure clothing is properly fastened
    C. Encouraging a man to shave off his beard
    D. Exposing the person when changing garments

## MOSBY'S NURSING ASSISTANT SKILLS VIDEOS EXERCISES

### Questions from the "Hair care, Shaving, Nail and Foot Care, and Dressing" Sections of the "Personal Hygiene and Grooming" Video

45. When you are delegated hair care, you need to follow the nurse's directions and the care plan for:

    A. _____

    B. _____

    C. _____

    D. _____

    E. _____

46. When shampooing Mr. Steele's hair in bed, the nursing assistant started from the

    _____

    and worked toward _____ .

47. When shaving with a blade razor, you need to:

    A. Shave in the direction of _____ .

    B. Apply _____ to cuts or nicks.

    C. Follow _____ and the

    _____ .

48. The nails and feet need special attention to:

    A. _____

    B. _____

49. The _____ and

    the _____ will

    tell you when to give nail and foot care.

50. When giving nail and foot care, you need to

    check the water temperature to prevent

    _____ .

51. When are clean clothes needed?

    A. _____

    B. _____

52. Assistance with dressing is needed when

    a person has _____ ,

    _____ ,

    _____ , or

    _____ .

53. Why is clothing removed from the strong or unaffected side first?

    _____

    _____

## CASE STUDY

*Ms. Angela Reid is recovering from surgery on her right knee. Today is her bath day. She also wants her hair shampooed. She has thick, long, curly hair, which she usually wears up. She dresses in regular clothes during the day and wears a nightgown to bed. She needs some assistance with dressing and undressing.*

*Answer the following questions.*

1. What information do you need from the nurse and the care plan before you assist Ms. Reid to shampoo her hair?

2. What safety measures will you practice when assisting Ms. Reid to shampoo her hair?

3. How will you brush or comb Ms. Reid's hair?

4. Who will choose what Ms. Reid wears?

5. What rules do you need to follow when assisting Ms. Reid to dress?

## ADDITIONAL LEARNING ACTIVITIES

1. List the grooming activities you perform every day. Answer these questions.
   A. How important are your grooming routines?

   B. How important is personal choice when you are performing your grooming activities?

   C. How important is privacy when you are performing your grooming activities?

   D. How would you feel if you were unable to perform your grooming activities?

   (1) How would you want to be treated?

2. View the CD Companion: Skills to help you learn and practice the following procedures:
   A. Brushing and Combing the Person's Hair

   B. Shampooing the Person's Hair

   C. Giving Nail and Foot Care

   D. Undressing the Person

   E. Dressing the Person

3. Carefully review the procedures in Chapter 14. Under the supervision of your instructor, use the procedure checklists on pages 270-287 to practice each procedure.
   A. Practice dressing and undressing procedures with classmates or family members.

   (1) Use different types of clothing. (For example: clothes that open in front and clothes that open in back; button and pullover shirts; pants with zippers and buttons; and pants that pull on.)

   (2) Role-play weakness on one side of the body.

   (3) Role-play that the person is not able to help.

   (4) Take your turn being the patient or resident.

   B. Did you feel safe and secure during the procedures?

   C. How will your experience affect how you help others with grooming and dressing activities?

# 15

# Assisting With Urinary Elimination

## OBJECTIVES

The questions and student activities in this chapter will help you meet these objectives.
- Define the key terms listed in this chapter
- Describe normal urine
- Describe the rules for normal urination

- Describe urinary incontinence and the care required
- Explain why catheters are used
- Explain how to care for persons with catheters
- Describe two methods of bladder training
- Perform the procedures described in this chapter

## STUDY QUESTIONS

*Crossword*

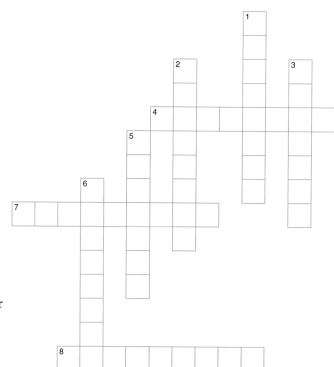

### Across

4. Scant amount of urine
7. Blood in the urine
8. The process of emptying urine from the bladder

### Down

1. Frequent urination at night
2. Abnormally large amounts of urine
3. Urination
5. Painful or difficult urination
6. A tube used to drain or inject fluid through a body opening

## Matching

*Match each term with the correct definition.*

1. _____ Urine leaks when the bladder is too full

2. _____ The loss of urine at predictable intervals when the bladder is full

3. _____ When urine leaks during exercise and certain movements

4. _____ Urine is lost in response to a sudden, urgent need to void

5. _____ The need to void at once

6. _____ The person has bladder control but cannot use the toilet in time

7. _____ Voiding at frequent intervals

8. _____ The loss of bladder control

A. Overflow incontinence

B. Urinary frequency

C. Functional incontinence

D. Urinary urgency

E. Stress incontinence

F. Reflex incontinence

G. Urge incontinence

H. Urinary incontinence

## Fill in the Blanks

9. The urinary system removes _____ from the blood and maintains the body's _____ _____.

10. List five factors affecting urine production.

    A. _____

    B. _____

    C. _____

    D. _____

    E. _____

11. When assisting with urination, you need to observe urine for:

    A. _____

    B. _____

    C. _____

    D. _____

    E. _____

12. Mr. Pete Andrews is recovering from hip replacement surgery. What type of bedpan will he use?

    _____

13. Explain how you will promote safety when handling bedpans and their contents.

    A. _____

    B. _____

14. Ms. Martha Lewis cannot assist in getting on the bedpan. How will you give her the bedpan?

    A. _____

    B. _____

    C. _____

    D. _____

    E. _____

    F. _____

15. You assist Ms. Martha Lewis with the bedpan. She is unable to clean her genital area. Describe how you will clean her genital area.

_____

_____

_____

16. Men use _____ to void.

17. Explain why you need to empty urinals promptly.

_____

_____

18. Mr. Lopez stands to use the urinal. How will you give him the urinal?

    A. _____

    B. _____

    C. _____

    D. _____

19. A _____ is a chair or wheelchair with an opening for a bedpan or container.

20. What information do you need from the nurse and the care plan when assisting with commodes?

    A. _____

    B. _____

    C. _____

    D. _____

    E. _____

21. You have transferred Mr. Brown to the commode. How can you provide warmth and promote privacy?

_____

_____

22. List seven causes of functional incontinence.

    A. _____

    B. _____

    C. _____

    D. _____

    E. _____

    F. _____

    G. _____

23. Ms. Jean Jensen has urge incontinence and overflow incontinence. This is called _____

_____.

24. Ms. Jean Jensen is incontinent of urine. You help prevent urinary tract infections by:

    A. _____

    B. _____

    C. _____

25. This type of urinary catheter is left in the bladder.

_____

_____

26. Persons with catheters are at high risk for

_____.

27. Ms. Ann Lopez has an indwelling catheter. Why do you need to keep her drainage bag below her bladder?

_____

_____

28. You have finished giving catheter care to Ms. Lopez. What observations do you need to report and record?

    A._____

    B._____

    C._____

    D._____

    E._____

29. What should you do if a urinary drainage system is accidentally disconnected?

    A. _____

    B. _____

    C. _____

    D. _____

    E. _____

    F. _____

    G. _____

30. You empty Ms. Lopez's urinary drainage bag at the end of your shift. What observations do you need to report and record?

    A. _____

    B. _____

    C. _____

    D. _____

    E. _____

31. A _____ is a soft sheath that slides over the penis.

32. Never use adhesive tape to secure a condom catheter because _____
    _____.

33. You should not apply a condom catheter if
    _____.

34. You are applying a condom catheter to Mr. Ray Spears. He becomes aroused. What should you do?

    _____

    _____

    _____

35. What is the goal of a bladder training program?

    _____

36. You need to remove bedpans promptly? Leaving a person sit on the bedpan is likely to cause

    _____.

37. If your state and agency allows you to do catheterizations:

    A. The procedure must _____

    _____.

    B. You must have the necessary _____

    _____.

    C. You must know how to use _____

    _____.

    D. A nurse must be available to _____

    _____.

*Multiple Choice*

Circle the **BEST** Answer

38. How much urine does the healthy adult produce each day?
    A. About 500 ml
    B. About 700 ml
    C. About 1500 ml
    D. About 3000 ml

39. Which is *not* a rule for normal elimination?
    A. Follow Standard Precautions and the Bloodborne Pathogen Standard.
    B. Limit the amount of fluid intake to 1500 ml daily.
    C. Follow the persons voiding routines and habits.
    D. Help the person to the bathroom when the request is made.

40. Normal urine
    A. Is pale yellow, straw colored, or amber
    B. Does not have an odor
    C. Is cloudy
    D. Contains particles

41. You promote normal elimination by
    A. Setting new voiding routines
    B. Asking the person to hurry
    C. Providing only small amounts of fluid
    D. Providing privacy

42. Remind men to place urinals on the overbed table after use.
    A. True
    B. False

43. Nervous system disorders and injuries are common causes of
    A. Stress incontinence
    B. Urge incontinence
    C. Functional incontinence
    D. Reflex incontinence

44. Which is *not* a nursing measure for persons with urinary incontinence?
    A. Increase fluid intake at bedtime.
    B. Provide good skin care.
    C. Answer signal lights promptly.
    D. Encourage voiding at scheduled intervals.

45. You feel impatient when caring for a person with incontinence. You must
    A. Tell a co-worker to take care of the person for you.
    B. Wait to provide care until you feel less stressed.
    C. Discuss the problem with the nurse at once.
    D. Tell the person how you feel.

46. Mr. Benson has dementia. You observe him voiding in his trash can. You should
    A. Remove the trash can from his room.
    B. Explain to him that he must void in the bathroom.
    C. Make him empty the trash can into the toilet.
    D. Check with the nurse and the care plan for measures to help him.

47. Catheters are used for all of the following reasons *except*:
    A. As a first choice to treat incontinence
    B. For persons who are too weak or disabled to use the bedpan, urinal, commode, or toilet
    C. To protect wounds and pressure ulcers from urine
    D. They allow hourly urinary output measurements

48. When caring for a person with an indwelling catheter, you need to do all of the following *except*:
    A. Keep the catheter connected to the drainage tube.
    B. Attach the drainage bag to the bed rail.
    C. Coil the drainage tubing on the bed. Secure it to the bottom linen.
    D. Report leaks to the nurse at once.

49. To apply a condom catheter correctly, you need to do all of the following *except*
    A. Roll the condom onto the penis.
    B. Leave a 1-inch space between the penis and the end of the catheter.
    C. Apply tape completely around the penis.
    D. Make sure the condom is not twisted.

## MOSBY'S NURSING ASSISTANT SKILLS VIDEOS EXERCISES

## Questions from the "Assisting with a Urinal, Assisting with a Bedpan, Providing Catheter Care, and Applying a Condom Catheter" Sections of the Normal Elimination Video

50. The passageway for the urine to leave the body is the
    A. Bladder
    B. Urethra
    C. Kidney
    D. Ureter

51. Do not place the urinal on the bedside stand

    because _____

    _____.

52. Before handling the urinal, you need to put on gloves.
    A. True
    B. False

53. _____

    are used for urine and bowel elimination when

    the person cannot get out of bed.

54. Before you assist the person off the bedpan, you need to:

    A. _____

    B. _____

    C. _____

55. Catheter care is required to reduce the potential

    for _____.

56. When delegated catheter care, the nurse and the care plan tell you:

    A. _____

    B. _____

57. Giving catheter care offers an important

    opportunity to observe _____

    _____

    and to make sure _____

    _____.

58. You need to hold the catheter during washing

    to prevent _____

    and _____.

59. When giving catheter care, clean from the urethral opening down the catheter about
    A. 2 inches
    B. 4 inches
    C. 8 inches
    D. 12 inches

60. Wear gloves and follow Standard Precautions

    and the Bloodborne Pathogen Standard when

    _____

    _____, and

    _____ condom catheters.

61. Every time you change a condom catheter you need to:

    A. _____

    B. _____

## CASE STUDY

*Ms. Ellen Gardner is a 70-year-old nursing center resident. She has an indwelling catheter.*

*Ms. Gardner is a private person. She is alert and can assist with her care. She likes to make her own decisions. She walks with a walker and is out of bed most of the day. Her husband visits every day at 1300.*

*Answer the following questions.*

1. What information do you need from the nurse and the care plan before giving catheter care?

2. What observations do you need to report and record?

3. What safety measures do you need to practice when giving catheter care?

4. How often do you need to give catheter care?

5. How will you protect Ms. Gardner's right to privacy?

6. How will you promote Ms. Gardner's independence?

## ADDITIONAL LEARNING ACTIVITIES

1. Think of your personal voiding patterns.
   A. List the factors that affect your daily patterns.

   B. Discuss how changes in your personal patterns affect your comfort.

2. View the CD Companion: Skills to help you learn and practice the following procedures:
   A. Giving the Bedpan

   B. Giving Catheter Care

3. Carefully review and practice the procedure for giving a bedpan. Work with a classmate. Use a regular bedpan and a fracture pan.
   A. Use the procedure checklist provided on pages 288-290 as a guide.

   B. Wear clothing to practice. Take your turn being the patient or resident. Discuss your experience.

(1) Did you have concerns about dignity and privacy?

(2) Was the experience physically comfortable? Explain.

(3) Was it difficult to position the bedpan correctly? Explain.

(4) Would you like to be left on a bedpan for 15 minutes or longer?

4. Carefully review and practice all the procedures in this chapter. Use a simulator when appropriate. Use the procedure checklists provided on pages 288-301. If you are embarrassed by any of these procedures, discuss your feelings with your instructor or a nurse.

# Assisting With Bowel Elimination

## OBJECTIVES

The questions and student activities in this chapter will help you meet these objectives.
- Define the key terms listed in this chapter
- Describe normal defecation and the observations to report
- Identify the factors that affect bowel elimination
- Describe common bowel elimination problems
- Explain how to promote comfort and safety during defecation

- Describe bowel training
- Explain why enemas are given
- Describe the common enema solutions
- Describe the rules for giving enemas
- Describe how to care for a person with an ostomy
- Perform the procedures described in this chapter

## STUDY QUESTIONS

*Crossword*

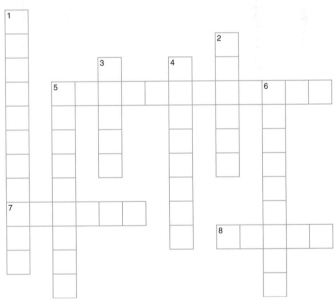

### Across

5. The passage of a hard, dry stool
7. A surgically created opening
8. An opening

### Down

1. A cone-shaped, solid drug that is inserted into a body opening; it melts at body temperature
2. Gas or air passed through the anus
3. The introduction of fluid into the rectum and lower colon
4. The frequent passage of liquid stools
5. A surgically created opening between the colon and abdominal wall
6. A surgically created opening between the ileum and the abdominal wall

## Matching

*Match each term with the correct definition.*

1. _____ The inability to control the passage of feces and gas through the anus

2. _____ The process of excreting feces from the rectum through the anus (bowel movement)

3. _____ The prolonged retention and buildup of feces in the rectum

4. _____ The semi-solid mass of waste products in the colon that are expelled through the anus

5. _____ The excessive formation of gas in the stomach and intestines

6. _____ Excreted feces

A. Flatulence

B. Stool

C. Fecal impaction

D. Fecal incontinence

E. Defecation

F. Feces

## Fill in the Blanks

7. Stools are normally _____,

_____,

_____,

and _____.

8. _____

causes black or tarry stools.

9. What observations about stools do you need to report to the nurse?

A. _____

B. _____

C. _____

D. _____

E. _____

F. _____

G. _____

H. _____

10. List eight factors that affect the frequency, consistency, color, and odor of stools?

A. _____

B. _____

C. _____

D. _____

E. _____

F. _____

G. _____

H. _____

11. Explain why providing privacy is important when meeting the person's elimination needs.

_____

_____

_____

12. Explain how aging affects bowel elimination.

_____

_____

_____

13. _____

results if constipation is not relieved.

14. You are caring for Mr. Leo Lawson. He has diarrhea. You need to:

A. _____

B. _____

C. _____

15. List seven causes of fecal incontinence.

A. _____

B. _____

C. _____

D. _____

E. _____

F. _____

G. _____

16. List six causes of flatulence.

A. _____

B. _____

C. _____

D. _____

E. _____

F. _____

17. What are the two goals of bowel training?

A. _____

B. _____

18. Doctors order enemas to _____

_____.

19. You are giving a cleansing enema to Mr. Paul Perkins. You need to stop tube insertion if

A. _____

B. _____

C. _____

20. Describe the following types of enemas.

A. Tap-water enema _____

_____

B. Soapsuds enema _____

_____

C. Saline enema _____

_____

21. You have given a saline enema to Mr. Jay Hart. What do you need to report and record?

A. _____

B. _____

C. _____

D. _____

E. _____

F. _____

22. Enemas are dangerous for _____

_____.

23. The doctor orders "enemas until clear." This means

_____

_____

_____.

24. To give a small volume enema, squeeze and roll up the plastic bottle from the bottom. You should not release pressure on the bottle because

_____

_____.

25. Describe the following:

A. A permanent colostomy _____

_____

B. A temporary colostomy _____

_____

_____

26. If a colostomy is near the start of the colon, stools

are _____.

27. List four measures that help prevent ostomy pouch odors.

A. _____

B. _____

C. _____

D. _____

28. Ms. Mann wears an ostomy pouch. You need to assist with her tub bath. Why should you delay her bath for 1 to 2 hours after applying a new pouch?

_____

_____

*Multiple Choice*

Circle the **BEST** Answer

29. Normal stools are
    A. Black in color
    B. Soft, formed, and moist
    C. Hard and marble sized
    D. Liquid and pale in color

30. Comfort and safety during bowel elimination are promoted by all of the following *except*
    A. Positioning the person in a normal sitting or squatting position
    B. Covering the person for warmth and privacy
    C. Allowing time for defecation
    D. Allowing visitors to stay in the room

31. Warm fluids decrease peristalsis.
    A. True
    B. False

32. Ms. Lopez has had a bowel movement. The stool is black in color and has a tarry consistency. You
    A. Ask Ms. Lopez if she has had anything unusual to eat.
    B. Ask the nurse to observe the stool.
    C. Dispose of the stool and report the color to the nurse.
    D. Ask a co-worker if this is normal for Ms. Lopez.

33. You need to follow Standard Precautions and the Bloodborne Pathogen Standard when in contact with stools.
    A. True
    B. False

34. Which is a common cause of constipation?
    A. A high fiber diet
    B. Regular exercise
    C. Increased fluid intake
    D. Ignoring the urge to defecate

35. Which is a sign of fecal impaction?
    A. Liquid feces seeping from the anus
    B. Black, tarry stools
    C. Increased flatulence
    D. Frequent passage of soft stools

36. Fecal incontinence is frustrating and embarrassing.
    A. True
    B. False

37. Ms. Jane Arnold has fecal incontinence. You know that
    A. She has dementia.
    B. A bowel training program will cure her incontinence.
    C. You need to provide good skin care.
    D. She has an intestinal disease.

38. Which action will *not* help produce flatus?
    A. Lying quietly in the supine position
    B. Walking
    C. Moving in bed
    D. The left-side lying position

39. Which measure does *not* promote comfort and safety when giving an enema to an adult?
    A. Have the person void first.
    B. Lubricate the enema tip before inserting it.
    C. Insert the enema tubing 7 inches.
    D. Give the solution slowly.

40. The preferred position for giving enemas is
    A. Fowler's or semi-Fowler's
    B. The left side-lying or Sims'
    C. Prone
    D. Dorsal recumbent

41. Nurses give enemas that contain drugs.
    A. True
    B. False

42. After giving an oil retention enema, do the following *except*
    A. Position the person in the supine position.
    B. Urge the person to retain the enema for the time ordered.
    C. Place extra waterproof pads on the bed if needed.
    D. Check the person often while the person retains the enema.

43. Mr. White has a colostomy. Which statement is *false*?
    A. Good skin care is very important.
    B. Colostomies can be permanent or temporary.
    C. Feces and flatus pass through a stoma located on the abdominal wall.
    D. The entire large intestine has been removed.

44. Ms. Mary Martin has an ileostomy. You know that
    A. Part of the colon is removed.
    B. Stool consistency ranges from liquid to solid.
    C. A skin barrier is not needed around the stoma.
    D. Good skin care is required.

45. Ostomy pouches are changed
    A. When completely full
    B. Every shift
    C. Every 3 to 7 days and when they leak
    D. After each meal

46. Stomas have nerve endings. They are painful.
    A. True
    B. False

47. Leaving a person sitting in feces is neglect. It is a form of physical abuse.
    A. True
    B. False

## MOSBY'S NURSING ASSISTANT SKILLS VIDEOS EXERCISES

## Questions from the "Administering a Cleansing Enema" Section of the *Normal Elimination* Video

48. Enemas are ordered to _____ and

    _____

    _____. An enema may also be used to

    _____

    _____.

49. When you are preparing to administer an enema, you need to follow the nurse's directions and the care plan for:

    A. _____

    B. _____

    C. _____

    D. _____

    E. _____

50. Why is the Sims' or left side-lying position used to administer an enema?

    _____

    _____

51. The enema tube is *never* inserted more than 6 inches.
    A. True
    B. False

52. Why should you ask the person to take a few deep breaths before inserting the lubricated enema tube?

    _____

    _____

53. When administering an enema solution, you should clamp the tube if the person:

    A. _____

    B. _____

    C. _____

54. Clamp the tube before the solution bag is empty

    to prevent _____

    _____ .

## CASE STUDY

*Mr. Bill Brown is a 50-year-old patient in Valley View Hospital. He is scheduled for bowel x-rays in the morning. His doctor ordered saline enemas until clear. He is also on NPO until after his x-rays in the morning. The RN has delegated the task of giving Mr. Brown the enemas to you.*

*Answer the following questions.*

1. How is a saline enema prepared?

2. Are enemas safe for all persons? Explain.

3. Does Mr. Brown need to give consent before you give the enema? Explain.

4. What comfort and safety measures must you practice when giving an enema?

5. How will you protect Mr. Brown's right to privacy?

6. What fears might Mr. Brown have?

7. You have finished giving the enema. What measures do you need to take to promote Mr. Brown's comfort and safety?

## ADDITIONAL LEARNING ACTIVITIES

1. Think of your personal elimination routines.
   A. Explain how important these routines are to your physical and psychological comfort.

   B. Are you aware of how your diet, fluid intake, and level of activity affect your bowel elimination routines? Explain.

   C. Have you had personal experience with constipation or diarrhea? How did the experience affect your comfort?

2. Do you know anyone with a colostomy or an ileostomy? If the person is willing, discuss how the ostomy has affected his or her daily life. Ask the following questions:
   A. How did the person adjust?

   B. What is the person's daily routine?

   C. How is the skin cared for?

3. If available at your school or place of work, examine several types of colostomy and ileostomy pouches. Read the manufacturers instructions. Practice handling the pouches and applying them on yourself and a willing classmate.

4. Handle the various types of enema equipment and become familiar with how each is used. This will increase your comfort and confidence.

5. Carefully review the procedures in Chapter 16.
   A. Under the supervision of your instructor, practice each procedure. Use a simulator when appropriate. Use the procedure checklists provided on pages 302-306 as a guide.

   B. If any of these procedures embarrass you, discuss your feelings with your instructor.

*NOTE:* **Remember that some states and agencies do not allow nursing assistants to give enemas.**

# 17 Assisting With Nutrition and Fluids

## OBJECTIVES

The questions and student activities in this chapter will help you meet these objectives.
- Define the key terms listed in this chapter
- Explain the purpose and use of the *MyPyramid Food Guidance System*
- Describe factors that affect eating and nutrition
- Describe the special diets and between-meal nourishments
- Identify the signs, symptoms, and precautions relating to aspiration and regurgitation
- Describe fluid requirements and the causes of dehydration
- Explain what to do when the person has special fluid orders
- Explain how to assist with food and fluid needs
- Explain how to assist with calories counts
- Explain how to assist with enteral nutrition and IV therapy
- Perform the procedures described in this chapter

## STUDY QUESTIONS

*Matching*

*Match each term with the correct definition.*

1. _____ Breathing fluid or an object into the lungs

2. _____ The amount of energy produced when the body burns food

3. _____ A decrease in the amount of water in body tissues

4. _____ The loss of appetite

5. _____ Difficulty swallowing

6. _____ Giving nutrients through the gastrointestinal tract

7. _____ Tube feeding

8. _____ The number of drops per minute (*gtt/min*)

9. _____ The swelling of body tissues with water

10. _____ The backward flow of food from the stomach into the mouth

11. _____ Giving fluids through a needle or catheter inserted into a vein

12. _____ A substance that is ingested, digested, absorbed, and used by the body

A. Dehydration

B. Gavage

C. Anorexia

D. Calorie

E. Regurgitation

F. Intravenous (IV) therapy

G. Aspiration

H. Nutrition

I. Edema

J. Flow rate

K. Nutrient

L. Dysphagia

13. _____ The processes involved in the ingestion, digestion, absorption, and use of foods and fluids by the body

M.  Enteral nutrition

## Fill in the Blanks

14. The amount and quality of food in the diet affects

_____.

15. Nutrients are grouped into _____,

_____, _____,

_____,

_____and _____.

16. The *MyPyramid Food Guidance System* encourages

_____

_____.

17. According to the *MyPyramid Food Guidance System*

A. The kind and amount of food eaten daily

depends on _____

_____.

B. For health benefits, at least _____

of physical activity are needed on most days of

the week.

C. For a 2000 calorie diet, _____

cups of vegetables are needed daily.

D. The best oil choices come from _____

_____.

18. _____ is the most

important nutrient.

19. _____ provide

energy and fiber for bowel elimination.

20. List six factors affecting eating and nutrition.

A. _____

B. _____

C. _____

D. _____

E. _____

F. _____

21. Explain how illness can affect eating and nutrition.

_____

_____

_____

_____.

22. Doctors order special diets for the following reasons:

A. _____

B. _____

23. Explain what happens when there is too much sodium in the body.

_____

_____

_____

24. _____

is produced and secreted by the pancreas. It lets

the body use sugar.

25. Explain why it is important for persons with diabetes to eat at regular times each day?

_____

26. Mr. Lane has dysphagia. You are feeding him his noon meal. What observations do you need to report at once?

    A. _____

    B. _____

27. Fluid balance is needed for health. The amount of

    _____ and the amount of

    _____

    must be equal.

28. List six common causes of dehydration.

    A. _____

    B. _____

    C. _____

    D. _____

    E. _____

    F. _____

29. Your assignment sheet tells you that Ms. Reed has an order to restrict fluids to 1500 ml per day. Explain what this means.

    _____

    _____

    _____

    _____

30. To provide for comfort, the meal setting must be

    free of _____

    _____.

31. You are preparing Ms. Hawthorne for breakfast. She will eat breakfast in bed. After you assist her with eyeglasses and hearing aids, oral hygiene, elimination, and hand washing you need to:

    A. _____

    B. _____

    C. _____

    D. _____

32. With _____,

    residents eat at a dinning room table with 4 to

    6 others. Tables have table clothes or placemats.

    Food is served as in a restaurant.

33. Describe low-stimulation dinning.

    _____

    _____

34. Explain why it is important to prepare the

    person for a meal before serving the meal tray.

    _____

    _____

    _____

35. What information do you need from the nurse and the care plan before serving meal trays?

    A. _____

    B. _____

    C. _____

    D. _____

36. You have finished feeding Ms. Gomez her noon meal. What observations do you need to report and record?

    A. _____

    B. _____

    C. _____

    D. _____

37. Mr. Harper eats slowly. He complains that food will not go down and he frequently coughs after swallowing. These are signs and symptoms of

    _____.

38. Mr. Harper has finished his noon meal. The nurse tells you to check him for pocketing. You need to check:

    A. _____

    B. _____

    C. _____

39. Mr. Grange has dysphagia. To prevent aspiration he is positioned in a chair or in the semi-Fowler's position for at least _____

    after eating.

40. Define the following terms:

    A. Nasogastirc (NG) tube _____

    _____

    B. Gastrostomy tube _____

    _____

41. Aspiration is _____

42. Why is it important for the RN to check tube placement before a tube feeding?

    _____

    _____

    _____

43. Why is the left side-lying position avoided after a tube feeding?

    _____

44. Ms. Blake is receiving nutrients through an NG tube. How often do you need to provide oral hygiene?

    _____

45. Explain why NG tubes are secured to the person's nose and gown.

    _____

    _____

46. Mrs. Adams is receiving IV therapy. When giving her a bath, you check the flow rate. You need to tell the nurse at once if:

    A. _____

    B. _____

    C. _____

*Labeling*

47. Using the numbers on a clock, describe each food item and where it is located on the plate.

    _____

    _____

    _____

    _____

48. Label the IV equipment.

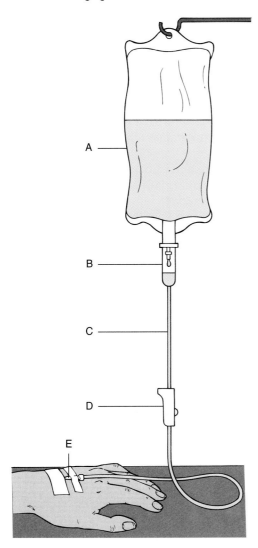

A._____

B. _____

C. _____

D. _____

E. _____

*Multiple Choice*

Circle the **BEST** Answer

49. One gram of protein has
    A. 4 calories
    B. 6 calories
    C. 8 calories
    D. 9 calories

50. The *MyPyramid Food Guidance System* encourages:
    A. The same kind and amount of food for all persons
    B. At least 30 minutes of physical activity on most days of the week
    C. Eating a diet high in solid fats and added sugars
    D. Eating at least 8 ounces of whole grain each day

51. Mr. John Jones is on a 2000 calorie diet. How much fruit does he need daily?
    A. 1 cup
    B. 2 cups
    C. About 3 servings
    D. At least 4 servings

52. Vegetables have the following health benefits *except*:
    A. Most vegetable are low in fat and calories.
    B. They contain no cholesterol.
    C. They contain potassium and fiber.
    D. They help build and maintain bone mass.

53. Remember the following when choosing foods from the meat and beans group:
    A. Choose lean and low-fat meat and poultry.
    B. Using fat for cooking decreases the caloric value of the food.
    C. Liver and other organ meats are low in cholesterol.
    D. Egg yolks are cholesterol free.

54. Remember the following when making oil choices:
    A. Vegetable oils are low in calories.
    B. The best oil choices are from fish, nuts, and vegetable oils.
    C. Oils from plant sources are high in cholesterol.
    D. Oils are a major source of vitamin C.

55. Protein is an important nutrient because:
    A. It provides fiber for bowel elimination.
    B. It is needed for tissue growth and repair.
    C. It helps the body use certain vitamins.
    D. It does not provide calories.

56. Which vitamins are stored by the body?
    A. The B complex vitamins
    B. Vitamin C and the B complex vitamins
    C. Vitamins A, D, E, and K
    D. Vitamin $B_{12}$ and the B complex vitamins

57. Beef is not eaten in:
    A. Poland
    B. India
    C. Mexico
    D. The Philippines

58. Which food is allowed on a clear liquid diet?
    A. Creamed cereal
    B. Plain puddings
    C. Gelatin
    D. Eggnog

59. Which is *not* an OBRA requirement for food served in nursing centers?
    A. Food is nourishing and tastes good.
    B. Hot food is served hot and cold food is served cold.
    C. Each person receives at least three meals and three snacks a day.
    D. The center provides any special eating equipment and utensils.

60. Diabetes is a chronic disease from a lack of insulin. Insulin lets the body use:
    A. Sugar
    B. Fat
    C. Protein
    D. Minerals

61. To promote safety when feeding a person with dysphagia, you must:
    A. Feed the person only liquids.
    B. Position the person in the semi-Fowler's position in bed.
    C. Give thickened liquids using a straw.
    D. Feed the person according to the care plan.

62. How many ml of fluid are needed per day for normal fluid balance?
    A. 1000 to 1500
    B. 1500 to 2000
    C. 2000 to 2500
    D. 2500 to 3000

63. Body water increases with age.
    A. True
    B. False

64. You notice an NPO sign above Mr. Juan's bed. This means:
    A. All of his fluids are given with a straw.
    B. He cannot eat or drink anything.
    C. Water is offered in small amounts.
    D. He cannot have solid food.

65. To prepare a person for meals, you need the following information from the nurse and the care plan *except*:
    A. How much help the person needs
    B. Where the person will eat
    C. A list of the person's favorite foods
    D. How to position the person

66. Ms. Jenson needs help eating. She eats at a horseshoe table in the dinning room. Two other residents also sit at her table. Which type of dinning program is this?
    A. Social dining
    B. Family dining
    C. Assistive dining
    D. Low-stimulation dining

67. When feeding a person do the following *except*:
    A. Serve food and fluids in the order the person prefers.
    B. Use a fork to feed the person.
    C. Offer fluids during the meal.
    D. Sit facing the person.

68. When feeding a visually impaired person you need to:
    A. Tell the person what is on the tray.
    B. Describe the aroma of each food item.
    C. Describe the color and consistency of each food item.
    D. Offer fluids only at the end of the meal.

69. Aspiration precautions include:
    A. Feeding the person liquids through a straw
    B. Positioning the person in Fowler's position or upright in a chair for meals and snacks
    C. Checking the person's mouth before each meal for pocketing
    D. Positioning the person supine after each meal and snack

70. Which action is *incorrect* when passing drinking water?
    A. Make sure the water pitcher is labeled with the person's name and room and bed number.
    B. Do not touch the rim or inside of the water glass or pitcher.
    C. Do not let the ice scoop touch the rim or inside of the water glass or pitcher
    D. Keep the ice scoop in the ice container or dispenser.

71. A calorie count is being kept for Mr. Lewis. You need to:
    A. On a flow sheet, note what he ate and how much.
    B. Weigh the food on his tray before and after eating.
    C. Measure the number of calories in each food item
    D. Ask the dietitian to check Mr. Lewis's tray after he finishes eating.

72. Ms. Blake is receiving nutrition through an NG tube. She complains of nausea and discomfort during the tube feeding. You should:
    A. Measure her vital signs.
    B. Report her complaints to the nurse at once.
    C. Stop the tube feeding until she feels better.
    D. Give her cool water orally.

73. Mr. Gomez is receiving IV therapy. The alarm on his infusion pump alarms . You should:
    A. Turn the pump off.
    B. Adjust the controls on the pump.
    C. Close the regulator clamp.
    D. Tell the nurse at once.

74. You are never responsible for starting or maintaining IV therapy.
    A. True
    B. False

75. Mrs. Adams has an IV in her right arm. She complains of pain at the IV site. The area around the IV site is swollen. What should you do?
    A. Turn off her IV infusion pump.
    B. Place a dressing over the IV insertion site.
    C. Apply heat to the area.
    D. Tell the nurse at once.

76. Mr. Hanson does not eat his pie for lunch. He offers it to you. You can eat it.
    A. True
    B. False

## MOSBY'S NURSING ASSISTANT SKILLS VIDEOS EXERCISES

### Questions from the "Nutrition and Fluids" video (*Sorrentino: Mosby's Nursing Assistant Skills Videos*)

77. List four factors that can interfere with meeting nutritional needs of patients and residents.

    A. _____

    B. _____

    C. _____

    D. _____

78. Always provide _____ and

    _____

    care when assisting patients and residents with

    meals.

79. _____

    are the most common causes of dysphagia in

    adults.

80. Dysphagia should be suspected when the person:

    A. _____

    B. _____

    C. _____

    D. _____

81. _____

    are the most difficult foods for a person with

    dysphagia to swallow.

82. Before helping a person with dysphagia with

    food and fluids, you need to _____

    _____

    _____.

83. When assisting a person with dysphagia with food and fluids, you need to report signs of difficulty swallowing to the nurse immediately.
    A. True
    B. False

84. List four factors that may affect a person's appetite and ability to eat.

    A. _____

    B. _____

    C. _____

    D. _____

85. You need to assist the person with hand washing before and after meals.
    A. True
    B. False

86. To prepare Mrs. Burger for meals, the nursing assistant did the following:

    A. _____

    B. _____

    C. _____

    D. _____

    E. _____

87. Serving food promptly ensures that _____

    _____.

88. Make sure the tray is complete by _____

    _____.

89. The _____ and the

    _____

    tell you what observations and measurements

    are needed.

90. To make sure the tray is complete, ask the patient or resident if the correct food and needed items are present.
    A. True
    B. False

91. Always explain what foods are on the tray and where they are located.
    A. True
    B. False

92. _____ can help to

    relieve feelings of helplessness and loss of control.

93. Letting the person help to the extent possible is

    important for _____.

94. Before feeding a person, you need to review:

    A. Precautions to prevent _____

    B. Signs and symptoms of _____

95. You need to report signs and symptoms of dysphagia to the nurse when you finish feeding the person.
    A. True
    B. False

96. Food is served in the order preferred by the person.
    A. True
    B. False

97. Checking for food that becomes pocketed in the

    mouth helps to prevent _____ and

    _____.

98. When the person has finished eating, you need to:

A. _____

B. _____

C. _____

D. _____

E. _____

F. _____

G. _____

H. _____

I. _____

J. _____

## CASE STUDY

*Mrs. Frieda Black is an 80-year-old resident of Pine View Nursing Center. She has diabetes and high blood pressure. She needs assistance to get ready for meals. She wears eyeglasses and wears a hearing aid in her right ear. She has upper and lower dentures, which she cares for herself. She is continent of bowel and bladder. She needs help with transfers to and from the toilet. She uses a wheelchair to get to the dining room and can push the wheelchair herself. She needs assistance preparing her food, but can eat by herself. She sits at a dining room table with three other residents. One of her tablemates also has diabetes.*

*Mrs. Black is a devout Christian. She always prays before meals.*

*Mrs. Black requires diabetes meal planning and a no added salt diet.*

*You assist Mrs. Black to get ready for her noon meal and help prepare her food when she is in the dining room. She complains that her food is not appetizing. She also tells you that her portions are too small. She tells you that she had bread and dessert for every meal when she was doing her own cooking.*

*Answer the following questions.*

1. What factors might affect Mrs. Blacks eating and nutrition?

2. What is involved in diabetes meal planning?

3. What dietary restriction does a no added salt diet require?

4. What important information will you find on Mrs. Blacks dietary card and care plan?

5. What information will you report to the nurse when Mrs. Black is finished eating? Why?

6. Who will you report Mrs. Black's complaints to? When will you report her complaints?
   A. How will this information be used in the care planning process?

## ADDITIONAL LEARNING ACTIVITIES

1. Discuss with a classmate the importance of food in your daily life. Besides meeting physical needs, what role does food play in your life?
   A. Discuss how your culture and religion affect the food you eat.

   B. Discuss the role food plays in your social life.

   C. Discuss why you enjoy some foods and dislike others.

2. Has illness ever affected your appetite or your ability to eat certain foods? Explain.
   A. Discuss your experience. How might your experience help you provide better care?

3. Review the *MyPyramid Food Guidance System* (pages 291-295 in the text).
   A. Based on the *MyPyramid Food Guidance System*, are you making wise food choices?

   B. Based on the *MyPyramid Food Guidance System*, is your diet well balanced?

4. Discuss the special needs of residents with dementia. List ways that you can help meet their nutritional needs.

5. View the CD Companion to help you learn and practice the Feeding the Person procedure.

6. Carefully review the procedures for Serving Meal Trays and Feeding the Person.
   A. Use the procedure checklists on pages 307-312 as a guide.

   B. Practice the procedures with a classmate using various food thicknesses.

   C. Take your turn being the patient or resident. Discuss your experience. Answer these questions:
   (1) How does it feel to be fed by another person?

   (2) Did you enjoy your meal? Explain.

   (3) Were you fed too fast or too slow?

(4) Was the amount given with each bite right for you?

(6) Did your food remain at the right temperature throughout the meal?

(5) Were liquids offered during the meal?

(7) How might your experience affect the care you give?

# 18 Assisting With Assessment

## OBJECTIVES

The questions and student activities in this chapter will help you meet these objectives.
- Define the key terms listed in this chapter
- Explain why vital signs are measured
- List the factors affecting vital signs
- Identify the normal ranges for each temperature site
- Know when to use each temperature site
- Identify the pulse sites
- Describe normal respirations
- Describe the practices followed when measuring blood pressure
- Explain why intake and output are measured
- Identify the fluids counted as intake and the fluids counted as output
- Explain how to prepare the person for weight and height measurements
- Explain how to assist with pain assessment
- Perform the procedures described in this chapter

## STUDY QUESTIONS

*Matching*

*Match each term with the correct definition.*

1. _____ The amount of heat in the body that is a balance between the amount of heat produced and the amount lost by the body

2. _____ A slow heart rate; the rate is less than 60 beats per minute

3. _____ The pressure in the arteries when the heart is at rest

4. _____ The amount of force exerted against the walls of an artery by the blood

5. _____ Blood pressure measurements that remain above a systolic pressure of 140 mm Hg or a diastolic pressure of 90 mm Hg

6. _____ When the systolic blood pressure is below 90 mm Hg and the diastolic pressure is below 60 mm Hg

7. _____ The beat of the heart felt at an artery as a wave of blood passes through the artery

8. _____ The number of heartbeats or pulses felt in 1 minute

9. _____ Breathing air into (inhalation) and out of (exhalation) the lungs

10. _____ An instrument used to listen to the sounds produced by the heart, lungs, and other body organs

A. Hypertension

B. Blood pressure

C. Respiration

D. Pulse

E. Stethoscope

F. Tachycardia

G. Hypotension

H. Diastolic pressure

I. Bradycardia

J. Pulse rate

K. Sphygmomanometer

L. Vital signs

11. _____ The amount of force needed to pump blood out of the heart into the arterial circulation

12. _____ A rapid heart rate; the heart rate is over 100 beats per minute

13. _____ Temperature, pulse, respirations, and blood pressure

14. _____ A cuff and measuring device used to measure blood pressure

15. _____ Means to ache, hurt, or be sore

M. Pain

N. Body temperature

O. Systolic pressure

### Fill in the Blanks

16. Vital signs reflect these three body processes:

    A. _____

    B. _____

    C. _____

17. Accuracy is essential when you _____,

    _____, and

    _____

    vital signs.

18. Vital signs show even minor changes in a person's condition. They also tell about response to treatment and often signal life-threatening events. Therefore you must report the following at once:

    A. _____

    B. _____

19. List the sites for measuring body temperature.

    A. _____

    B. _____

    C. _____

    D. _____

20. List the normal range for body temperature for the:

    A. Rectal site _____

    B. Oral site _____

    C. Tympanic membrane site _____

    D. Axillary site _____

21. Oral temperatures are *not* taken if the person:

    A. _____

    B. _____

    C. _____

    D. _____

    E. _____

    F. _____

    G. _____

    H. _____

    I. _____

    J. _____

22. Mr. Lewis has heart disease. Which temperatures sites can you use?

    _____

    _____

23. Which temperature site is *not* used for infants and children under 6 years of age?

_____

24. How should you shake down a glass thermometer?

_____

_____

_____

_____

25. What do the short lines on a Fahrenheit thermometer mean?

_____

26. What does each long line on a centigrade thermometer mean?

_____

27. List four special measures needed when taking a rectal temperature with a glass thermometer.

A. _____

B. _____

C. _____

D. _____

28. Tympanic membrane thermometers are gently inserted into the _____.

29. You have finished measuring Mr. Abbot's temperature. What observations do you need to report and record?

A. _____

B. _____

30. How is the person positioned when measuring a rectal temperature?

_____

31. Which site is used most often for taking a pulse?

_____

32. Which pulse is taken with a stethoscope?

_____

33. List the rules to follow when using a stethoscope.

A. _____

_____

B. _____

_____

C. _____

_____

D. _____

_____

34. The normal adult pulse rate is between _____ beats per minute.

35. The rhythm of the pulse should be regular. This means _____

_____.

36. Where is the radial artery located?

_____

37. You should not use your thumb to take a pulse because _____

_____

_____.

38. Apical pulses are taken for persons who:

A. _____

B. _____

C. _____

39. Describe normal respirations.

   _____

   _____

40. The healthy adult has _____

   respirations per minute.

41. When are respirations usually counted?

   _____

42. You have counted Mr. Wilson's respirations. What observations do you need to report and record?

   A. _____

   B. _____

   C. _____

   D. _____

   E. _____

   F. _____

43. _____ and

   _____

   are used to measure blood pressure.

44. What should you do if a mercury manometer breaks?

   _____

   _____

45. Before measuring blood pressure, what information do you need from the nurse and the care plan?

   A. _____

   B. _____

   C. _____

   D. _____

   E. _____

   F. _____

46. When taking a blood pressure, how should you position the person's arm?

   _____

   _____

47. Intake and output (I&O) records are used to

   _____

   _____.

   They also are kept when _____

   _____.

48. Output includes _____

   _____.

49. Define the following types of pain.

   A. Acute pain _____

   _____

   _____

   B. Chronic pain _____

   _____

   _____

50. Ms. Laura Frank complains of pain in her lower abdomen. What other information about Ms. Frank's pain does the nurse need?

   A. _____

   B. _____

   C. _____

   D. _____

   E. _____

   F. _____

*Labeling*

51. Label the pulse sites.

52. Label the parts of a stethoscope.

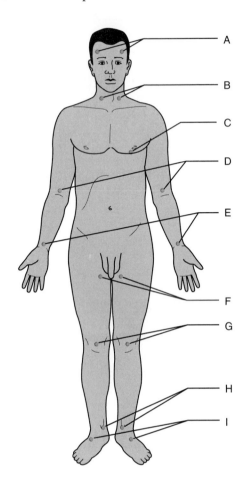

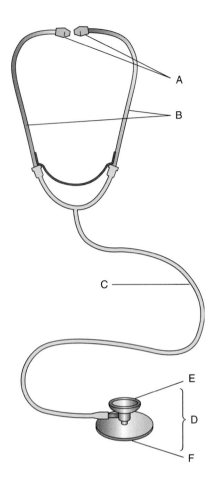

A. _____

B. _____

C. _____

D. _____

E. _____

F. _____

G. _____

H. _____

I. _____

A. _____

B. _____

C. _____

D. _____

E. _____

F. _____

53. Place an X at the apical pulse site.

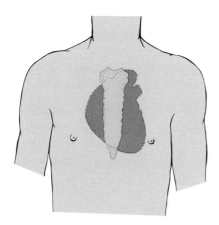

*Multiple Choice*

Circle the **BEST** Answer

54. Unless otherwise ordered, vital signs are taken
    A. After the person's bath
    B. With the person lying or sitting
    C. After breakfast
    D. After performing ROM exercise

55. Do *not* take a rectal temperature if
    A. The person is unconscious.
    B. The person has just had a bath.
    C. The person is receiving oxygen.
    D. The person has diarrhea.

56. The least reliable temperature site is the
    A. Oral site
    B. Axillary site
    C. Tympanic membrane site
    D. Rectal site

57. When using a glass thermometer, do the following to prevent infection
    A. Use only the person's thermometer.
    B. Rinse the thermometer under warm running water.
    C. Dry the thermometer from the bulb to the stem with tissue.
    D. After cleaning, store the thermometer in the person's bedside stand.

58. You are taking a rectal temperature with a glass thermometer. Which is *incorrect*?
    A. Privacy is important.
    B. The thermometer is lubricated before insertion.
    C. The thermometer is held in place.
    D. The thermometer remains in the rectum for 1 minute.

59. Axillary temperatures
    A. Are more reliable than oral temperatures.
    B. Are taken right after bathing the person.
    C. Are taken for 3 minutes.
    D. Are used when other routes cannot be used.

60. The force of a pulse relates to
    A. How regular the pulse is
    B. The strength of the pulse
    C. The number of beats per minute
    D. The number of skipped beats

61. Which pulse rate would you report to the nurse at once?
    A. 60 beats per minute
    B. 72 beats per minute
    C. 90 beats per minute
    D. 104 beats per minute

62. The apical pulse is located
    A. In the middle of the sternum
    B. On the right side of the chest slightly above the nipple
    C. On the left side of the chest slightly below the nipple
    D. One inch below and to the left of the sternum

63. An apical pulse is counted for
    A. 30 seconds
    B. 1 minute
    C. 2 minutes
    D. 5 minutes

64. The period of heart muscle contraction is called
    A. Systole
    B. Diastole
    C. Blood pressure
    D. Aneroid

65. The normal range for diastolic blood pressure is
    A. Greater than 80 mm Hg
    B. Less than 80 mm Hg
    C. Greater than 120 mm Hg
    D. Less than 120 mm Hg

66. Which is *not* a guideline for measuring blood pressure?
    A. Avoid taking blood pressure on an injured arm.
    B. Let the person rest for 10 to 20 minutes before measuring blood pressure.
    C. Measure blood pressure with the person sitting or lying.
    D. Apply the cuff over clothing.

67. Blood pressure is normally measured
    A. In the radial artery
    B. At the apical site
    C. In the brachial artery
    D. In the popliteal artery

68. One ounce equals
    A. 30 ml
    B. 50 ml
    C. 90 ml
    D. 100 ml

69. Which is *not* measured as intake?
    A. Gravy
    B. Milk
    C. Gelatin
    D. Orange juice

70. Which is *correct* when measuring weight and height?
    A. The person wears pajamas, a robe, and shoes for warmth and comfort.
    B. After breakfast is the best time to weigh the person.
    C. Balance the scale at zero before weighing the person.
    D. The person voids after being weighed.

71. Pain is personal. It differs for each person.
    A. True
    B. False

72. Pain felt in a body part that is no longer there is
    A. Chronic pain
    B. Radiating pain
    C. False pain
    D. Phantom pain

73. You are having problems hearing Mr. Reed's blood pressure measurement. What should you do?
    A. Report what you think you heard.
    B. Ask a co-worker what Mr. Reed's usual blood pressure is.
    C. Ask Mr. Reed what his usual blood pressure is.
    D. Tell the nurse.

## MOSBY'S NURSING ASSISTANT SKILLS VIDEOS EXERCISES

### Questions from the *Measurements* Video

74. How did the nursing assistant aide Mr. Bernardo's stability while measuring his weight?

    _____

75. Calibrated containers are used to measure intake and output. They are measured at eye level.
    A. True
    B. False

76. If you are careful, there is no need to wear gloves when measuring output.
    A. True
    B. False

77. When measuring intake, you need to follow these steps:

    A. _____

    B. _____

    C. _____

    D. _____

78. Intake and output has been ordered for Mr. Bernardo. Why is it important to remind him to use the signal light when the specimen container or urinal needs emptying?

    _____

    _____

    _____

    _____

79. What procedure guidelines are followed for these measurements:

    A. Body temperature _____

    _____

    B. Pulse _____

    _____

    C. Respirations _____

    _____

    D. Blood pressure _____

    _____

80. Body temperature is the same at all temperature sites.
    A. True
    B. False

81. When using an electronic thermometer, you need to use a new probe cover each time.
    A. True
    B. False

82. A rectal temperature must be performed skillfully and with attention to _____,

    _____, and

    _____.

83. Note the pulse _____,

    _____, and

    _____

    before you count the pulse rate.

84. You need to clean the _____ and

    _____

    of the stethoscope with alcohol wipes before and

    after measuring the apical pulse.

85. Count each rise of the chest as one respiration and each fall of the chest as one respiration.
    A. True
    B. False

## CASE STUDY

*Ms. Jane Lane is an 80-year-old resident of Valley View Nursing Center. She shares a room with Mrs. Bloom. Ms. Lane has the bed by the door. She is receiving continuous oxygen by mask. She has a dressing on her lower left arm. Ms. Lane is able to communicate her needs. The nurse has delegated measuring and recording Ms. Lane's vital signs to you. When you enter her room, you notice that she is drinking a cup of coffee.*

*Answer the following questions.*

1. What sites can you use to measure Ms. Lane's temperature?

2. Which arm will you use to measure Ms. Lane's pulse and blood pressure?

3. What observations about Ms. Lane's respirations do you need to report and record?

4. What pulse rates do you need to report at once?

5. How can you promote Ms Lane's right to personal choice?

6. How can you protect Ms. Lane's right to privacy?

## ADDITIONAL LEARNING ACTIVITIES

1. View the CD Companion Skills to help you practice the following procedures:
   A. Taking Temperatures With Glass and Electronic Thermometers.

   B. Taking a Radial Pulse and Counting Respirations

   C. Measuring Blood Pressure

   D. Measuring Intake and Output

   E. Measuring Weight and Height

2. Practice the procedures in Chapter 18 with a classmate. Use the procedure checklists on pages 313-330 as a guide. Practice with various partners. Take your turn being the patient or resident.
   *Use a simulator for practicing rectal temperature.*
   A. Temperature
      (1) Practice reading a glass thermometer.

      (2) If available, practice taking temperatures with different types of thermometers. Discuss the advantages and disadvantages of each.

   B. Pulse
      (1) Practice with various classmates. Locate the following pulse sites: carotid, apical, brachial, radial, femoral, popliteal, and dorsalis pedis.

   (2) Take radial pulses on various persons. Do you notice differences in rate, rhythm, and force?

   (3) Take a person's pulse before and after exercise. Notice and record the differences in rate, rhythm, and force.

   C. Respirations
      (1) Practice with various people. Note differences in respiratory rates. Does the respiratory rate and depth of respirations change with exercise?

   D. Blood pressure
      (1) Practice with various people.

      (2) Take and record blood pressure before and after exercise.

      (3) Take and record blood pressures with the person lying, sitting, and standing.

      (4) If available, practice using different types of blood pressure equipment.

# 19 Assisting With Specimens

## OBJECTIVES

The questions and student activities in this chapter will help you meet these objectives.
- Define the key terms listed in this chapter
- Explain why specimens are collected

- Describe the different types of urine specimens
- Explain why urine specimens are tested
- Explain the rules for collecting specimens
- Perform the procedures described in this chapter

## STUDY QUESTIONS

### Matching

*Match each term with the correct definition.*

1. _____ Sugar in the urine; glycosuria

2. _____ Blood in the urine

3. _____ Bloody sputum

4. _____ Acetone; ketone

5. _____ Samples collected and tested to prevent, detect, and treat disease

6. _____ A substance that appears in urine from rapid breakdown of fat for energy

7. _____ Mucus from the respiratory system that is expectorated through the mouth

A. Hematuria

B. Ketone body

C. Sputum

D. Glucosuria

E. Hemoptysis

F. Acetone

G. Specimens

### Fill in the Blanks

8. What information do you need from the nurse before collecting a urine specimen?

   A. _____

   B. _____

   C. _____

   D. _____

   E. _____

9. To identify the person when collecting a specimen,

   you need to _____

   _____

   _____.

10. The midstream specimen is also called _____

_____

_____ .

11. The nurse asks you to collect a midstream specimen from Mrs. Peterson. What equipment and supplies do you need to collect?

     A. _____

     B. _____

     C. _____

     D. _____

     E. _____

     F. _____

     G. _____

12. _____

     is another term for a double-voided specimen.

13. Fresh-fractional specimens are used to test urine

     for _____ .

14. _____ measures if urine

     is acidic or alkaline.

15. _____ specimens are best

     for testing urine for glucose and ketones.

16. Unseen blood is called _____ .

17. When testing urine specimens, what observations do you need to report and record?

     A. _____

     B. _____

     C. _____

     D. _____

     E. _____

18. How can you make sure that you use reagent strips correctly?

_____

19. What information do you need from the nurse before collecting a stool specimen?

     A. _____

     B. _____

     C. _____

20. Stool specimens are studied for _____ ,

_____ ,

_____ ,

_____ and

_____ .

21. When collecting specimens, you must follow

_____ , and

     the _____ .

22. Sputum specimens are studied for _____ ,

_____ ,

     and _____ .

23. Mouth wash is not used to rinse the mouth before collecting a sputum specimen because

_____ .

24. The nurse asks you to collect a sputum specimen from Mr. Juarez. What observations do you need to report and record?

A. _____

B. _____

C. _____

D. _____

E. _____

F. _____

G. _____

H. _____

I. _____

25. When collecting a sputum specimen from a person who has or may have TB, you need to follow Standard Precautions, and the Bloodborne Pathogen Standard, The doctor may order

_____.

26. You promote comfort when collecting specimens by _____

_____.

27. You made an error in procedure when collecting a stool specimen from Ms. Rita Jones. What should you do?

_____

_____

_____

*Multiple Choice*

Circle the **BEST** Answer

28. Which is *not* a rule for collecting specimens?
    A. Follow the rules of medical asepsis.
    B. Use the correct container.
    C. Label the container accurately.
    D. Collect the specimen when you have time.

29. What type of specimen is collected for a routine urinalysis?
    A. A random specimen
    B. A midstream specimen
    C. A 24-hour specimen
    D. A double-voided specimen

30. A random urine specimen is collected in the morning before breakfast.
    A. True
    B. False

31. A sterile container is used for a midstream specimen.
    A. True
    B. False

32. A double-voided specimen is needed to test urine pH.
    A. True
    B. False

33. The body needs insulin to
    A. Maintain fluid balance
    B. Use protein for tissue repair
    C. Produce urine
    D. Use sugar for energy

34. What kind of urine specimen is needed to test for blood?
    A. A clean-catch specimen
    B. A double-voided specimen
    C. A routine specimen
    D. An early morning specimen

35. The normal pH of urine is between
    A. 2.0 and 3.5
    B. 4.6 and 8.0
    C. 10.2 and 10.8
    D. 10.5 and 12.2

36. When testing urine with reagent strips, you need to wear gloves.
    A. True
    B. False

37. Stool specimens must not be contaminated with urine.
    A. True
    B. False

38. Which statement about collecting sputum specimens is *false*?
    A. It is easier to collect a specimen in the evening.
    B. The person coughs up sputum from the bronchi and trachea.
    C. The person rinses the mouth with water before coughing up sputum.
    D. Privacy is important.

## CASE STUDY

*Mr. Granger is a 60-year-old patient on third floor medical. You have been assigned to assist with his care. Your assignment includes collecting:*
- *A urine specimen to check for blood*
- *A stool specimen to check for occult blood*
  *Mr. Granger is able to assist in obtaining the specimens. The RN will test the urine and stool specimens.*

*Answer the following questions.*

1. What information do you need from the nurse before collecting each specimen?

2. What safety measures do you need to practice when collecting each specimen?

3. What instructions do you need to give Mr. Granger about the urine specimen?

4. What type of urine specimen do you need to collect?

---

## ADDITIONAL LEARNING ACTIVITIES

1. Read the following situation. Then answer the questions that follow.
   *The nurse asks you to collect a double-voided specimen from Mrs. Smith.*
   A. What additional information do you need from the nurse before you collect the specimen?

   B. What equipment and supplies do you need to collect?

   C. How will you explain the procedure to Mrs. Smith?

D. What are the steps involved in collecting the specimen?

E. What observations do you need to report and record?

2. Under the supervision of your instructor, practice the procedures in Chapter 19. Use the procedure checklists on pages 331-342 as a guide.

# 20 Assisting With Exercise and Activity

## OBJECTIVES

The questions and student activities in this chapter will help you meet these objectives.
- Define the key terms listed in this chapter
- Describe bedrest and how to prevent related complications
- Describe the devices used to support and maintain body alignment
- Describe range-of-motion exercises
- Explain how to help a falling person
- Describe four walking aids
- Perform the procedures described in this chapter

## STUDY QUESTIONS

### Matching

*Match each term with the correct definition.*

1. _____ Moving a body part away from the midline of the body

2. _____ Moving a body part toward the midline of the body

3. _____ The lack of joint mobility caused by abnormal shortening of a muscle

4. _____ Bending the toes and foot up at the ankle

5. _____ Straightening a body part

6. _____ Turning the joint outward

7. _____ The act of walking

8. _____ Turning the joint inward

9. _____ The decrease in size or a wasting away of tissue

10. _____ Bending a body part

11. _____ Excessive straightening of a body part

12. _____ The foot falls down at the ankle; permanent plantar flexion

13. _____ Abnormally low blood pressure when the person suddenly stands up; postural hypotension

A. Adduction

B. Dorsiflexion

C. Hyperextension

D. Orthostatic hypotension

E. Pronation

F. Internal rotation

G. Abduction

H. Postural

I. External rotation

J. Contracture

K. Flexion

L. Plantar flexion

M. Supination

N. Atrophy

14. _____ The foot is bent; bending the foot down at the ankle

15. _____ Turning the joint downward

16. _____ The movement of a joint to the extent possible without causing pain

17. _____ Turning the joint upward

18. _____ Turning the joint

19. _____ Relates to posture or standing

O. Extension

P. Range of motion (ROM)

Q. Rotation

R. Footdrop

S. Ambulation

## Fill in the Blanks

20. List five reasons why bedrest is ordered.

   A. _____

   B. _____

   C. _____

   D. _____

   E. _____

21. Define these types of bedrest.

   A. Bedrest _____

   _____

   B. Strict bedrest _____

   _____

   C. Bedrest with commode privileges _____

   _____

   D. Bedrest with bathroom privileges _____

   _____

22. List seven complications of bedrest.

   A. _____

   B. _____

   C. _____

   D. _____

   E. _____

   F. _____

   G. _____

23. _____

   is key to preventing orthostatic hypotension.

24. Trochanter rolls keep the hips and legs from

   _____.

25. What is the purpose of foot boards?

   _____

   _____

26. Splints keep the _____,

    _____,

    _____,

    _____,

    _____, and

    _____ in

    normal position.

27. _____

    keep the weight of top linens off the feet and toes.

28. _____

    range-of-motion exercises are done by the

    person.

29. You have been delegated range-of-motion exercises for Miss Mary Adams. What information do you need from the nurse and the care plan?

    A. _____

    B. _____

    C. _____

    D. _____

    E. _____

30. When can you perform range-of-motion exercises to a person's neck?

    _____

    _____

31. List and describe the range-of-motion exercises performed to the hips.

    A. _____

    B. _____

    C. _____

    D. _____

    E. _____

    F. _____

32. The nurse asks you to assist Mr. Green with ambulation. Mr. Green is weak and unsteady. What safety measures are needed?

    _____

    _____

    _____

33. What observations do you need to report and record after assisting Mr. Green with ambulation?

    A. _____

    B. _____

    C. _____

    D. _____

    E. _____

34. Why should you ease a person to the floor if the person starts to fall?

    A. _____

    B. _____

35. Mr. Reese lost his balance while you were assisting him with ambulation. You eased him to the floor. What must you report to the nurse?

    A. _____

    B. _____

    C. _____

    D. _____

    E. _____

36. Explain why loose clothes are unsafe for a person using crutches.

    _____

    _____

    _____

37. Canes help provide _____ and

    _____.

38. Braces are used to:

    A. _____

    B. _____

    C. _____

39. You are applying a knee brace to Mr. Reese's left knee. What observations do you need to report to the nurse at once?

    A. _____

    B. _____

40. The _____

    tells you when to apply and remove a brace.

41. OBRA requires activity programs for nursing center residents. Activities must _____

    _____

    _____.

*Multiple Choice*

Circle the **BEST** Answer

42. Exercise and activity are promoted in all persons to the extent possible.
    A. True
    B. False

43. Complications of bedrest include all of the following *except*
    A. Pneumonia
    B. Muscle atrophy
    C. Pressure ulcers
    D. Dorsiflexion

44. Bed boards are used to
    A. Prevent the mattress from sagging
    B. Prevent plantar flexion
    C. Prevent orthostatic hypotension
    D. Strengthen the feet

45. Where are hip abduction wedges placed?
    A. At the foot of the bed
    B. Between the person's legs
    C. Alongside the person's body
    D. Under the mattress

46. Who performs active-assistive range-of-motion exercises?
    A. The person
    B. The person with some help from another person
    C. A health team member
    D. The physical therapist

47. You are assisting Miss Mary Adams with range-of-motion exercises. Which is *incorrect*?
    A. Exercise only the joints the nurse tells you to exercise.
    B. Expose only the body part being exercised.
    C. Move the joint slowly, smoothly, and gently.
    D. Move the joint slightly beyond the point of pain.

48. You are assisting Mr. Green with ambulation. Which is *incorrect*?
    A. He needs to wear nonskid foot wear.
    B. Encourage him to stand erect with his head up and his back straight.
    C. Encourage him to use the hand rails on his strong side.
    D. Encourage him to walk slowly and to slide his feet.

49. Ms. Saunders started to fall while you were assisting her with ambulation. You eased her to the floor. She is confused and tries to get up. You should hold her down until the nurse arrives.
    A. True
    B. False

50. You must complete an incident report after a patient or resident falls.
    A. True
    B. False

51. Which is *not* a safety measure for using crutches?
    A. Replace worn or torn crutch tips.
    B. Check wooden crutches for cracks.
    C. Have the person wear comfortable bedroom slippers.
    D. Keep crutches within the person's reach.

52. When using a cane to walk
    A. The cane tip is about 16 inches to the side of the foot.
    B. The grip is level with the waist.
    C. The cane is held on the strong side.
    D. The strong leg is moved forward first.

53. A walker gives more support than a cane.
    A. True
    B. False

54. To promote mental comfort during exercise, you need to
    A. Provide for privacy.
    B. Do as much as possible for the person.
    C. Discuss the person's exercise program with the person's family.
    D. Tell the person everything will be OK.

55. OBRA requires activity programs for nursing center residents. Which is *false*?
    A. Activities are important for physical and mental well-being.
    B. The right to personal choice is protected.
    C. The person must participate in at least one activity each day.
    D. You help residents to activities as needed.

## MOSBY'S NURSING ASSISTANT SKILLS VIDEOS EXERCISES

### Questions from the Body Mechanics and Exercise Video

56. Being active is important for _____

    and _____

    well-being.

57. Inactivity affects normal function of every body system and the person's mental well-being.
    A. True
    B. False

58. You are performing range-of-motion exercise on a patient. How many times do you need to repeat ROM to each joint?

    _____

    _____

59. Signs and symptoms of orthostatic hypotension include:

    A. _____

    B. _____

    C. _____

    D. _____

## CASE STUDY

*Mr. Joe White is a resident at Long Meadow Nursing Center. You have received the following information from the end of shift report and your assignment sheet:*
- *Mr. White is in bed most of the day. He needs help to get out of bed. He is often unsteady when he gets out of bed.*
- *Mr. White needs help to walk three times a day. He uses a wheeled walker. He also wears a brace over his right ankle.*

- *Mr. White receives active-assistive range-of-motion exercises to both knees and ankles. He is able to move up in bed and turn using a trapeze.*

*Answer the following questions.*

1. Mr. White is at risk for which conditions?

   A. What measures can help decrease these risks?

2. What information do you need from the nurse and the care plan before you
   A. Help Mr. White to walk?

   B. Assist with range-of-motion exercises?

3. What safety measures are practiced when getting Mr. White out of bed?

4. What safety measures are practiced when helping Mr. White to ambulate?

5. What information do you need to report and record about range-of-motion exercises?

6. When putting on and removing Mr. White's brace, what do you need to report to the nurse at once?

7. How will you promote personal choice when providing care for Mr. White?

8. How will you promote Mr. White's right to privacy when assisting him with range-of-motion exercises?

---

## ADDITIONAL LEARNING ACTIVITIES

1. Make a list of activities in your daily life which provide range-of-motion exercises.
   A. How do these activities promote your physical, social, and emotional well-being?

   B. How can you use daily activities to promote ROM for patients and residents?

2. View the CD Companion Skills to help you learn and practice the following procedures:
   A. Performing Range-of-Motion Exercises

   B. Helping the Person to Walk

3. Practice active range-of-motion exercises. Use the procedure checklist on pages 343-347 as a guide. This will help you better understand the ROM of each joint.

4. Under the supervision of your instructor, practice the procedures in Chapter 20. Use the procedure checklists on pages 343-350 as a guide.

   A. Take your turn being the patient or resident.

   B. Discuss your experience.

# Assisting With Wound Care

## OBJECTIVES

The questions and student activities in this chapter will help you meet these objectives.
- Define the key terms listed in this chapter
- Describe skin tears, pressure ulcers, and circulatory ulcers and how to prevent them
- Identify the pressure points in each body position
- Describe what to observe about wounds

- Explain how to secure dressings
- Explain the rules for applying dressings
- Explain the purpose, effects, and complications of heat and cold applications
- Describe the rules for applying heat and cold
- Perform the procedures described in this chapter

## STUDY QUESTIONS

### Matching

Match each term with the correct definition.

1. _____ A soft pad applied over a body area

2. _____ To narrow

3. _____ To expand or open wider

4. _____ An open wound on the lower legs and feet caused by decreased blood flow through arteries or veins

5. _____ Scraping the skin, causing an open area

6. _____ When the skin sticks to a surface while deeper tissues move downward

7. _____ Any injury caused by unrelieved pressure

8. _____ A break or rip in the skin; the epidermis separates from underlying tissues

9. _____ A blood clot

10. _____ A break in the skin or mucous membrane

11. _____ A blood clot that travels through the vascular system until it lodges in a distant vessel

A. Constrict

B. Shearing

C. Pressure ulcer (decubitus ulcer)

D. Dilate

E. Thrombus

F. Friction

G. Circulatory ulcer

H. Wound

I. Skin tear

J. Embolus

K. Compress

*Fill in the Blanks*

12. _____

is an accident or violent act that injures the skin,

mucous membranes, bones, and internal organs.

13. Pressure ulcers occur from _____ and

_____

_____ .

14. Wound care involves _____

_____ .

15. Skin tears are caused by _____

_____ .

16. List five measures that prevent skin tears.

  A. _____

  _____

  B. _____

  _____

  C. _____

  _____

  D. _____

  _____

  E. _____

  _____

17. _____,

_____, and

_____

are common causes of skin breakdown and

pressure ulcers. Other factors include

_____,

_____,

_____,

_____,

and _____ .

18. Persons at risk for pressure ulcers are those who:

  A. _____

  B. _____

  C. _____

  D. _____

  E. _____

  F. _____

  G. _____

  H. _____

19. The first sign of a pressure ulcer is _____

_____ .

20. Where do pressure ulcers usually occur?

  _____

21. List four common sites for pressure ulcers in
obese persons.

  A. _____

  B. _____

  C. _____

  D. _____

22. _____

    is a condition in which there is death of tissue.

23. How do elastic stockings help prevent blood clots?

    _____

    _____

    _____

24. Persons at risk for thrombi include those who:

    A. _____

    B. _____

    C. _____

    D. _____

25. What information do you need from the nurse and the care plan before you apply elastic stockings?

    A. _____

    B. _____

    C. _____

    D. _____

26. Explain why elastic stockings are applied before the person gets out of bed.

    _____

    _____

27. When applying elastic bandages, you need to

    start at _____

    _____.

28. You are applying an elastic bandage to Mr. John

    Hansen's right leg. You should expose his toes

    because _____.

29. Mrs. Rita Monk has an elastic bandage on her left arm. She complains of pain and tingling in her fingers. What should you do?

    _____

    _____

30. List five purposes for wound dressings.

    A. _____

    B. _____

    C. _____

    D. _____

    E. _____

31. Mr. Paul Bloom has an abdominal dressing. The nurse tells you that he has a lot of pain during dressing changes. What measure will help promote Mr. Bloom's comfort?

    _____

    _____

    _____

32. An incorrectly applied binder can cause:

    A. _____

    B. _____

    C. _____

33. You need to reapply a binder if _____

    _____

    _____.

34. You need to change binders that are _____,

    _____, or

    _____.

35. When heat is applied to the skin, blood vessels in

    the area _____.

36. When applying heat to an area, you need to observe for pale skin because _____

    _____

    _____

    _____.

37. Which persons are at risk for burns from heat applications?

    A. _____

    B. _____

    C. _____

38. A hot soak involves _____

    _____.

39. Provide the temperature range in Fahrenheit and Centigrade for each of the following.

    A. Hot _____

    B. Tepid _____

    C. Cold _____

40. Cold applications are used to:

    A. _____

    B. _____

    C. _____

41. Explain what happens when cold is applied for a long time.

    _____

    _____

    _____

42. List seven observations you need to report and record when applying heat and cold applications.

    A. _____

    B. _____

    C. _____

    D. _____

    E. _____

    F. _____

    G. _____

43. You are assisting Ms. Luna with a sitz bath. How will you promote her safety?

    _____

    _____

    _____

44. An aquathermia pad is placed in a flannel cover because _____

    _____

    _____.

45. Before applying an elastic bandage, changing a dressing, or applying heat and cold, you need to make sure that:

    A. _____

    B. _____

    C. _____

    D. _____

    E. _____

    F. _____

## Labeling

46. Place an x on the pressure points for each position.

**A.**

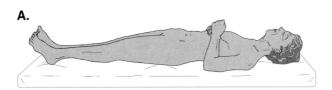

**B.**

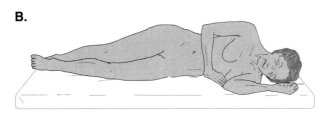

**C.**

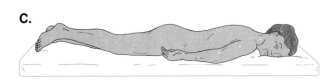

**D.**

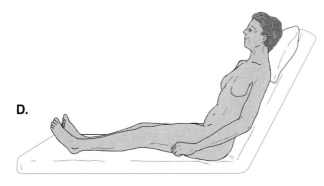

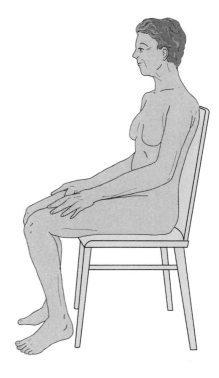

## Multiple Choice

Circle the **BEST** Answer

47. Any injury caused by unrelieved pressure is
    A. A skin tear
    B. An intentional wound
    C. A decubitus ulcer
    D. A chronic wound

48. Miss Paul has a stage 2 pressure ulcer. This means
    A. The skin is red but intact.
    B. The skin is cracked and there is a shallow crater.
    C. The skin is gone. The underlying tissue is gone.
    D. Muscle and bone are exposed and damaged.

49. Which measure helps prevent pressure ulcers?
    A. Repositioning the person every 4 hours
    B. Raising the head of the bed 45 to 60 degrees when the person is in bed
    C. Vigorously rubbing the skin dry after bathing
    D. Positioning the person in the 30-degree lateral position

50. Remind persons sitting in chairs to shift their positions
    A. Whenever they think about it
    B. *Before* and after meals
    C. Every hour
    D. Every 15 minutes

51. A frame placed on the bed and over the person to keep top linens off the feet is called a
    A. Bed cradle
    B. Heel elevator
    C. Flotation pad
    D. Trochanter frame

52. Open wounds on the lower legs and feet caused by poor blood return through the veins are called
    A. Arterial ulcers
    B. Pressure ulcers
    C. Epidermal ulcers
    D. Stasis ulcers

53. Which action will *not* help prevent circulatory ulcers?
    A. Having the person use elastic type garters to hold socks in place
    B. Keeping linens clean, dry, and wrinkle-free
    C. Keeping pressure off the heels
    D. Reporting changes in skin color

54. When applying a non-sterile dressing to Mr. Roland's abdomen, you need to
    A. Tell him how you feel about his wound.
    B. Remove the dressing so Mr. Roland can see the soiled side. He should know what the drainage looks like.
    C. Tell Mr. Roland that he needs to look at his wound so he can observe the healing process.
    D. Remove tape by pulling it toward the wound.

55. After applying an elastic bandage to Mr. Hansen's right leg, you need to check the color and temperature of the leg:
    A. Every 15 minutes
    B. Every hour
    C. Every 2 hours
    D. Every shift

56. Which is *correct* when applying tape to secure a dressing?
    A. Tape is applied to secure the top and bottom of the dressing.
    B. Tape should encircle the entire body part whenever possible.
    C. The tape extends 1 inch on each side of the dressing.
    D. Tape is applied to secure the top, middle, and bottom of the dressing.

57. Montgomery ties are used to secure a dressing. Which is *incorrect*?
    A. The adhesive strips are removed with each dressing change.
    B. Cloth ties are secured over the dressing.
    C. The cloth ties are undone for dressing changes.
    D. The adhesive strips are removed when soiled.

58. Heat is *not* applied to a joint replacement site.
    A. True
    B. False

59. Moist heat has greater and faster effects than dry heat.
    A. True
    B. False

60. Which is a moist, cold application?
    A. Ice bag
    B. Ice collar
    C. Ice glove
    D. Cold compress

61. The prolonged application of cold has the same effects as heat applications.
    A. True
    B. False

62. You have applied an ice pack to Mr. Wilson's left knee. How often do you need to check the skin at the application site?
    A. Every 5 minutes
    B. Every 10 minutes
    C. Every 15 minutes
    D. Frequently

63. Heat and cold are applied for no longer than
    A. 1 hour
    B. 30 minutes
    C. 15 to 20 minutes
    D. 5 to 10 minutes

64. To safely apply an aquathermia pad
    A. Keep the heating unit below the pad and connecting hoses.
    B. Check the device for damage or flaws.
    C. Place the pad under the person.
    D. Secured the pad with pins.

65. Cold applications are used for all of the following *except*
    A. To reduce pain
    B. To cool the body when fever is present
    C. To increase circulation to an area
    D. To prevent swelling

## MOSBY'S NURSING ASSISTANT SKILLS VIDEOS EXERCISES

### Questions from the Preventing and Treating Pressure Ulcers Video

66. A pressure ulcer can be life-threatening.
    A. True
    B. False

67. Nursing assistants play an important role in helping to prevent pressure ulcers.
    A. True
    B. False

68. A bony prominence is _____

    _____.

69. Pressure ulcers never develop when preventive care measures are practiced.
    A. True
    B. False

70. List the factors that place Mr. Raider at risk for pressure ulcers.

    A. _____

    B. _____

    C. _____

    D. _____

    E. _____

71. Which factors place Mrs. Jensen at risk for pressure ulcers?

    A. _____

    B. _____

    C. _____

    D. _____

72. When you are delegated measures to prevent pressure ulcers, you need to obtain specific instructions from _____

    _____.

## CASE STUDY

*Ms. Adele Raines is a 50 year-old patient at Valley View Hospital. She has red hair and very fair skin. Her doctor has ordered sitz baths following rectal surgery. The doctor has also ordered elastic stockings for both legs. The RN has assigned you to apply the elastic stockings and to assist Ms. Raines with her sitz bath.*

*Answer the following questions.*

1. What additional information do you need before you apply the elastic stockings?

2. When should you apply the elastic stockings?

3. What safety measures are needed when applying elastic stockings?

4. After applying the elastic stockings, what observations do you need to report and record?

5. What complications from the sitz bath is Ms. Raines at risk for?

A. What measures can help prevent these complications?

B. What questions might you ask Ms. Raines to promote her comfort and safety during the sitz bath?

## ADDITIONAL LEARNING ACTIVITIES

1. If available, handle the various types of dressings commonly used for wound care. Practice opening packages and applying various types of dressings. Also practice applying and removing various types of tape. The greater your skill, the better care you can provide.

2. If available, handle the various types of heat and cold applications commonly used in health care agencies. Practice opening packages and applying various types of applications. The greater your skill, the better care you can provide.

3. View the CD Companion Skills to help you learn and practice the Applying Elastic Stockings procedure.

4. Under the supervision of your instructor, practice the procedures in this chapter. Use the procedure checklists on pages 351 and 352 as a guide. Take your turn being the patient or resident.
   A. Discuss ways to promote the person's safety, comfort, and dignity when performing each procedure.

# 22 Assisting With Oxygen Needs

## OBJECTIVES

The questions and student activities in this chapter will help you meet these objectives.
- Define the key terms listed in this chapter
- Describe hypoxia and abnormal respirations
- Explain the measures that promote oxygenation
- Describe the devices used in oxygen therapy
- Explain how to safely assist with oxygen therapy
- Perform the procedure described in this chapter

## STUDY QUESTIONS

### Matching

*Match each term with the correct definition.*

1. _____ Slow breathing; respirations are less than 12 per minute

2. _____ Respirations gradually increase in rate and depth and then become shallow and slow; breathing may stop for 10 to 20 seconds

3. _____ Respirations are rapid and deeper than normal

4. _____ Respirations are slow, shallow, and sometimes irregular

5. _____ The lack or absence of breathing

6. _____ Breathing deeply and comfortably only when sitting

7. _____ Sitting up and leaning over a table to breathe

8. _____ Rapid breathing; respirations are 24 or more per minute

9. _____ Cells do not have enough oxygen

10. _____ Difficult, labored, or painful breathing

A. Tachypnea

B. Cheyne-Stokes

C. Orthopnea

D. Dyspnea

E. Hypoventilation

F. Hyperventilation

G. Bradypnea

H. Orthopneic position

I. Hypoxia

J. Apnea

*Fill in the Blanks*

11. Describe normal respirations.

   _____

   _____

12. Breathing is usually easier in these positions.

   A. _____

   B. _____

13. Mr. Jenson has difficulty breathing. He prefers the orthopneic position. What can you do to increase his comfort?

   _____

14. How do coughing and deep-breathing exercises help persons with respiratory problems?

   A. _____

   B. _____

15. The nurse delegates coughing and deep-breathing exercises to you. What information do you need from the nurse and the care plan?

   A. _____

   B. _____

   C. _____

16. Oxygen is treated as a _____.

17. List and briefly describe four ways that oxygen is supplied.

   A. _____

   _____

   B. _____

   _____

   C. _____

   _____

   D. _____

   _____

18. Describe the following devices used to give oxygen.

   A. Nasal cannula _____

   _____

   _____

   B. Simple facemask _____

   _____

   _____

19. List two complications that can occur when using a nasal cannula.

   A. _____

   B. _____

20. The amount of oxygen given is called _____

   _____.

*Multiple Choice*

Circle the **BEST** Answer.

21. Oxygen is a gas. It has no taste, odor, or color.
    A. True
    B. False

22. *Early* signs of hypoxia include:
    A. Breathing comfortably only when sitting
    B. Restlessness, dizziness, and disorientation
    C. Cyanosis and increased pulse rate
    D. Increased temperature and decreased respiratory rate

23. How often do normal respirations occur in a healthy adult?
    A. 12 to 20 times per minute
    B. 20 to 30 times per minute
    C. 5 to 10 times per minute
    D. 35 times per minute

24. A bluish color to the skin, lips, mucous membranes, and nail beds is:
    A. Dyspnea
    B. Cannula
    C. Cyanosis
    D. Oxygen concentration

25. To promote oxygenation, position changes are needed:
    A. When the person complains of difficulty breathing
    B. When the person requests a position change
    C. At least every 2 hours
    D. As often as you have time

26. You are assisting Mrs. Lopez with coughing and deep-breathing exercises. Which is *incorrect*?
    A. Have her place her hands over her rib cage.
    B. Have her take a deep breath in through her nose.
    C. Ask her to hold the breath for 3 seconds.
    D. Ask her to exhale slowly through her nose.

27. Which is *not* a safety rule for oxygen therapy?
    A. Remove the oxygen device when assisting the person with ambulation.
    B. Make sure the oxygen device is secure but not tight.
    C. Check for signs of irritation from the device.
    D. Make sure there are no kinks in the tubing.

28. The nurse tells you that Mrs. Dunn's oxygen flow rate needs to be at 2 liters per minute. When getting her up to sit in the chair you note that her flow rate is 4 liters per minute. You should:
    A. Ask Mrs. Dunn if she changed the flow rate.
    B. Tell the nurse at once.
    C. Change the oxygen flow rate to 2 liters per minute.
    D. Check the care plan as soon as you have time.

## CASE STUDY

*Mrs. Edna Larson is a 55 year-old patient on 3 West Medical. She is in a private room. Mrs. Dunn has pneumonia, which is causing difficult and painful breathing (dyspnea). Mrs. Dunn's doctor has ordered:*
- *Bedrest with bathroom privileges*
- *Oxygen by nasal cannula at 3 liters per minute*
- *Position changes every 2 hours*
- *Coughing and deep-breathing exercises every 2 hours while awake*
  *You have been assigned to care for Mrs. Dunn today.*

*Answer the following questions.*

1. What information do you need from the nurse and the care plan before providing care for Mrs. Dunn?

2. What observations do you need to report and record when assisting Mrs. Dunn with coughing and deep-breathing exercises?

3. How will you promote Mrs. Dunn's comfort?

4. How will you promote Mrs. Dunn's safety?

5. How will you protect Mrs. Dunn's right to privacy?

## ADDITIONAL LEARNING ACTIVITIES

1. If available, handle the various types of oxygen administration devices.

2. Position yourself in the orthopneic position and note how it feels.

3. Review the following:
   A. The safety measures to prevent equipment accidents in Chapter 8

   B. The safety measures for fire and the use of oxygen in Chapter 8

C. The safety rules for oxygen therapy in this chapter
   • Knowing and following these rules is needed to provide safe and effective care.

4. Under the supervision of your instructor, practice the procedure in this chapter. Use the procedure checklist on pages 359-360 as a guide. Take your turn being the patient or resident.
   A. Discuss ways to promote the person's safety, comfort, and dignity when performing the procedure.

# 23 Assisting With Rehabilitation and Restorative Care

## OBJECTIVES

The questions and student activities in this chapter will help you meet these objectives.
- Define the key terms listed in this chapter
- Describe how rehabilitation involves the whole person

- Identify the complications to prevent
- Explain your role in rehabilitation and restorative care
- Explain how to promote quality of life

## STUDY QUESTIONS

*Matching*

*Match each term with the correct definition.*

1. _____ The inability to speak.

2. _____ The activities usually done during a normal day in a person's life

3. _____ Any lost, absent, or impaired physical or mental function

4. _____ An artificial replacement for a missing body part

5. _____ Difficulty swallowing

6. _____ The process of restoring the person to his or her highest possible level of physical, psychological, social, and economic function

7. _____ A nursing assistant with special training in restorative nursing and rehabilitation skills

8. _____ Care that helps persons regain their health, strength, and independence

A. Prosthesis

B. Restorative nursing care

C. Activities of daily living (ADL)

D. Aphasia

E. Rehabilitation

F. Disability

G. Restorative aide

H. Dysphagia

*Fill in the Blanks*

9. The focus of rehabilitation is on _____

   _____ .

   When improved function is not possible, the goal

   is to _____ .

10. Restorative nursing programs prevent _____

    _____ .

11. The person with a disability needs to adjust ___,

    _____ ,

    _____ ,

    _____ ,

    and _____ .

12. Explain why rehabilitation usually takes longer
    in older persons.

    _____

    _____

13. List three complications that need to be
    prevented for rehabilitation to be successful.

    A. _____

    B. _____

    C. _____

14. Mr. John Reece is learning how to use an artificial

    left arm. The goal is for the prosthesis to

    _____ .

15. All members of the rehabilitation team help the

    person regain _____

    and _____ .

16. Explain why family members are key members
    of the team.

    _____

    _____

    _____

17. Every part of your job focuses on _____

    _____ .

18. Successful rehabilitation and restorative care
    improve the person's quality of life. To promote
    the person's quality of life, you need to:

    A. _____

    B. _____

    C. _____

    D. _____

    E. _____

    F. _____

    G. _____

19. You are assisting Mr. Clark apply a leg brace.
    Why should you practice applying the brace
    on yourself?

    _____

*Multiple Choice*

Circle the **BEST** Answer

20. Restorative nursing and rehabilitation both
    focus on
    A. The person's strengths
    B. Promoting independence
    C. Regaining physical abilities
    D. The whole person

21. When does rehabilitation start?
    A. When the person enters a rehabilitation
       hospital
    B. When the person goes home with home care
    C. When the person seeks health care
    D. When it is ordered by the doctor

22. Successful rehabilitation depends on the person's attitude.
    A. True
    B. False

23. You promote a person's rehabilitation by
    A. Doing as much as possible for the person
    B. Helping the person focus on abilities
    C. Telling the person to work harder
    D. Focusing on what the person cannot do

24. Mr. Clark is feeling discouraged with his slow progress. You need to do all of the following *except*
    A. Remind him of his progress.
    B. Give support and encouragement.
    C. Give him sympathy.
    D. Stress his strengths and abilities.

25. Mr. Clark is receiving physical therapy. You hear a caregiver shouting at him in an angry voice. You must
    A. Report what you heard to the nurse at once.
    B. Tell the caregiver to stop shouting.
    C. Tell Mr. Clark's family what you heard.
    D. Do nothing. It's none of your business.

26. Mrs. Beal wants to skip her exercises scheduled for 1400 hours because she is tired. You should
    A. Let her take a nap.
    B. Allow her to do only half the amount required.
    C. Check her care plan.
    D. Report the problem to the nurse.

27. Mr. Clark is making slow progress learning how to use a transfer board. He says he is tired and is not going to work today. You feel yourself getting impatient. You should
    A. Tell Mr. Clark that he will never get better if he does not keep trying.
    B. Ask a co-worker to work with Mr. Clark today.
    C. Leave the room and come back when you are less impatient.
    D. Discuss your feelings with the nurse.

28. Nursing teamwork involves providing emotional support to each other.
    A. True
    B. False

## CASE STUDY

*Mrs. Barbara Brown is 60 years old. She is a widow. She works as a secretary for a lawyer. Mrs. Brown had a stroke. Her right side is paralyzed. She has facial drooping. Her speech is affected. She has trouble expressing herself. She needs assistance with all ADL. She is receiving rehabilitation in a skilled nursing center. Her goal is to learn to walk and to care for herself, so she can go home. She is afraid she will never be able to work as a secretary again.*

*Mrs. Brown is motivated and works hard with the rehabilitation team. She tells you that she is embarrassed by her appearance. She wants to eat in her room as she feels she is messy. She told the nurse that she does not want visitors until she is doing better.*

*Answer the following questions.*

1. How does Mrs. Brown's stroke affect her physically, psychologically, socially, and financially?

2. What effect does the stroke have on Mrs. Brown's self-image?

3. What health team members might be involved in Mrs. Brown's rehabilitation?

4. How can the health team promote Mrs. Brown's right to
   A. Privacy

   B. Personal choice

C. Be free from abuse and mistreatment

5. What measures will promote her safety?

---

## ADDITIONAL LEARNING ACTIVITIES

1. Do you have a family member or a friend with a physical disability? Interview the person if he or she is willing.
   A. Discuss how the disability affects activities of daily living.

   B. Is the person involved in rehabilitation?

   C. Are community programs available when needed?

   D. Does the person use self-help devices?

   E. Have any changes been made in the person's home to help maintain independence?

   F. Has the person's job been affected by the disability?

2. If available, handle various self-help devices used in the rehabilitation process. Becoming familiar with these devices will help you provide effective and safe care. You may want to go to a medical supply business and look at the self-help devices and other rehabilitation equipment available.

# 24 Caring For Persons With Common Health Problems

## OBJECTIVES

The questions and student activities in this chapter will help you meet these objectives.
- Define the key terms listed in this chapter
- Describe how cancer is treated
- Describe musculoskeletal disorders and the care required
- Describe hearing loss and the care required
- Describe eye disorders and the care required
- Describe respiratory disorders and the care required
- Describe cardiovascular disorders and the care required
- Describe urinary system disorders and the care required
- Describe digestive disorders and the care required
- Describe diabetes and the care required
- Describe communicable diseases and the care required
- Describe mental health disorders and the care required

## STUDY QUESTIONS

*Crossword*

### Across

1. A bladder infection
7. A broken bone
9. Joint inflammation
10. Hair loss

### Down

2. A new growth of abnormal cells
3. Loss of appetite
4. The spread of cancer to other body parts
5. A vague, uneasy feeling in response to stress
6. A tumor that grows fast and invades other tissues
8. The inability to speak

## Matching

*Match each term with the correct definition.*

1. _____ The surgical replacement of a joint

2. _____ Difficulty expressing or sending out thoughts

3. _____ Paralysis on one side of the body

4. _____ High sugar in the blood

5. _____ Low sugar in the blood

6. _____ Paralysis from the waist down

7. _____ Paralysis from the neck down

8. _____ Difficulty receiving information

9. _____ Inflammation of the mouth

A. Receptive aphasia

B. Quadriplegia

C. Paraplegia

D. Hemiplegia

E. Hypoglycemia

F. Hyperglycemia

G. Stomatitis

H. Expressive aphasia

I. Arthroplasty

## Fill in the Blanks

10. List the eight cancer risk factors cited by the National Cancer Institute.

    A. _____

    B. _____

    C. _____

    D. _____

    E. _____

    F. _____

    G. _____

    H. _____

11. List and briefly describe three common cancer treatments.

    A. _____

    _____

    _____

    B. _____

    _____

    _____

    C. _____

    _____

    _____

12. List and briefly describe the two types of arthritis.

   A. _____

   _____

   _____

   B. _____

   _____

   _____

13. Treatment goals for rheumatoid arthritis are to:

   A. _____

   B. _____

   C. _____

14. With _____,

   the bone becomes porous and brittle. Bones are

   fragile and break easily.

15. List seven risk factors for osteoporosis.

   A. _____

   B. _____

   C. _____

   D. _____

   E. _____

   F. _____

   G. _____

16. Describe these types of fractures:

   A. Closed fracture _____

   _____

   B. Open fracture _____

   _____

17. The signs and symptoms of a fracture include:

   A. _____

   B. _____

   C. _____

   D. _____

   E. _____

   F. _____

18. A new cast has been applied to Ms. Roberta

   Jensen's right leg. You must not cover the cast

   with blankets or other material because _____

   _____

   _____.

19. Mr. Bob Andrews has a cast on his left arm.

   He complains of numbness in his fingers. This

   signals _____

   _____.

20. A hip fracture is fixed in position with a _____,

   _____,

   _____,

   _____,

   _____, or

   _____.

21. Ms. Burt had surgery to repair a fractured right hip. List three life-threatening problems that can occur.

   A. _____

   B. _____

   C. _____

22. Stroke is _____

   _____.

23. What are the two main causes of stroke (cerebrovascular accident [CVA])?

    A. _____

    B. _____

24. List five warning signs of stroke.

    A. _____
    _____

    B. _____
    _____

    C. _____
    _____

    D. _____
    _____

    E. _____
    _____

25. Briefly describe Parkinson's disease.

    _____
    _____
    _____.

26. _____
    is a chronic disease in which the myelin in the brain
    and spinal cord are destroyed.

27. Common causes of spinal cords injuries are:

    A. _____

    B. _____

    C. _____

    D. _____

28. Deafness is _____
    _____.

29. List five signs of hearing loss.

    A. _____

    B. _____

    C. _____

    D. _____

    E. _____

30. List four simple measures to try when a hearing aid does not seem to be working properly.

    A. _____

    B. _____

    C. _____

    D. _____

31. Briefly describe what occurs with glaucoma.

    _____
    _____
    _____

32. Treatment for glaucoma involves _____
    _____.

33. With _____
    the lens of the eye becomes cloudy. Light cannot
    enter the eye.

34. _____
    is the only treatment for a cataract.

35. How can you protect a person's eyeglasses from breakage or other damage?

    _____
    _____
    _____

36. To properly care for a person's contact lenses, you need to _____ _____.

37. What two aids are used worldwide to assist blind person's to move about safely?

    A._____

    B._____

38. _____ is a writing system that uses raised dots.

39. List the three disorders grouped under chronic obstructive pulmonary disease (COPD).

    A. _____

    B. _____

    C. _____

40. _____ is the major cause of chronic bronchitis.

41. In emphysema, the _____ enlarge and become less elastic.

42. The most common cause of emphysema is _____.

43. Pneumonia is _____ _____.

    It is caused by _____ _____.

44. Tuberculosis (TB) is spread by _____ with coughing, sneezing, speaking, and singing.

45. List seven signs and symptoms of TB.

    A. _____

    B. _____

    C. _____

    D. _____

    E. _____

    F. _____

    G. _____

46. With hypertension the _____ is too high.

47. Prehypertension is _____ _____.

48. List four risk factors for hypertension you *cannot* change.

    A. _____

    B. _____

    C. _____

    D. _____

49. The _____ supply the heart with blood.

50. The most common cause of coronary artery disease is _____.

51. Major complications of coronary artery disease (CAD) are _____ and _____.

52. Angina pectoris is chest pain from _____ _____.

53. With _____,
blood flow to the heart muscle is suddenly blocked.
Part of the heart muscle dies.

54. _____
occurs when the heart cannot pump blood
normally. Blood backs up and tissue congestion
occurs.

55. With left-sided heart failure, blood backs up into

the_____. The

person has _____

_____.

56. List four common causes of urinary tract infections.

A. _____

B. _____

C. _____

D. _____

57. Cystitis is _____.

58. _____ is inflammation

of the kidney pelvis.

59. _____ is the most common endocrine

disorder.

60. List and briefly describe the three types of diabetes.

A. _____

_____

_____

B. _____

_____

_____

C. _____

_____

61. Type 1 diabetes is treated with:

A. _____

B. _____

C. _____

62. Causes of hypoglycemia include:
A. _____

B. _____

C. _____

D. _____

E. _____

F. _____

63. Many people have small pouches in the colon.

Each pouch is called a _____.

64. The condition of having pouches in the colon is

called _____.

The pouches can become inflamed. This is called

_____.

65. Vomiting means _____.

66. Mr. Drew is vomiting. You turn his head well to

one side to prevent _____.

67. _____ and

_____

are followed when caring for persons with

communicable diseases.

68. _____ is an inflammation of

the liver.

69. Hepatitis A is spread by _____.

70. The hepatitis B virus is present in _____

_____.

71. The AIDS virus (HIV) is transmitted mainly by:

A. _____

_____

B. _____

_____

C. _____

_____

72. Sexually transmitted diseases are spread by

_____.

73. Using _____

helps prevent the spread of sexually transmitted

diseases, especially HIV and AIDS.

74. Mental relates to the _____.

75. Stress is _____

_____.

76. Define the following terms:

A. Mental health _____

_____

B. Mental illness _____

_____

77. List five causes of mental health disorders.

A. _____

B. _____

C. _____

D. _____

E. _____

78. Defense mechanisms are _____

_____.

79. _____means split mind.

80. Define the following terms.

A. Psychosis _____

_____

B. Hallucination _____

C. Paranoia _____

_____

81. Affect relates to _____.

82. The person with bipolar disorder has _____

_____.

83. Personality disorders involve _____

_____.

84. Maladaptive means _____

_____.

85. Describe an antisocial personality.

_____

_____

_____

86. Ms. Green has an abusive personality. This means

_____

_____.

*Multiple Choice*

Circle the **BEST** Answer

87. When caring for a person in traction, do the following *except*
   A. Keep the person in good alignment.
   B. Remove the traction when making the person's bed.
   C. Keep the weights off the floor.
   D. Complete a safety check before leaving the room.

88. When caring for a person with a stroke, do the following *except*
    A. Perform range-of-motion exercises to prevent contractures.
    B. Give good skin care to prevent pressure sores.
    C. Keep the bed in the flat position to promote breathing.
    D. Encourage coughing and deep breathing.

89. Ms. Burt had surgery to repair her fractured right hip. You need to do the following *except*
    A. Keep the operated leg adducted at all times.
    B. Give good skin care.
    C. Prevent external rotation of the right hip.
    D. Apply elastic stockings as directed.

90. The leading cause of disability in adults in the United States is
    A. Cancer
    B. Heart attack
    C. Stroke
    D. Parkinson's disease

91. When caring for a person with a stroke, you need to
    A. Keep the bed in the flat position.
    B. Turn and reposition the person every 4 hours.
    C. Do all ADL for the person.
    D. Assist with range-of-motion exercises as directed.

92. A person has Parkinson's disease. It is important to do everything for the person.
    A. True
    B. False

93. A person has multiple sclerosis. Which is *false*?
    A. There is no known cure.
    B. Muscle weakness and difficulty with balance occur.
    C. Symptoms usually start after age 65.
    D. The person's condition worsens over time.

94. With spinal cord injuries, the higher the level of injury, the less function is lost.
    A. True
    B. False

95. A person who wears a hearing aid hears better because
    A. The hearing problem is cured.
    B. Background noise is decreased.
    C. The person's ability to hear improves.
    D. The hearing aid makes sounds louder.

96. To care for a hearing aid properly, do the following *except*
    A. Follow the manufacturer's instructions.
    B. Wash the mold in soapy water every day.
    C. Remove the battery at night.
    D. When not in use, turn the hearing aid off.

97. To communicate with a hearing impaired person
    A. Shout loudly.
    B. Approach the person from behind.
    C. Speak clearly, distinctly, and slowly.
    D. Stand or sit in dim light.

98. When caring for a blind person, you must avoid using the words *see*, *look*, or *read*.
    A. True
    B. False

99. Which action will *not* promote safety when caring for a blind person?
    A. Provide lighting as the person prefers.
    B. Orient the person to the room.
    C. Keep doors partly open.
    D. Tell the person when you are leaving the room.

100. When assisting a blind person to walk, you need to
    A. Walk slightly in front of the person.
    B. Walk slightly behind the person.
    C. Guide the person in front of you.
    D. Walk very slowly.

101. Allergies and emotional stress are common causes of
    A. Emphysema
    B. Chronic bronchitis
    C. Asthma
    D. Pneumonia

102. Standard Precautions and Isolation Precautions are followed when caring for a person with TB.
    A. True
    B. False

103. The leading causes of death in the United States are
    A. Infections
    B. Pulmonary diseases
    C. Cardiovascular disorders
    D. Cancers

104. Which is *not* a risk factor for hypertension?
    A. Cigarette smoking
    B. A high-sodium diet
    C. Regular exercise
    D. Obesity

105. Angina pectoris is relieved by
    A. Exercise and fresh air
    B. Food and fluids
    C. Continuous oxygen
    D. Rest and nitroglycerin

106. Which is *not* a sign or symptom of myocardial infarction?
    A. Sudden, severe chest pain
    B. Indigestion and nausea
    C. Warm, dry, flushed skin
    D. Fear, apprehension, and a feeling of doom

107. Mr. Benson has right-sided heart failure. You know that
    A. Blood backs up into his lungs.
    B. Swelling of the feet and ankles is a sign.
    C. A high-sodium diet is needed.
    D. The dorsal recumbent position is preferred for breathing.

108. Heart failure cannot be treated.
    A. True
    B. False

109. Renal calculi are
    A. Particles in the urine
    B. Kidney stones
    C. Waste products
    D. Pus in the urine

110. Mrs. Rita Moore has renal failure. Which statement is *false*?
    A. She has urinary frequency and urgency.
    B. Her kidneys do not function or are severely impaired.
    C. Waste products are not removed from her blood.
    D. Her body retains fluid.

111. Mrs. Smith has diabetes. Which is *true*?
    A. Her body cannot produce or use insulin properly.
    B. She is obese.
    C. She cannot eat a balanced diet.
    D. She needs a diet low in protein.

112. Which is a cause of hyperglycemia?
    A. Vomiting
    B. Too much insulin
    C. Eating too much food
    D. Increased exercise

113. Vomitus is measured as output.
    A. True
    B. False

114. Hepatitis C is spread by
    A. Food contaminated with feces
    B. Poor hygiene
    C. Blood contaminated with the virus
    D. Water contaminated with feces

115. The AIDS virus is spread through
    A. Sneezing and coughing
    B. Holding hands and hugging
    C. Insects
    D. Blood, semen, vaginal secretions, and breast milk

116. All persons infected with the HIV virus have symptoms.
    A. True
    B. False

117. Mr. Paul Gibbons is infected with the HIV virus. He does not have symptoms. He cannot spread the disease.
    A. True
    B. False

118. Persons over age 50 are *not* at risk for AIDS.
    A. True
    B. False

119. Which statement about anxiety is *false*?
    A. Anxiety is an abnormal response to stress.
    B. Often anxiety occurs when a person's needs are not met.
    C. Signs and symptoms depend on the degree of anxiety.
    D. Defense mechanisms are used to relieve anxiety.

120. Mr. Peter Granby had a disagreement with his boss. When he gets home he shouts at his son. Which defense mechanism is he using?
    A. Projection
    B. Displacement
    C. Regression
    D. Denial

121. This is an intense and sudden feeling of fear, anxiety, terror, or dread.
    A. Phobia
    B. Compulsion
    C. Obsession
    D. Panic

122. Ms. Green believes she is the mother of Christ. This is
    A. An hallucination
    B. A delusion
    C. Paranoia
    D. A phobia

123. Depression is common in older people.
    A. True
    B. False

124. You can share information about a resident's or patient's health problems with his or her family.
    A. True
    B. False

## CASE STUDIES

*Mr. Adam Lane is 55 years old. He is married and has 2 teenage children. He is a teacher at the high school. He enjoys hiking and camping with his family. He attends church every Sunday with his family. His wife works part time as a check out clerk at the local grocery store. Mr. Lane is being treated for colon cancer. He had surgery to remove a tumor and is now receiving radiation therapy.*

*Answer the following questions.*

1. What fears might Mr. Lane have?

2. What physical, psychological, and spiritual needs might Mr. Lane have?

3. What members of the health team might be involved in meeting Mr. Lane's needs?

4. What are the side effects of radiation therapy?

*Mrs. Ann Lopez is a 75-year-old retired nurse. She lives alone in her home. She does volunteer work at the hospital 2 days a week. She is teaching her granddaughter how to quilt. She has a small flower garden and enjoys working in it every day. Mrs. Lopez fell in her driveway and fractured her right hip. She had a hip pinning and is receiving rehabilitation at a skilled nursing center.*

*Answer the following questions.*

1. What are the signs and symptoms of a fracture?

2. What fears might Mrs. Lopez have?

3. What care measures are practiced after surgery to repair a fractured hip?

4. What complications is Mrs. Lopez at risk for?

    A. What nursing measures can help prevent these complications?

*Miss Rita Reed is an 80-year-old resident of Green Valley Nursing Center. She is hearing impaired in both ears. She wears hearing aids and lip reads. She needs assistance putting her hearing aids in and taking them out. Miss Reed also has glaucoma, which is controlled with drugs. She wears eyeglasses. She can see well enough to read large print. She also listens to talking books.*

*Answer the following questions.*

1. How might Miss Reed's hearing and vision impairments affect her ability to care for herself?

2. How might Miss Reed's social life be affected by her hearing and vision impairments?

3. How can you promote Miss Reed's safety?

4. What measures will you practice when caring for Miss Reed's eyeglasses and hearing aids?

5. What measures will you practice when communicating with Miss Reed?

## ADDITIONAL LEARNING ACTIVITIES

1. Review each of the health problems discussed in this chapter.
   A. Identify how each problem affects the indivitual's physical, psychological, social and spritual needs.

   B. List the risk factors for each of the health problems discussed in this chapter.
      (1) Which risk factors can be controlled and which cannot?

   (2) List any life-style changes you can make to decrease your risks for any of the health problems discussed in this chapter?

# 25 Caring For Persons With Confusion and Dementia

## OBJECTIVES

The questions and student activities in this chapter will help you meet these objectives.
- Define the key terms listed in this chapter
- Describe confusion and its causes
- List the measures that help confused persons
- Explain the differences between delirium, (depression), and dementia

- Describe Alzheimer's disease (AD)
- Describe the signs, symptoms, and behaviors of AD
- Explain the care required by persons with AD and other dementias
- Describe the effects of AD on the family

## STUDY QUESTIONS

*Matching*

*Match each term with the correct definition.*

1. _____ A false belief

2. _____ The loss of cognitive function and social function caused by changes in the brain

3. _____ Signs, symptoms, and behaviors of AD increase during hours of darkness

4. _____ Seeing, hearing, or feeling something that is not real

5. _____ False dementia

6. _____ A state of temporary but acute mental confusion

A. Pseudodementia

B. Dementia

C. Delirium

D. Sundowning

E. Hallucination

F. Delusion

*Fill in the Blanks*

7. Cognitive function involves:

   A. _____

   B. _____

   C. _____

   D. _____

   E. _____

   F. _____

8. The treatment of acute confusion (delirium) is

   aimed at _____.

9. List eight early warning signs of dementia.

   A. _____

   B. _____

   C. _____

   D. _____

   E. _____

   F. _____

   G. _____

   H. _____

10. Treatable causes of dementia include:

   A. _____

   B. _____

   C. _____

   D. _____

   E. _____

   F. _____

   G. _____

11. Multi-infarct dementia is caused by _____

   _____.

12. _____

   is the most common type of permanent dementia.

13. _____

   is the most common mental health problem in

   older persons.

14. The classic sign of AD is _____

   _____.

15. What is the purpose of the Alzheimer's
    Association's "Safe Return Program"?

   _____

   _____

16. Briefly describe catastrophic reactions.

   _____

   _____

17. Explain how caregivers can cause agitation and
    restlessness when caring for a person with
    Alzheimer's disease.

   _____

   _____

18. Sexual behaviors are labeled abnormal because of

   _____.

19. Persons with AD are not oriented to person,

   place, and time. Therefore sexual behaviors

   may involve _____

   _____.

20. What are some nonsexual reasons a person with dementia may touch or rub the genitals?

    A. _____

    B. _____

    C. _____

21. Mr. John Kane has AD. He is a resident at Valley View Nursing Center. Why is it important to report any changes in his usual behavior to the nurse?

    _____

    _____

22. Some nursing centers have special secured units for persons with AD and other dementias. What is the purpose of these units?

    _____

    _____

    _____

23. Persons in the early stages of AD may live at home with family. Long-term care is needed when:

    A. _____

    B. _____

    C. _____

    D. _____

    E. _____

24. Many adult children are in the *sandwich generation.*

    This means _____

    _____

    _____.

25. Many caregivers join AD support groups. What is the purpose of these groups?

    _____

    _____

    _____

26. Maintaining the day-night cycle is important when caring for persons with AD. List measures that might help maintain the day-night cycle.

    A. _____

    B. _____

    C. _____

## Multiple Choice

Circle the **BEST** Answer

27. Cognitive relates to
    A. Beliefs
    B. Changes in the brain
    C. Social function
    D. Knowledge

28. Which is *not* a change in the nervous system from aging?
    A. Reaction times are slower.
    B. Delirium occurs.
    C. Taste and smell decrease.
    D. Sleep patterns change.

29. Which statement about acute confusion is *false*?
    A. Treatment is aimed at the cause.
    B. It occurs suddenly.
    C. It usually is permanent.
    D. It can occur from infection.

30. Dementia is a normal part of aging.
    A. True
    B. False

31. Delirium is an emergency.
    A. True
    B. False

32. The most common mental health problem in older persons is
    A. Alcohol abuse
    B. Delusions
    C. Schizophrenia
    D. Depression

33. Which statement about Alzheimer's disease is *true?*
    A. It is usually diagnosed before age 65.
    B. The disease is sudden in onset.
    C. The cause is unknown.
    D. It is a normal part of aging.

34. A person in stage 1 of AD
    A. Is disoriented to time and place
    B. Has fecal and urinary incontinence
    C. Has problems with movement and gait
    D. Cannot swallow

35. Mr. Jones is confused. Which of the following measures is *not* helpful?
    A. Provide care in a calm, relaxed manner.
    B. Explain everything in great detail.
    C. Use touch to communicate.
    D. Tell him the date and time each morning.

36. Mrs. Adams has AD. You promote her safety by
    A. Keeping her restrained
    B. Explaining safety rules to her
    C. Changing her room frequently
    D. Placing safety plugs in electrical outlets

37. You are caring for a person with AD. Which action causes increased agitation?
    A. Rushing the person
    B. Keeping noise levels low
    C. Speaking in a calm, gentle voice
    D. Using touch to calm the person

38. Mrs. Adams has AD. She is screaming in the dining room. You can help by
    A. Firmly asking her to stop
    B. Taking her to her room and closing the door
    C. Turning on loud music
    D. Having a favorite caregiver comfort and calm her

39. Which measure is *not* helpful when caring for a person having hallucinations?
    A. Make sure the person is wearing eyeglasses and hearing aids as needed.
    B. Distract the person with some item or activity.
    C. Use touch to calm and reassure the person.
    D. Calmly explain that the hallucinations are not real.

40. Mr. Reed resists your efforts to help him into the bathtub. He starts to scream. Which action might be helpful?
    A. Explain why he needs a bath.
    B. Get help from two co-workers to force him into the tub.
    C. Try bathing him later, when he is calm.
    D. Step into the tub yourself, to show him that there is nothing to be afraid of.

41. Repetitive behaviors are usually harmless.
    A. True
    B. False

42. The person with AD
    A. Chooses to be incontinent
    B. Needs your support and understanding
    C. Has control over his or her actions
    D. Can understand and follow instructions

43. Proper use of validation therapy requires special training.
    A. True
    B. False

44. The right to privacy and confidentiality is *not* important for persons with dementia.
    A. True
    B. False

45. Restraints can make confusion and demented behaviors worse.
    A. True
    B. False

46. According to OBRA, secured units are physical restraints.
    A. True
    B. False

## CASE STUDY

*Mrs. Mary Schmitt is a resident on the secured unit at Maywood Nursing Center. She was diagnosed with AD 3 years ago. Before coming to the nursing center she lived with her daughter. Mrs. Schmitt's daughter admitted her to the nursing center after she was found wandering three blocks from home at 9 o'clock at night. Mrs. Schmitt's daughter lives a few blocks from the nursing center and visits at least three times a week. She often brings her 3-year-old son with her. She has left a picture album with family pictures for her mother.*

*Mrs. Schmitt frequently gets up at night and wanders about the unit. She tells you that she is looking for her baby. She repeats the question "Where is my baby?" over and over. Sometimes she wanders into other resident rooms looking for her baby.*

*Answer the following questions.*

1. What stage of AD might Mrs. Schmitt be in?
   A. What signs and symptoms does she have?

2. What measures might be part of Mrs. Schmitt's care plan to:
   A. Promote safety

   B. Promote dignity

3. What measures might help with the wandering situation?

4. What can you do to protect Mrs. Schmitt's right to confidentiality and privacy?

5. What feelings might Mrs. Schmitt's daughter have about admitting her mother to a nursing center?

6. How might Mrs. Schmitt's daughter be involved in her mother's care?

## ADDITIONAL LEARNING ACTIVITIES

1. Compare the signs and symptoms of delirium, depression, and early Alzheimer's disease.
   Answer the following questions.
   A. How are the signs and symptoms similar?

   B. Why is a correct diagnosis needed?

Copyright © 2006, 2001 by Mosby, Inc. All rights reserved.

# 26 Assisting With Emergency Care

## OBJECTIVES

The questions and student activities in this chapter will help you meet these objectives.
- Define the key terms listed in this chapter
- Describe the general rules of emergency care
- Identify the signs of cardiac arrest and obstructed airway
- Describe the signs, symptoms, and emergency care for hemorrhage
- Identify the signs, symptoms, and emergency care for shock
- Describe the types of seizures and how to care for a person during a seizure
- Identify the common causes and emergency care for fainting
- Describe the signs, symptoms, and emergency care for stroke
- Perform the procedures described in this chapter

## STUDY QUESTIONS

### Matching

*Match each term with the correct definition.*

1. _____ The heart and breathing stop suddenly and without warning

2. _____ The excessive loss of blood in a short time

3. _____ The sudden loss of consciousness from an inadequate blood supply to the brain

4. _____ Breathing stops but heart action continues for several minutes

5. _____ Violent and sudden contractions or tremors of muscle groups; convulsion

6. _____ Results when organs and tissues do not get enough blood

A. Hemorrhage

B. Respiratory arrest

C. Cardiac arrest

D. Fainting

E. Shock

F. Seizure

*Fill in the Blanks*

7. In an emergency, the _____

_____ is activated.

8. You have activated the EMS system. What information do you need to give the operator?

   A. _____

   B. _____

   C. _____

   D. _____

   E. _____

   F. _____

9. When the heart and breathing stops, the person

   is _____.

10. Mr. Brown is in respiratory arrest. If breathing in

    not restored, _____

    will occur.

11. The American Heart Association's basic life support courses teach the adult Chain of Survival. Chain of Survival actions are:

    A. _____

    B. _____

    C. _____

    D. _____

12. What are the three major signs of cardiac arrest?

    A. _____

    B. _____

    C. _____

13. _____ must be started

    at once when a person is in cardiac arrest.

14. What are the three basic parts of cardiopulmonary resuscitation (CPR)?

    A. _____

    B. _____

    C. _____

15. Describe how to perform the head-tilt/chin-lift maneuver.

    A. _____

    _____

    B. _____

    _____

    C. _____

    _____

    D. _____

    _____

    E. _____

    _____

    F. _____

    _____

16. To check for adequate breathing, you need to take no more than 10 seconds to do the following:

    A. _____

    B. _____

    C. _____

    D. _____

    E. _____

    F. _____

17. When giving mouth-to-mouth breathing, you need to pinch the person's nostrils shut. Why is this done?

_____

_____

18. What is the purpose of the barrier device used in mouth-to-barrier device rescue breathing?

_____

_____

19. During CPR, _____

breaths are given after every _____

chest compressions.

20. Before starting chest compressions, check for

_____.

21. Before staring CPR in an adult, you check to see

if the person is responding by _____

_____

_____.

22. How should your hands and arms be positioned to give chest compressions?

_____

_____

_____

_____

23. How far is the sternum depressed when doing chest compressions on an adult?

_____

24. Chest compressions are given at a rate of

_____.

25. What is the most common cause of FBAO?

_____

26. The Heimlich maneuver involves _____

_____.

27. The _____

is used with the Heimlich maneuver when an

adult becomes unconscious.

28. The Heimlich maneuver is not effective for:

A. _____

B. _____

29. The recovery position is used when _____

_____.

30. Do not use the recovery position if _____

_____.

31. Briefly describe ventricular fibrillation.

_____

_____

_____

32. What is the purpose of an automated external defibrillator (AED)?

_____

_____

_____

33. List five signs and symptoms of internal hemorrhage.

A. _____

B. _____

C. _____

D. _____

E. _____

34. For internal bleeding, you need to:

    A. _____

    B. _____

35. What should you do if direct pressure over the bleeding site does not control external bleeding?

    _____

36. List the signs and symptoms of shock.

    A. _____

    B. _____

    C. _____

    D. _____

    E. _____

    F. _____

    G. _____

37. List and briefly describe the two major types of seizures.

    A. _____

    B. _____

38. Describe the two phases of a generalized tonic-clonic seizure (grand mal seizure).

    A. _____

    _____

    _____

    B. _____

    _____

    _____

39. Stroke occurs when _____

    _____

40. Signs of stroke depend on _____

    _____

41. Emergency care for stroke includes the following:

    A. _____

    B. _____

    C. _____

    D. _____

    E. _____

    F. _____

    G. _____

    H. _____

42. During an emergency, your main concern is

    _____.

*Multiple Choice*

Circle the **BEST** Answer

43. When providing emergency care, it is important to do the following *except*
    A. Check for signs of life-threatening problems.
    B. Move the person to a comfortable position.
    C. Call for help.
    D. Keep the person warm.

44. The airway is opened by
    A. Turning the head to the side
    B. Lifting the head up and tilting it forward
    C. Sitting the person up
    D. The head-tilt/chin-lift maneuver

45. During two person cardiopulmonary resuscitation, which is *correct*?
    A. Give 1 breath after every 10 chest compressions.
    B. Give 2 breaths after every 15 chest compressions.
    C. Give 1 breath after every 5 chest compressions.
    D. Give 1 breath at the same rate as chest compressions.

46. Which artery is used to check for a pulse before starting chest compressions?
    A. The radial artery
    B. The carotid artery
    C. The brachial artery
    D. The femoral artery

47. For chest compressions to be effective, the person:
    A. Must be in a sitting position
    B. Must be flat and on a soft surface
    C. Must be supine and on a hard, flat surface
    D. Is positioned with pillows

48. The Heimlich maneuver can be performed with the person standing, sitting, or lying down.
    A. True
    B. False

49. This method is used to relieve FBAO in very obese persons and in pregnant women.
    A. The Heimlich maneuver
    B. Chest thrusts
    C. Back blows
    D. Abdominal thrusts

50. If you find a person unconscious, you can assume the person is choking.
    A. True
    B. False

51. Mr. Jones is in ventricular fibrillation. Defibrillation as soon as possible increases his chance of survival.
    A. True
    B. False

52. To control external hemorrhage, do the following *except*
    A. Have the person lie down.
    B. Remove any objects that have pierced or stabbed the person.
    C. Place a sterile dressing directly over the wound.
    D. Apply pressure with your hand directly over the bleeding site.

53. To prevent or treat shock, do the following *except*
    A. Maintain an open airway.
    B. Control hemorrhage.
    C. Keep the person warm.
    D. Keep the person in Fowler's position.

54. Which action will protect the person from injury during a generalized tonic-clonic seizure?
    A. Lower the person to the floor.
    B. Turn the person on his or her back.
    C. Restrain body movements during the seizure.
    D. Put your fingers or an object between the person's teeth.

55. Emergency care for fainting includes the following *except*
    A. Have the person sit or lie down.
    B. Loosen clothing.
    C. If the person is lying down, elevate the legs.
    D. Give the person sips of cool water.

56. There is no need to protect the person's right to privacy and confidentiality during an emergency.
    A. True
    B. False

## CASE STUDY

*Ms. Morris is a resident of Valley View Nursing Center. While she is eating lunch in the dining room, you notice that the left side of her face is drooping and she is leaning to the left. She is having difficulty swallowing and has slurred speech.*

*Answer the following questions.*

1. You know that Ms. Morris is having signs of

   _____.

2. What are some possible causes?

3. What does emergency care involve?

4. How would you protect Ms. Morris's right to privacy and confidentiality?

## ADDITIONAL LEARNING ACTIVITIES

1. Identify the EMS system in your community.
   A. Check the phone book yellow pages.



   B. Do you know how to activate the EMS system in an emergency?



   C. If you have children, do they know how to activate the EMS system in your community?



2. Are you and your family prepared to respond to emergency situations in your home?
   A. Are emergency phone numbers easily found?



   B. Do members of your family know what information to give the operator in an emergency?



   C. Do you and your family know basic life support procedures?



3. Do you know which agencies in your community offer classes in basic life support procedures and first aid? The list below may be helpful.
   A. Hospitals

B. Nursing centers

C. Community colleges

D. The American Heart Association

E. The American Red Cross

F. The National Safety Council

4. If possible, enroll in a basic life support class. Your instructor can help you with this process.

# 27 Caring For the Dying Person

## OBJECTIVES

The questions and student activities in this chapter will help you meet these objectives.
- Define the key terms listed in this chapter
- Explain the factors that affect attitudes about death
- Describe the five stages of dying
- Explain how to meet the needs of the dying person and family
- Describe hospice care
- Describe three advance directives and their purposes
- Identify the signs of approaching death and the signs of death
- Perform the procedure described in this chapter

## STUDY QUESTIONS

*Matching*

*Match each term with the correct definition.*

1. _____ Care that focuses on physical, emotional, social, and spiritual needs; it is not concerned with cure or life-saving measures

2. _____ After death

3. _____ The belief that the spirit or soul is reborn in another human body or in another form of life

4. _____ A document about measures that support or maintain life when death is likely

5. _____ The stiffness or rigidity of skeletal muscles that occurs after death

6. _____ An illness or injury for which there is no reasonable expectation of recovery

7. _____ A document stating a person's wishes about health care when that person cannot make his or her own decisions

8. _____ Gives the power to make health care decisions to another person

A. Postmortem

B. Rigor mortis

C. Hospice care

D. Durable power of attorney

E. Living will

F. Advance directive

G. Terminal illness

H. Reincarnation

*Fill in the Blanks*

9. Explain why it is important for you to understand the dying process.

    _____

    _____

    _____

10. In the _____

    culture, persons are often accepting of God's will.

    The person's desire to be clearheaded as death

    nears must be assessed in planning medical

    treatment.

11. List four fears adults may have when facing death.

    A. _____

    B. _____

    C. _____

    D. _____

12. Adults often resent death because it affects ____,

    _____,

    _____, and

    _____.

13. Why might some older people welcome death?

    _____

    _____

    _____

14. List the five stages of dying described by Dr. Elizabeth Kübler-Ross.

    A. _____

    B. _____

    C. _____

    D. _____

    E. _____

15. How can you use listening and touch to help meet the dying person's psychological, social, and spiritual needs?

    A. Listening-_____

    _____

    B. Touch-_____

    _____

16. _____ is one of the last

    functions lost.

17. Which position is usually best for breathing problems?

    _____

18. You can promote comfort to the dying person by providing:

    A. _____

    B. _____

    C. _____

    D. _____

    E. _____

    F. _____

    G. _____

19. The goal of hospice care is to _____

    _____.

20. _____ and

    _____

    give persons the right to accept or refuse medical

    treatment and to make advance directives.

21. A living will may instruct doctors:

    A. _____

    B. _____

22. The doctor has written a "Do Not Resuscitate" order for Miss Lake. What does this mean?

    _____

    _____

23. List six signs that signal death is near.

    A. _____

       _____

    B. _____

       _____

    C. _____

       _____

    D. _____

       _____

    E. _____

       _____

    F. _____

       _____

24. The signs of death include:

    A. _____

    B. _____

25. Postmortem care is done to _____

    _____.

26. What information do you need from the nurse when assisting with postmortem care?

    A. _____

    B. _____

    C. _____

    D. _____

27. A patient you are caring for has an advance directive that is against your religious values. What should you do?

    _____

*Multiple Choice*

Circle the **BEST** Answer

28. Attitudes and beliefs about death usually stay the same throughout a person's life.
    A. True
    B. False

29. Infants and toddlers have no concept of death.
    A. True
    B. False

30. Children between the ages of 3 and 5 years
    A. Know that death is final
    B. Often think they will die
    C. Often blame themselves when someone dies
    D. Are not curious about death

31. The person in the bargaining stage of dying
    A. Is very sad
    B. Makes promises in exchange for more time
    C. Is calm and at peace
    D. Feels anger and rage

32. Ms. Mary Andrews is dying. She asks you to stay and talk in the middle of the night. Which is *correct*?
    A. Tell Ms. Andrews that she needs to sleep.
    B. Call Ms. Andrews' family to stay with her.
    C. Call a pastor to talk with Ms. Andrews.
    D. Being there and listening help meet Ms. Andrews' psychological and social needs.

33. Ms. Andrews is receiving hospice care. Her pastor is visiting her at 11:00 PM. You need to
    A. Stay in the room while the pastor visits.
    B. Provide for privacy.
    C. Tell the nurse at once.
    D. Ask Ms. Andrews why her pastor is visiting so late.

34. Mr. Jason Parks is unconscious. When providing care, you need to do the following *except*
    A. Assume that he can hear you.
    B. Speak in a whisper.
    C. Offer words of comfort.
    D. Avoid topics that could upset him.

35. You promote comfort when caring for a dying person by
    A. Playing cheerful music
    B. Asking a lot of questions to keep the person talking
    C. Providing care quickly, so the person can be alone
    D. Providing good skin care and personal hygiene

36. A darkened room is comforting to the dying person.
    A. True
    B. False

37. The dying person has the right to receive kind and respectful care before and after death.
    A. True
    B. False

38. Postmortem care involves the following *except*
    A. Pronouncing the person dead
    B. Positioning the body in normal alignment before rigor mortis sets in
    C. Preparing the body for viewing by the family
    D. Bathing soiled areas

39. When providing postmortem care you must practice Standard Precautions and follow the Bloodborne Pathogen Standard.
    A. True
    B. False

40. The right to confidentiality does not apply after death.
    A. True
    B. False

## CASE STUDY

*Mr. Paul Clark is a patient on the inpatient hospice unit at Valley View Hospital. He is 59 years old and has a terminal illness. Mr. Clark currently sleeps most of the time and does not respond verbally. He occasionally opens his eyes. His wife stays with him most of the day and has spent the night the past two nights. She says prayers and talks to him about important events in their lives. His son from another state arrived 3 days ago. Mr. Clark's daughter lives in the same town and visits several times a day. She often washes his face and applies lotion to his feet. She tells him that she loves him and that she will miss him.*

*After Mr. Clark's son arrived, Mr. Clark told his wife that he was ready to die and that he was at peace with his family and with God. He discussed his will and his funeral arrangements with his wife. Mr. and Mrs. Clark are of the Catholic faith. The day after his son arrived, Mr. Clark asked for the priest to administer the sacrament of the anointing of the sick (Last Rites). An hour after he received Last Rites, Mr. Clark became unresponsive. Mr. Clark's son is often tearful. He states that he wishes he had more time to spend with his father. He often sits and holds his fathers hand.*

*Answer the following questions.*

1. According to Elizabeth Kübler Ross's stages of dying, what stage is Mr. Clark in? Explain.

2. What physical care needs does Mr. Clark have?

3. What measures will help meet Mr. Clark's psychological, social, and spiritual needs?

4. What role do Mr. Clark's religious beliefs have in his attitude toward death?

5. How will you promote Mr. Clark's rights?

6. What measures will help meet the family's needs?

---

## ADDITIONAL LEARNING ACTIVITIES

1. List your thoughts and feelings about death and dying. Answers these questions:
   A. How do your religion, culture, and age affect your feelings about death?

   B. Have you had experience with the death of a family member or friend that affects your feelings about death and dying? Explain.

   C. How do you feel about advance directives?

2. If you have fears about caring for dying persons, discuss them with your instructor.

# Procedure Checklists

## Using a Fire Extinguisher

Name: _____          Date: _____

| Procedure | S | U | Comments |
|---|---|---|---|
| 1. Pulled the fire alarm. | _____ | _____ | _____ |
| 2. Got the nearest fire extinguisher. | _____ | _____ | _____ |
| 3. Carried it upright. | _____ | _____ | _____ |
| 4. Took it to the fire. | _____ | _____ | _____ |
| 5. Removed the safety pin. | _____ | _____ | _____ |
| 6. Directed the hose at the base of the fire. | _____ | _____ | _____ |
| 7. Pushed the top handle down. | _____ | _____ | _____ |
| 8. Swept the hose slowly back and forth at the base of the fire. | _____ | _____ | _____ |

Date of Satisfactory Completion _____          Instructor's Initials_____

## Applying Restraints

Name: _____          Date: _____

| Quality of Life | S | U | Comments |
|---|---|---|---|

- Knocked before entering the person's room.    _____ _____ _____
- Addressed the person by name.    _____ _____ _____
- Introduced yourself by name and title.    _____ _____ _____
- Explained the procedure to the person
  before beginning and during the procedure.    _____ _____ _____
- Protected the person's rights during the procedure.    _____ _____ _____
- Handled the person gently during the procedure.    _____ _____ _____

### Pre-Procedure

1. Followed "Delegation Guidelines: Applying Restraints."
   Reviewed "Promoting Safety and Comfort: Applying
   Restraints."    _____ _____ _____
2. Collected the following:
   - Correct type and size of restraints    _____ _____ _____
   - Padding for bony areas    _____ _____ _____
   - Bed rail pads or gap protectors (if needed)    _____ _____ _____
3. Practiced hand hygiene.    _____ _____ _____
4. Identified the person. Checked the ID bracelet against
   the assignment sheet. Called the person by name.    _____ _____ _____
5. Provided for privacy.    _____ _____ _____

### Procedure

6. Made sure the person was comfortable and in
   good body alignment.    _____ _____ _____
7. Put the bed rail pads or gap protectors on the bed
   if the person was in bed, if needed. Followed
   the manufacturer's instructions.    _____ _____ _____
8. Padded bony areas according to the nurse's instructions
   and the care plan.    _____ _____ _____
9. Read the manufacturer's instructions. Noted the front
   and back of the restraint.    _____ _____ _____
10. For wrist restraints:
    a. Applied the restraint following the manufacturer's
       instructions. Placed the soft part toward the skin.    _____ _____ _____
    b. Secured the restraint so it was snug but not tight.
       Made sure you could slide 1 or 2 fingers under
       the restraint. Followed the manufacturer's instructions.
       Adjusted the straps if the restraint was too loose
       or too tight. Checked for snugness again.    _____ _____ _____
    c. Tied the straps to the movable part of the bed frame
       out of the person's reach. Used an agency-approved
       tie. Left 1 to 2 inches of slack in the straps.    _____ _____ _____
    d. Repeated steps 10 a, b, and c for the other wrist.    _____ _____ _____

*Continued*

| Procedure—cont'd | S | U | Comments |
|---|---|---|---|

11. For mitt restraints:

    a. Made sure the person's hands were clean and dry.  \_\_\_\_\_ \_\_\_\_\_ _____

    b. Applied the mitt restraint. Followed the manufacturer's instructions.  \_\_\_\_\_ \_\_\_\_\_ _____

    c. Tied the straps to the movable part of the bed frame. Used an agency-approved tie. Left 1 to 2 inches of slack in the straps.  \_\_\_\_\_ \_\_\_\_\_ _____

    d. Made sure the restraint was snug. Slid 1 or 2 fingers between the restraint and the wrist. Followed the manufacturer's instructions. Adjusted the straps if the restraint was too loose or too tight. Checked for snugness again.  \_\_\_\_\_ \_\_\_\_\_ _____

    e. Repeated steps 11b, c, and d for the other hand.  \_\_\_\_\_ \_\_\_\_\_ _____

12. For a belt restraint:

    a. Assisted the person to a sitting position.  \_\_\_\_\_ \_\_\_\_\_ _____

    b. Applied the restraint with your free hand. Followed the manufacturer's instructions.  \_\_\_\_\_ \_\_\_\_\_ _____

    c. Removed wrinkles or creases from the front and back of the restraint.  \_\_\_\_\_ \_\_\_\_\_ _____

    d. Brought the ties through the slots in the belt.  \_\_\_\_\_ \_\_\_\_\_ _____

    e. Helped the person lie down if he or she was in bed.  \_\_\_\_\_ \_\_\_\_\_ _____

    f. Made sure the person was comfortable and in good alignment.  \_\_\_\_\_ \_\_\_\_\_ _____

    g. Secured the straps to the movable part of the bed frame out of the person's reach or to the chair or wheelchair. Used an agency-approved tie. Left 1 to 2 inches of slack in the straps.  \_\_\_\_\_ \_\_\_\_\_ _____

    h. Made sure the belt was snug. Slid an open hand between the restraint and the person. Adjusted the restraint if it was too loose or too tight. Checked for snugness again.  \_\_\_\_\_ \_\_\_\_\_ _____

13. For a vest restraint:

    a. Assisted the person to a sitting position.  \_\_\_\_\_ \_\_\_\_\_ _____

    b. Applied the restraint with your free hand. Followed the manufacturer's instructions. The "V" part of the vest crossed in front.  \_\_\_\_\_ \_\_\_\_\_ _____

    c. Made sure the vest was free of wrinkles in the front and back.  \_\_\_\_\_ \_\_\_\_\_ _____

    d. Helped the person lie down if he or she was in bed.  \_\_\_\_\_ \_\_\_\_\_ _____

    e. Brought the straps through the slots.  \_\_\_\_\_ \_\_\_\_\_ _____

    f. Made sure the person was comfortable and in good alignment.  \_\_\_\_\_ \_\_\_\_\_ _____

    g. Secured the straps to the chair or to the movable part of the bed frame. If secured to the bed frame, the straps were secured at waist level out of the person's reach. Used an agency-approved tie. Left 1 to 2 inches of slack in the straps.  \_\_\_\_\_ \_\_\_\_\_ _____

*Continued*

| Procedure—cont'd | S | U | Comments |
|---|---|---|---|

    h. Made sure the vest was snug. Slid an open hand between the restraint and the person. Adjusted the restraint if it was too loose or too tight. Checked for snugness again.  _____ _____ _____

14. For a jacket restraint:

    a. Assisted the person to a sitting position.  _____ _____ _____

    b. Applied the restraint with your free hand. Followed the manufacturer's instructions. (The jacket opening was in back.)  _____ _____ _____

    c. Closed the back with the zipper, ties, or hook and loop closures.  _____ _____ _____

    d. Made sure the side seams were under the arms. Removed any wrinkles in the front and back.  _____ _____ _____

    e. Helped the person lie down if he or she was in bed.  _____ _____ _____

    f. Made sure the person was comfortable and in good alignment.  _____ _____ _____

    g. Secured the straps to the chair or to the movable part of the bed frame. If secured to the bed frame, the straps were secured at waist level out of the person's reach. Used an agency-approved knot. Left 1 to 2 inches of slack in the straps.  _____ _____ _____

    h. Made sure the jacket was snug. Slid an open hand between the restraint and the person. Adjusted the restraint if it was too loose or too tight. Checked for snugness again.  _____ _____ _____

## Post-Procedure

15. Positioned the person as the nurse directed.  _____ _____ _____
16. Provided for comfort as noted on the inside of the front book cover.  _____ _____ _____
17. Placed the signal light within the person's reach.  _____ _____ _____
18. Raised or lowered bed rails. Followed the care plan and the manufacturer's instructions for the restraint.  _____ _____ _____
19. Unscreened the person.  _____ _____ _____
20. Completed a safety check of the room as indicated on the inside of the front book cover.  _____ _____ _____
21. Decontaminated hands.
22. Checked the person and the restraints at least every 15 minutes. Reported and recorded observations.  _____ _____ _____

    a. For wrist and mitt restraints: checked the pulse, color, and temperature of the restrained parts.  _____ _____ _____

    b. For vest, jacket, and belt restraints: checked the person's breathing. Called the nurse at once if there were problems breathing. Made sure the restraint was properly positioned in the front and back.  _____ _____ _____

*Continued*

| Procedure—cont'd | S | U | Comments |
|---|---|---|---|

23. Did the following at least every 2 hours:
    - Removed the restraint. _____ _____ _____
    - Repositioned the person. _____ _____ _____
    - Met food, fluid, hygiene, and elimination needs. _____ _____ _____
    - Gave skin care. _____ _____ _____
    - Performed range-of-motion exercises or helped the person walk. Followed the care plan. _____ _____ _____
    - Provided for comfort as noted on the inside of the front book cover. _____ _____ _____
    - Reapplied the restraints. _____ _____ _____
24. Completed a safety check of the room as noted on the inside of the front book cover. _____ _____ _____
25. Reported and recorded observations and the care given. _____ _____ _____

Date of Satisfactory Completion _____    Instructor's Initials_____

# Hand Washing (NNAAP™)

Name: _____          Date: _____

| Procedure | S | U | Comments |
|---|---|---|---|
| 1. Reviewed "Promoting Safety and Comfort: Hand Hygiene." | ____ | ____ | _____ |
| 2. Made sure you had soap, paper towels, orange stick or nail file, and a wastebasket. Collected missing items. | ____ | ____ | _____ |
| 3. Pushed watch up 4 to 5 inches. Pushed up uniform sleeves (if sleeves were long). | ____ | ____ | _____ |
| 4. Stood away from the sink so that clothes did not touch the sink. Stood so the soap and faucet were easy to reach. | ____ | ____ | _____ |
| 5. Turned on and adjusted the water until it felt warm. | ____ | ____ | _____ |
| 6. Wet wrists and hands. Kept hands lower than elbows. Made sure to wet the area 3 to 4 inches above the wrists. | ____ | ____ | _____ |
| 7. Applied about 1 teaspoon of soap to hands. | ____ | ____ | _____ |
| 8. Rubbed palms together and interlaced fingers to work up a good lather for at least 15 seconds. (Some state competency tests require that you wash your hands for 20 seconds.) | ____ | ____ | _____ |
| 9. Washed each hand and wrist thoroughly. Cleaned well between the fingers. | ____ | ____ | _____ |
| 10. Cleaned under the fingernails. Rubbed the finger-tips against the palms. | ____ | ____ | _____ |
| 11. Cleaned under fingernails with a nail file or orange stick. | ____ | ____ | _____ |
| 12. Rinsed wrists and hands well. Water flowed from the arms to the hands. | ____ | ____ | _____ |
| 13. Repeated steps 7 through 12, if needed. | ____ | ____ | _____ |
| 14. Dried wrists and hands with paper towels. Patted dry starting at the fingertips. | ____ | ____ | _____ |
| 15. Discarded the paper towels. | ____ | ____ | _____ |
| 16. Turned off faucets with clean paper towels. Used a clean paper towel for each faucet. | ____ | ____ | _____ |
| 17. Discarded paper towels into a wastebasket. | ____ | ____ | _____ |

Date of Satisfactory Completion _____ Instructor's Initials_____

## Removing Gloves

Name: _____    Date: _____

| Procedure | S | U | Comments |
|---|---|---|---|
| 1. Reviewed "Promoting Safety and Comfort: Gloves." | _____ | _____ | _____ |
| 2. Made sure that glove only touched glove. | _____ | _____ | _____ |
| 3. Grasped a glove just below the cuff. Grasped it on the outside. | _____ | _____ | _____ |
| 4. Pulled the glove down over the hand so it was inside out. | _____ | _____ | _____ |
| 5. Held the removed glove with the other gloved hand. | _____ | _____ | _____ |
| 6. Reached inside the other glove. Used the first 2 fingers of the ungloved hand. | _____ | _____ | _____ |
| 7. Pulled the glove down (inside out) over the hand and the other glove. | _____ | _____ | _____ |
| 8. Discarded the gloves. Followed agency policy. | _____ | _____ | _____ |
| 9. Decontaminated hands. | _____ | _____ | _____ |

Date of Satisfactory Completion _____    Instructor's Initials_____

# Donning and Removing a Gown

Name: _____          Date: _____

| Procedure | S | U | Comments |
|---|---|---|---|
| 1. Removed the watch and all jewelry. | ___ | ___ | _____ |
| 2. Rolled up uniform sleeves. | ___ | ___ | _____ |
| 3. Practiced hand hygiene. | ___ | ___ | _____ |
| 4. Held a clean gown out in front of you. Let it unfold. Did not shake the gown. | ___ | ___ | _____ |
| 5. Put the hands and arms through the sleeves. | ___ | ___ | _____ |
| 6. Made sure the gown covered you from your neck to your knees. It covered the arms to the end of your wrists. | ___ | ___ | _____ |
| 7. Tied the strings at the back of the neck. | ___ | ___ | _____ |
| 8. Overlapped the back of the gown. Made sure it covered the uniform. The gown was snug, not loose. | ___ | ___ | _____ |
| 9. Tied the waist strings at the back or the side. | ___ | ___ | _____ |
| 10. Put on the gloves. Provided care. | ___ | ___ | _____ |
| 11. Removed and discarded the gloves. Decontaminated hands. | ___ | ___ | _____ |
| 12. Removed and discarded the goggles or face shield if worn. (Did this at the door.) | ___ | ___ | _____ |
| 13. Removed the gown. | | | |
|   a. Untied the neck and waist strings. Did not touch the front of the gown. | ___ | ___ | _____ |
|   b. Pulled the gown down from each shoulder toward the same hand. | ___ | ___ | _____ |
|   c. Turned the gown inside out as it was removed. Held it at the inside shoulder seams and brought hands together. | ___ | ___ | _____ |
| 14. Held and Rolled up the gown away from you. Kept it inside out. | ___ | ___ | _____ |
| 15. Discarded the gown. Followed agency policy. | ___ | ___ | _____ |
| 16. Removed and discarded the mask if worn. (A respirator was removed outside the room.) | ___ | ___ | _____ |
| 17. Decontaminated hands. | ___ | ___ | _____ |
| 18. Opened the door using a paper towel. Discarded it as you left. | ___ | ___ | _____ |

Date of Satisfactory Completion _____          Instructor's Initials_____

# Donning and Removing a Mask

Name: _____     Date: _____

| Procedure | S | U | Comments |
|---|---|---|---|
| 1. Practiced hand hygiene. | _____ | _____ | _____ |
| 2. Put on a gown if required. | _____ | _____ | _____ |
| 3. Picked up the mask by its upper ties. Did not touch the part that would cover the face. | _____ | _____ | _____ |
| 4. Placed the mask over the nose and mouth. | _____ | _____ | _____ |
| 5. Placed the upper strings above the ears. Tied them at the back in the middle of the head. | _____ | _____ | _____ |
| 6. Tied the lower strings at the back of the neck. The lower part of the mask was under the chin. | _____ | _____ | _____ |
| 7. Pinched the metal band around the nose. The top of the mask was snug over the nose. If eyeglasses were worn, the mask was snug under the bottom of the eyeglasses. | _____ | _____ | _____ |
| 8. Made sure the mask was snug over the face and under the chin. | _____ | _____ | _____ |
| 9. Put on goggles or a face shield if needed and if not part of the mask. | _____ | _____ | _____ |
| 10. Decontaminated hands. Put on gloves. | _____ | _____ | _____ |
| 11. Provided care. Avoided coughing, sneezing, and unnecessary talking. | _____ | _____ | _____ |
| 12. Changed the mask if it became moist or contaminated. | _____ | _____ | _____ |
| 13. Removed the mask at the doorway. (Note: a respirator is removed outside the door.) Removed the mask as follows: | _____ | _____ | _____ |
| a. Removed the gloves. Removed the goggles or face shield and gown if worn. | _____ | _____ | _____ |
| b. Untied the lower strings of the mask. | _____ | _____ | _____ |
| c. Untied the top strings. | _____ | _____ | _____ |
| d. Held the top strings. Removed the mask. | _____ | _____ | _____ |
| 14. Discarded the mask. Followed agency policy. | _____ | _____ | _____ |
| 15. Decontaminated hands. | _____ | _____ | _____ |

Date of Satisfactory Completion _____     Instructor's Initials_____

## Moving the Person Up in Bed

Name: _____          Date: _____

| Quality of Life | S | U | Comments |
|---|---|---|---|

- Knocked before entering the person's room.
- Addressed the person by name.
- Introduced yourself by name and title.
- Explained the procedure to the
  person before beginning and during the procedure.
- Protected the person's rights during the procedure.
- Handled the person gently during the procedure.

### Pre-Procedure

1. Followed "Delegation Guidelines:
   Moving Persons in Bed." Reviewed "Promoting
   Safety and Comfort:
   - Moving Persons in Bed"
   - Moving the Person up in Bed"
2. Asked a co-worker to assist.
3. Practiced hand hygiene.
4. Identified the person. Checked the ID bracelet against
   the assignment sheet. Called the person by name.
5. Provided for privacy.
6. Locked the bed wheels.
7. Raised the bed for body mechanics. Bed rails
   were up if used.

### Procedure

8. Lowered the head of the bed to a level appropriate
   for the person. It was as flat as possible.
9. Stood on one side of the bed. The co-worker stood
   on the other side.
10. Lowered the bed rails if up.
11. Removed the pillow as directed by the nurse.
    Placed a pillow upright against the headboard
    if the person could be without it.
12. Stood with a wide base of support. Pointed the foot
    near the head of the bed toward the head of the bed.
    Faced the head of the bed.
13. Bent your hips and knees. Kept your back straight.
14. Placed one arm under the person's shoulder and one
    arm under the thighs. Your co-worker did the same.
    Grasped each other's forearms.
15. Asked the person to grasp the trapeze.

*Continued*

| Procedure—cont'd | S | U | Comments |
|---|---|---|---|

16. Had the person flex both knees.
17. Explained that:
    - You would count "1, 2, 3."
    - The move would be on "3."
    - On "3," the person would push against the bed with the feet if able. And the person would pull up with the trapeze.
18. Moved the person to the head of the bed on the count of "3." Shifted weight from your rear leg to the front leg. The co-worker did the same.
19. Repeated steps 12 through 18, if necessary.

## Post-Procedure

20. Put the pillow under the person's head and shoulders. Straightened linens.
21. Positioned the person in good alignment.
22. Provided for comfort as noted on the inside on the front book cover.
23. Placed the signal light within reach.
24. Raised the head of the bed to a level appropriate for the person.
25. Lowered the bed to its lowest position.
26. Raised or lowered bed rails. Followed the care plan.
27. Unscreened the person.
28. Completed a safety check of the room as noted on the inside of the front book cover.
29. Decontaminated hands.
30. Reported and recorded observations.

Date of Satisfactory Completion _____    Instructor's Initials_____

## Moving the Person Up in Bed With an Assist Device

Name: _____    Date: _____

| Quality of Life | S | U | Comments |
|---|---|---|---|

**Quality of Life**

- Knocked before entering the person's room.
- Addressed the person by name.
- Introduced yourself by name and title.
- Explained the procedure to the person before beginning and during the procedure.
- Protected the person's rights during the procedure.
- Handled the person gently during the procedure.

**Pre-Procedure**

1. Followed "Delegation Guidelines: Moving Persons in Bed." Reviewed "Promoting Safety and Comfort: Moving Persons in Bed."
2. Asked a co-worker to help.
3. Practiced hand hygiene.
4. Identified the person. Checked the ID bracelet against the assignment sheet. Called the person by name.
5. Provided for privacy.
6. Locked the bed wheels.
7. Raised the bed for body mechanics. Bed rails were up if used.

**Procedure**

8. Lowered the head of the bed to a level appropriate for the person. It was as flat as possible.
9. Stood on one side of the bed. The co-worker stood on the other side.
10. Lowered the bed rails if up.
11. Removed pillows as directed by the nurse. Placed a pillow against the headboard if the person could be without it.
12. Stood with a broad base of support. Pointed the foot near the head of the bed toward the head of the bed. Faced that direction.
13. Rolled the sides of the assist device up close to the person. (Omitted this step if device had handles.)
14. Grasped the rolled-up assist device firmly near the person's shoulders and hips or grasped it by the handles.) Supported the head.
15. Bent your hips and knees.
16. Moved the person up in bed on the count of "3." Shifted your weight from the rear leg to the front leg.
17. Repeated steps 12 through 16 if necessary.
18. Unrolled the assist device (omitted this step if the device had handles.)

*Continued*

| Post-Procedure | S | U | Comments |
|---|---|---|---|
| 19. Put the pillow under the person's head and shoulders. | ___ | ___ | _____ |
| 20. Positioned the person in good alignment. | ___ | ___ | _____ |
| 21. Provided for comfort as noted on the inside of the front book cover. | ___ | ___ | _____ |
| 22. Placed the signal light within reach. | ___ | ___ | _____ |
| 23. Raised the head of the bed to a level appropriate for the person. | ___ | ___ | _____ |
| 24. Lowered the bed to its lowest position. | ___ | ___ | _____ |
| 25. Raised or lowered bed rails. Followed the care plan. | ___ | ___ | _____ |
| 26. Unscreened the person. | ___ | ___ | _____ |
| 27. Completed a safety check of the room as noted on the inside of the front book cover. | ___ | ___ | _____ |
| 28. Decontaminated hands. | ___ | ___ | _____ |
| 29. Reported and recorded observations. | ___ | ___ | _____ |

Date of Satisfactory Completion _____ Instructor's Initials_____

## Moving the Person to the Side of the Bed

Name: _____     Date: _____

| Quality of Life | S | U | Comments |
|---|---|---|---|

- Knocked before entering the person's room.
- Addressed the person by name.
- Introduced yourself by name and title.
- Explained the procedure to the person before beginning and during the procedure.
- Protected the person's rights during the procedure.
- Handled the person gently during the procedure.

### Pre-Procedure

1. Followed "Delegation Guidelines: Moving Persons in Bed." Reviewed "Promoting Safety and Comfort:
   - Moving Persons in Bed"
   - Moving the Person to the Side of the Bed"
2. Asked a co-worker to help if using an assist device.
3. Practiced hand hygiene.
4. Identified the person. Checked the ID bracelet against the assignment sheet. Called the person by name.
5. Provided for privacy.
6. Locked the bed wheels.
7. Raised the bed for body mechanics. Bed rails were up if used.

### Procedure

8. Lowered the head of the bed to a level appropriate for the person. It was as flat as possible.
9. Stood on the side of the bed to which you would move the person.
10. Lowered the bed rail near you if bed rails were used. (Both bed rails are lowered for step 15.)
11. Removed pillows as directed by the nurse.
12. Stood with your feet about 12 inches apart. One foot was in front of the other. Flexed your knees.
13. Crossed the person's arms over the person's chest.
14. Method 1: Moving the person in segments
    a. Placed your arm under the person's neck and shoulders. Grasped the far shoulder.
    b. Placed your other arm under the mid-back.
    c. Moved the upper part of the person's body toward you. Rocked backward and shifted weight to your rear leg.

*Continued*

| Procedure—cont'd | S | U | Comments |
|---|---|---|---|

    d. Placed one arm under the person's waist and one under the thighs.

    e. Rocked backward to move the lower part of the person toward you.

    f. Repeated the procedure for the legs and feet. Your arms were under the person's thighs and calves.

15. Method 2: Moving the person with a drawsheet

    a. Rolled the drawsheet up close to the person.

    b. Grasped the rolled-up drawsheet near the person's shoulders and hips. The co-worker did the same. Supported the head.

    c. Rocked backward on the count of "3," moving the person toward you. The co-worker rocked backward slightly and then forward toward you while keeping the arms straight.

    d. Unrolled the drawsheet. Removed any wrinkles.

## Post-Procedure

16. Positioned the person in good alignment. Followed the nurse's directions and the care plan.

17. Provided for comfort as noted on the inside of the front book cover.

18. Placed the signal light within reach.

19. Lowered the bed to its lowest position.

20. Raised or lowered bed rails. Followed the care plan.

21. Unscreened the person.

22. Completed a safety check of the room as noted on the inside of the front book cover.

23. Decontaminated hands.

24. Reported and recorded observations.

Date of Satisfactory Completion _____ Instructor's Initials_____

# Turning and Positioning the Person (NNAAP™)

Name: _____     Date: _____

## Quality of Life

|  | S | U | Comments |
|---|---|---|---|

- Knocked before entering the person's room.
- Addressed the person by name.
- Introduced yourself by name and title.
- Explained the procedure to the person before beginning and during the procedure.
- Protected the person's rights during the procedure.
- Handled the person gently during the procedure.

## Pre-Procedure

1. Followed "Delegation Guidelines: Turning Persons." Reviewed "Promoting Safety and Comfort: Turning Persons."
2. Practiced hand hygiene.
3. Identified the person. Checked the ID bracelet against the assignment sheet. Called the person by name.
4. Provided for privacy.
5. Locked the bed wheels.
6. Raised the bed for body mechanics. Bed rails were up if used.

## Procedure

7. Lowered the head of the bed to a level appropriate for the person. It was as flat as possible.
8. Stood on the side of the bed opposite to where you would turn the person. The far bed rail was up if used.
9. Lowered the bed rail near you if used.
10. Moved the person to the side near you.
11. Crossed the person's arms over his or her chest. Crossed the leg near you over the far leg.
12. Turning the person away from you:
    a. Stood with a wide base of support. Flexed your knees.
    b. Placed one hand on the person's shoulder. Placed the other on the hip near you.
    c. Pushed the person gently toward the other side of the bed. Shifted your weight from the rear leg to the front leg.
13. Turning the person toward you:
    a. Raised the bed rail if used.
    b. Went to the other side. Lowered the bed rail if used.
    c. Stood with a wide base of support. Flexed your knees.

*Continued*

| Procedure—cont'd | S | U | Comments |
|---|---|---|---|

   d. Placed one hand on the person's far shoulder. Placed the other on the far hip.

   e. Rolled the person toward you gently.

14. Positioned the person. Followed the nurse's directions and the care plan. The following is common:

   a. Placed a pillow under the head and neck.

   b. Adjusted the shoulder. The person did not lie on an arm.

   c. Placed a small pillow under the upper hand and arm.

   d. Positioned a pillow against the back.

   e. Flexed the upper knee. Positioned the upper leg in front of the lower leg.

   f. Supported the upper leg and thigh on pillows. Made sure the ankle was supported.

## Post-Procedure

15. Provided for comfort as noted on the inside of the front book cover.

16. Placed the signal light within reach.

17. Lowered the bed to its lowest position.

18. Raised or lowered bed rails. Followed the care plan.

19. Unscreened the person.

20. Completed a safety check of the room as noted on the inside of the front book cover.

21. Decontaminated hands.

22. Reported and recorded observations.

Date of Satisfactory Completion _____    Instructor's Initials_____

## Logrolling the Person

Name: _____     Date: _____

| Quality of Life | S | U | Comments |
|---|---|---|---|
| • Knocked before entering the person's room. | _____ | _____ | _____ |
| • Addressed the person by name. | _____ | _____ | _____ |
| • Introduced yourself by name and title. | _____ | _____ | _____ |
| • Explained the procedure to the person before beginning and during the procedure. | _____ | _____ | _____ |
| • Protected the person's rights during the procedure. | _____ | _____ | _____ |
| • Handled the person gently during the procedure. | _____ | _____ | _____ |

### Pre-Procedure

| | S | U | Comments |
|---|---|---|---|
| 1. Followed "Delegation Guidelines: Turning Persons." Reviewed "Promoting Safety and Comfort: | _____ | _____ | _____ |
|    • Turning Persons" | _____ | _____ | _____ |
|    • Logrolling Persons" | _____ | _____ | _____ |
| 2. Asked a co-worker to help. | _____ | _____ | _____ |
| 3. Practiced hand hygiene. | _____ | _____ | _____ |
| 4. Identified the person. Checked the ID bracelet against the assignment sheet. Called the person by name. | _____ | _____ | _____ |
| 5. Provided for privacy. | _____ | _____ | _____ |
| 6. Locked the bed wheels. | _____ | _____ | _____ |
| 7. Raised the bed for body mechanics. Bed rails were up if used. | _____ | _____ | _____ |

### Procedure

| | S | U | Comments |
|---|---|---|---|
| 8. Made sure the bed was flat. | _____ | _____ | _____ |
| 9. Stood on the side opposite to which you would turn the person. A co-worker stood on the other side. | _____ | _____ | _____ |
| 10. Lowered the bed rails if used. | _____ | _____ | _____ |
| 11. Moved the person as a unit to the side of the bed near you. Used the assist device. | _____ | _____ | _____ |
| 12. Placed the person's arms across the chest. Placed a pillow between the knees. | _____ | _____ | _____ |
| 13. Raised the bed rail if used. | _____ | _____ | _____ |
| 14. Went to the other side. | _____ | _____ | _____ |
| 15. Stood near the shoulders and chest. A co-worker stood near the hips and thighs. | _____ | _____ | _____ |
| 16. Stood with a broad base of support. One foot was in front of the other. | _____ | _____ | _____ |
| 17. Asked the person to hold his or her body rigid. | _____ | _____ | _____ |
| 18. Rolled the person toward you or used the assist device. Turned the person as a unit. | _____ | _____ | _____ |

*Continued*

Post-Procedure                                      S        U              Comments

19. Positioned the person in good alignment. Used pillows
    as directed by the nurse and care plan: (The following
    is common unless the spinal cord is involved.)

    a.  One pillow against the back for support.         _____  _____  _____

    b.  One pillow under the head and neck if allowed.   _____  _____  _____

    c.  One pillow or folded bath blanket between the legs.  _____  _____  _____

    d.  A small pillow under the arm and hand.           _____  _____  _____

20. Provided for comfort as noted on the inside of the   _____  _____  _____
    front book cover.

21. Placed the signal light within reach.                _____  _____  _____

22. Lowered the bed to its lowest position.              _____  _____  _____

23. Raised or lowered bed rails. Followed the care plan. _____  _____  _____

24. Unscreened the person.                               _____  _____  _____

25. Completed a safety check of the room as noted on the _____  _____  _____
    inside of the front book cover.

26. Decontaminated hands.                                _____  _____  _____

27. Reported and recorded observations.                  _____  _____  _____

Date of Satisfactory Completion _____    Instructor's Initials_____

## Helping the Person Sit on the Side of the Bed (Dangle)

Name: _____     Date: _____

| Quality of Life | S | U | Comments |
|---|---|---|---|

- Knocked before entering the person's room.
- Addressed the person by name.
- Introduced yourself by name and title.
- Explained the procedure to the person before beginning and during the procedure.
- Protected the person's rights during the procedure.
- Handled the person gently during the procedure.

### Pre-Procedure

1. Followed "Delegation Guidelines: Dangling" Reviewed "Promoting Safety and Comfort: Dangling."
2. Practiced hand hygiene.
3. Identified the person. Checked the ID bracelet against the assignment sheet. Called the person by name.
4. Provided for privacy.
5. Decided what side of the bed to use.
6. Moved furniture to provide moving space.
7. Locked the bed wheels.
8. Raised the bed for body mechanics. Bed rails were up if used.
9. Lowered the bed rail if up.

### Procedure

10. Positioned the person in the side-lying position facing you. The person laid on the strong side.
11. Raised the head of the bed to a sitting position.
12. Stood by the person's hips. Faced the foot of the bed.
13. Stood with the feet apart. The foot near the head of the bed was in front of the other foot.
14. Slid one arm under the person's neck and shoulders. Grasped the far shoulder. Placed your other hand over the thighs near the knees.
15. Pivoted toward the foot of the bed while moving the person's legs and feet over the side of the bed. As the legs went over the edge of the mattress, the trunk was upright.
16. Asked the person to hold onto the edge of the mattress. This supported the person in the sitting position.
17. Did not leave the person alone. Provided support if necessary.

*Continued*

| Procedure—cont'd | S | U | Comments |
|---|---|---|---|
| 18. Checked the person's condition: | | | |
| a. Asked how the person felt. Asked if the person felt dizzy or light-headed. | \_\_\_\_\_ | \_\_\_\_\_ | _____ |
| b. Checked pulse and respirations. | \_\_\_\_\_ | \_\_\_\_\_ | _____ |
| c. Checked for difficulty breathing. | \_\_\_\_\_ | \_\_\_\_\_ | _____ |
| d. Noted if the skin was pale or bluish in color. | \_\_\_\_\_ | \_\_\_\_\_ | _____ |
| 19. Helped the person lie down if necessary. | \_\_\_\_\_ | \_\_\_\_\_ | _____ |
| 20. Reversed the procedure to return the person to bed. | \_\_\_\_\_ | \_\_\_\_\_ | _____ |
| 21. Lowered the head of the bed after the person returned to bed. Helped him or her move to the center of the bed. | \_\_\_\_\_ | \_\_\_\_\_ | _____ |
| 22. Positioned the person in good alignment. | \_\_\_\_\_ | \_\_\_\_\_ | _____ |

## Post-Procedure

| | S | U | Comments |
|---|---|---|---|
| 23. Provided for comfort as noted on the inside of the front book cover. | \_\_\_\_\_ | \_\_\_\_\_ | _____ |
| 24. Placed the signal light within reach. | \_\_\_\_\_ | \_\_\_\_\_ | _____ |
| 25. Lowered the bed to its lowest position. | \_\_\_\_\_ | \_\_\_\_\_ | _____ |
| 26. Raised or lowered bed rails. Followed the care plan. | \_\_\_\_\_ | \_\_\_\_\_ | _____ |
| 27. Returned furniture to its proper place. | \_\_\_\_\_ | \_\_\_\_\_ | _____ |
| 28. Unscreened the person. | \_\_\_\_\_ | \_\_\_\_\_ | _____ |
| 29. Completed a safety check of the room as noted on the inside of the front book cover. | \_\_\_\_\_ | \_\_\_\_\_ | _____ |
| 30. Decontaminated hands. | \_\_\_\_\_ | \_\_\_\_\_ | _____ |
| 31. Reported and recorded observations. | \_\_\_\_\_ | \_\_\_\_\_ | _____ |

Date of Satisfactory Completion _____    Instructor's Initials_____

## Applying a Transfer Belt

Name: _____          Date: _____

| Quality of Life | S | U | Comments |
|---|---|---|---|

- Knocked before entering the person's room.            _____ _____ _____
- Addressed the person by name.                          _____ _____ _____
- Introduced yourself by name and title.                 _____ _____ _____
- Explained the procedure to the person
  before beginning and during the procedure.             _____ _____ _____
- Protected the person's rights during the procedure.    _____ _____ _____
- Handled the person gently during the procedure.        _____ _____ _____

### Procedure

1. Reviewed "Promoting Safety and Comfort: Transfer Belts."   _____ _____ _____
2. Practiced hand hygiene.                                     _____ _____ _____
3. Identified the person. Checked the ID bracelet against
   the assignment sheet. Called the person by name.            _____ _____ _____
4. Provided for privacy.                                       _____ _____ _____
5. Assisted the person to a sitting position.                  _____ _____ _____
6. Applied the belt around the person's waist over
   clothing. Did not apply it over bare skin.                  _____ _____ _____
7. Tightened the belt so it was snug. It did not cause
   discomfort or impair breathing. You were able to slide
   4 fingers (your open hand) under the belt.                  _____ _____ _____
8. Made sure that a woman's breasts were
   not caught under the belt.                                  _____ _____ _____
9. Placed the buckle off center in the front or in the
   back for the person's comfort. The buckle was not
   over the spine.                                             _____ _____ _____

Date of Satisfactory Completion _____     Instructor's Initials_____

# Transferring the Person to a Chair or Wheelchair (NNAAP™)

Name: _____    Date: _____

| Quality of Life | S | U | Comments |
|---|---|---|---|
| • Knocked before entering the person's room. | _____ | _____ | _____ |
| • Addressed the person by name. | _____ | _____ | _____ |
| • Introduced yourself by name and title. | _____ | _____ | _____ |
| • Explained the procedure to the person before beginning and during the procedure. | _____ | _____ | _____ |
| • Protected the person's rights during the procedure. | _____ | _____ | _____ |
| • Handled the person gently during the procedure. | _____ | _____ | _____ |

**Pre-Procedure**

1. Followed "Delegation Guidelines: Transferring Persons."Reviewed "Promoting Safety and Comfort:
   - Transferring Persons"
   - Transfer Belts"
   - Chair or Wheelchair Transfers"
2. Collected:
   - Wheelchair or arm chair
   - Bath blanket
   - Lap blanket
   - Robe and non-skid footwear
   - Paper or sheet
   - Transfer belt (if needed)
   - Seat cushion (if needed)
3. Practiced hand hygiene.
4. Identified the person. Checked the ID bracelet against the assignment sheet. Called the person by name.
5. Provided for privacy.
6. Decided which side of the bed to use. Moved furniture for a safe transfer.

**Procedure**

7. Placed the chair near the bed on the person's strong side. The arm of the chair almost touched the bed.
8. Placed a folded bath blanket or cushion on the seat (if needed).
9. Locked wheelchair wheels. Raised the footplates. Removed or swung the front rigging out of the way.
10. Lowered the bed to its lowest position. Locked the bed wheels.
11. Fan-folded top linens to the foot of the bed.

| Procedure—cont'd | S | U | Comments |
|---|---|---|---|

12. Placed the paper or sheet under the person's feet. Put footwear on the person.   _____ _____ _____

13. Helped the person sit on the side of the bed. His or her feet touched the floor.   _____ _____ _____

14. Helped the person put on a robe.   _____ _____ _____

15. Applied the transfer belt (if needed).   _____ _____ _____

16. Method 1: Using a transfer belt

   a. Stood in front of the person.   _____ _____ _____

   b. Had the person hold onto the mattress.   _____ _____ _____

   c. Made sure the person's feet were flat on the floor.   _____ _____ _____

   d. Had the person lean forward.   _____ _____ _____

   e. Grasped the transfer belt at each side. Grasped the belt from underneath.   _____ _____ _____

   f. Prevented the person from sliding or falling by doing one of the following:

     (1) Braced your knees against the person's knees. Blocked the person's feet with your feet.   _____ _____ _____

     (2) Used the knee and foot of one leg to block the person's weak foot. Placed your other foot slightly behind you for balance.   _____ _____ _____

     (3) Straddled your legs around the person's weak leg.   _____ _____ _____

   g. Explained the following:

     (1) You would count "1, 2, 3."   _____ _____ _____

     (2) The move would be on "3."   _____ _____ _____

     (3) On "3" the person would push down on the mattress and stand.   _____ _____ _____

   h. Asked the person to push down on the mattress and to stand on the count of "3."   _____ _____ _____

   i. Pulled the person in to a standing position as you straightened your knees.   _____ _____ _____

17. Method 2: No transfer belt

   a. Followed steps 16a-16c.   _____ _____ _____

   b. Placed your hands under the person's arms. Your hands were around the person's shoulder blades.   _____ _____ _____

   c. Had the person lean forward.   _____ _____ _____

   d. Prevented the person from sliding or falling by doing one of the following:   _____ _____ _____

     (1) Braced your knees against the person's knees. Blocked the person's feet with your feet.   _____ _____ _____

     (2) Used the knee and foot of one leg to block the person's weak foot. Placed your other foot slightly behind you for balance.   _____ _____ _____

     (3) Straddled your legs around the person's weak leg.   _____ _____ _____

   e. Explained the count of "3" as in step 16-g.   _____ _____ _____

   f. Asked the person to push down on the mattress and to stand on the count of "3." Pulled the person into a standing position as you straightened your knees.   _____ _____ _____

*Continued*

| Procedure—cont'd | S | U | Comments |
|---|---|---|---|
| 18. Supported the person in the standing position. Held the transfer belt or kept your hands around the person's shoulder blades. Continued to prevent the person from falling. | _____ | _____ | _____ |
| 19. Turned the person so he or she could grasp the far arm of the chair. The person's legs touched the edge of the chair. | _____ | _____ | _____ |
| 20. Continued to turn the person until the other armrest was grasped. | _____ | _____ | _____ |
| 21. Lowered the person into the chair as you bent your hips and knees. The person assisted by leaning forward and bending the elbows and knees. | _____ | _____ | _____ |
| 22. Made sure the buttocks were to the back of the seat. Positioned the person in good alignment. | _____ | _____ | _____ |
| 23. Attached the wheelchair front rigging. Positioned the person's feet on the wheelchair footplates. | _____ | _____ | _____ |
| 24. Covered the person's lap and legs with a lap blanket. Kept the blanket off the floor and the wheels. | _____ | _____ | _____ |
| 25. Removed the transfer belt if used. | _____ | _____ | _____ |
| 26. Positioned the chair as the person preferred. Locked the wheelchair wheels according to the care plan. | _____ | _____ | _____ |

**Post-Procedure**

| | S | U | Comments |
|---|---|---|---|
| 27. Provided for comfort as noted on the inside of the front book cover. | _____ | _____ | _____ |
| 28. Placed the signal light and other needed items within reach. | _____ | _____ | _____ |
| 29. Unscreened the person. | _____ | _____ | _____ |
| 30. Completed a safety check of the room as noted on the inside of the front book cover. | _____ | _____ | _____ |
| 31. Decontaminated hands. | _____ | _____ | _____ |
| 32. Reported and recorded observations. | _____ | _____ | _____ |

Date of Satisfactory Completion _____    Instructor's Initials_____

# Transferring the Person From a Chair or Wheelchair to Bed

Name: _____     Date: _____

| Quality of Life | S | U | Comments |
|---|---|---|---|

- Knocked before entering the person's room.
- Addressed the person by name.
- Introduced yourself by name and title.
- Explained the procedure to the person before beginning and during the procedure.
- Protected the person's rights during the procedure.
- Handled the person gently during the procedure.

## Pre-Procedure

1. Followed "Delegation Guidelines: Transferring Persons." Reviewed "Promoting Safety and Comfort:
   - Transferring Persons"
   - Transfer Belts"
   - Chair or Wheelchair Transfers"
2. Collected transfer belt (if needed).
3. Practiced hand hygiene.
4. Identified the person. Checked the ID bracelet against the assignment sheet. Called the person by name.
5. Provided for privacy.

## Procedure

6. Moved furniture for moving space.
7. Raised the head of the bed to a sitting position. The bed was in the lowest position.
8. Moved the signal light so it was on the strong side when the person was in bed.
9. Positioned the chair or wheelchair so the person's strong side was next to the bed. Had a co-worker help if necessary.
10. Locked the wheelchair and bed wheels.
11. Removed and folded the lap blanket.
12. Removed the person's feet from the footplates. Raised the footplates. Removed or swung the front rigging out of the way.
13. Applied the transfer belt (if needed).
14. Made sure the person's feet were flat on the floor.
15. Stood in front of the person.

*Continued*

| Procedure—cont'd | S | U | Comments |
|---|---|---|---|

16. Asked the person to hold onto the armrests or placed your arms under the person's arms. Your hands were around the shoulder blades. _____ _____ _____

17. Had the person lean forward. _____ _____ _____

18. Grasped the transfer belt on each side if using it. Grasped underneath the belt. _____ _____ _____

19. Prevented the person from sliding or falling by doing one of the following: _____ _____ _____

   a. Braced your knees against the person's knees. Blocked his or her feet with your feet. _____ _____ _____

   b. Used the knee and foot of one leg to block the person's weak leg or foot. Placed your other foot slightly behind you for balance. _____ _____ _____

   c. Straddled your legs around the person's weak leg. _____ _____ _____

20. Explained the count of "3" as in procedure "Transferring the Person to a Chair or Wheelchair." _____ _____ _____

21. Asked the person to push down on the armrests on the count of "3." Pulled the person into a standing position as you straightened your knees. _____ _____ _____

22. Supported the person in the standing position. Held the transfer belt or kept your hands around the person's shoulder blades. Continued to prevent the person from sliding or falling. _____ _____ _____

23. Turned the person so he or she could reach the edge of the mattress. The person's legs touched the mattress. _____ _____ _____

24. Continued to turn the person until he or she could reach the mattress with both hands. _____ _____ _____

25. Lowered the person onto the bed as you bent your hips and knees. The person assisted by leaning forward and bending the elbows and knees. _____ _____ _____

26. Removed the transfer belt. _____ _____ _____

27. Removed the robe and footwear. _____ _____ _____

28. Helped the person lie down. _____ _____ _____

## Post-Procedure

29. Provided for comfort as noted on the inside of the front book cover. _____ _____ _____

30. Placed the signal light and other needed items within reach. _____ _____ _____

31. Raised or lowered bed rails. Followed the care plan. _____ _____ _____

32. Arranged furniture to meet the person's needs. _____ _____ _____

33. Unscreened the person. _____ _____ _____

34. Completed a safety check of the room as noted on the inside of the front book cover. _____ _____ _____

35. Decontaminated hands. _____ _____ _____

36. Reported and recorded observations. _____ _____ _____

Date of Satisfactory Completion _____ Instructor's Initials_____

## Transferring the Person Using A Mechanical Lift

Name: _____    Date: _____

| Quality of Life | S | U | Comments |
|---|---|---|---|

- Knocked before entering the person's room.
- Addressed the person by name.
- Introduced yourself by name and title.
- Explained the procedure to the person before beginning and during the procedure.
- Protected the person's rights during the procedure.
- Handled the person gently during the procedure.

### Pre-Procedure

1. Followed "Delegation Guidelines: Transferring Persons." Reviewed "Promoting Safety and Comfort:
   - Transferring Persons"
   - Mechanical Lifts"
2. Asked a co-worker to help.
3. Collected:
   - Mechanical lift
   - Arm chair or wheelchair
   - Footwear
   - Bath blanket or cushion
   - Lap blanket
4. Practiced hand hygiene.
5. Identified the person. Checked the ID bracelet against the assignment sheet. Called the person by name.
6. Provided for privacy.

### Procedure

11. Centered the sling under the person. To position the sling, turned the person from side to side as if making an occupied bed. Positioned the sling according to the manufacturer's instructions.
12. Positioned the person in semi-Fowler's position.
13. Placed the chair at the head of the bed. It was even with the headboard and about 1 foot away from the bed. Placed a folded bath blanket or cushion in the chair.
14. Locked the bed wheels. Lowered the bed to its lowest position.
15. Raised the lift so it could be positioned over the person.
16. Positioned the lift over the person.
17. Locked the lift wheels in position.
18. Attached the sling to the swivel bar.
19. Raised the head of the bed to a sitting position.

*Continued*

Procedure—cont'd                                  S       U         Comments

20. Crossed the person's arms over the chest. The person
held onto the straps or chains but not the swivel bar.      \_\_\_\_    \_\_\_\_    _____

21. Raised the lift high enough until the person and
sling were free of the bed.                                \_\_\_\_    \_\_\_\_    _____

22. Had a co-worker support the person's legs as you
moved the lift and person away from the bed.               \_\_\_\_    \_\_\_\_    _____

23. Positioned the lift so that the person's back
was toward the chair.                                      \_\_\_\_    \_\_\_\_    _____

24. Positioned the chair so the person could be lowered into it.   \_\_\_\_    \_\_\_\_    _____

25. Lowered and guided the person into the chair.          \_\_\_\_    \_\_\_\_    _____

26. Lowered the swivel bar to unhook the sling. Removed the   \_\_\_\_    \_\_\_\_    _____
sling from under the person unless otherwise indicated.

27. Put footwear on the person. Positioned the person's
feet on wheelchair footplates.                            \_\_\_\_    \_\_\_\_    _____

28. Covered the person's lap and legs with a lap blanket.
Kept it off the floor and wheels.                         \_\_\_\_    \_\_\_\_    _____

29. Positioned the chair as the person preferred. Locked the   \_\_\_\_    \_\_\_\_    _____
wheelchair wheels according to the care plan.

Post-Procedure

30. Provided for comfort as noted on the inside
of the front book cover.                                  \_\_\_\_    \_\_\_\_    _____

31. Placed the signal light and other needed items
within reach.                                             \_\_\_\_    \_\_\_\_    _____

32. Unscreened the person.                                 \_\_\_\_    \_\_\_\_    _____

33. Completed a safety check of the room as noted on the   \_\_\_\_    \_\_\_\_    _____
inside of the front book cover.

34. Decontaminated hands.                                  \_\_\_\_    \_\_\_\_    _____

35. Reported and recorded observations.                    \_\_\_\_    \_\_\_\_    _____

36. Reversed the procedure to return the person to bed.    \_\_\_\_    \_\_\_\_    _____

Date of Satisfactory Completion _____    Instructor's Initials_____

# Transferring the Person to and From the Toilet

Name: _____     Date: _____

| Quality of Life | S | U | Comments |
|---|---|---|---|

- Knocked before entering the person's room.
- Addressed the person by name.
- Introduced yourself by name and title.
- Explained the procedure to the person before beginning and during the procedure.
- Protected the person's rights during the procedure.
- Handled the person gently during the procedure.

## Pre-Procedure

1. Followed "Delegation Guidelines: Transferring Persons." Reviewed "Promoting Safety and Comfort:
   - Transfer Belts"
   - Chair or Wheelchair Transfers"
2. Practiced hand hygiene.
3. Made sure the person had an elevated toilet seat. The toilet seat and wheelchair were at the same level.
4. Checked the grab bars by the toilet. If they were loose, told the nurse. Did not transfer the person to the toilet if the grab bars were not secure.

## Procedure

5. Had the person wear non-skid footwear.
6. Positioned the wheelchair next to the toilet if there was enough room. If not, positioned the wheelchair at a right angle to the toilet. (If possible, the person's strong side was near the toilet.)
7. Locked the wheelchair wheels.
8. Raised the footplates. Removed or swung front rigging out of the way.
9. Applied the transfer belt.
10. Helped the person unfasten clothing.
11. Used the transfer belt to help the person stand and to turn to the toilet. (See procedure "Transferring the Person to a Chair or Wheelchair.") The person used the grab bars to turn to the toilet.
12. Supported the person with the transfer belt while he or she lowered clothing. Or had the person hold onto the grab bars for support. Lowered the person's pants and undergarments.
13. Used the transfer belt to lower the person onto the toilet seat.

*Continued*

| Procedure—cont'd | S | U | Comments |
|---|---|---|---|
| 14. Removed the transfer belt. | ___ | ___ | _____ |
| 15. Told the person you would stay nearby. Reminded the person to use the signal light or call for help when needed. Stayed with the person if required by the care plan. | ___ | ___ | _____ |
| 16. Closed the bathroom door to provide for privacy. | ___ | ___ | _____ |
| 17. Stayed near the bathroom. Completed other tasks in the person's room. Checked on the person every 5 minutes. | ___ | ___ | _____ |
| 18. Knocked on the bathroom door when the person called. | ___ | ___ | _____ |
| 19. Helped with wiping, perineal care, flushing, and hand washing as needed. Wore glove and practiced hand hygiene. | ___ | ___ | _____ |
| 20. Applied the transfer belt. | ___ | ___ | _____ |
| 21. Used the transfer belt to help the person stand. | ___ | ___ | _____ |
| 22. Helped the person raise and secure clothing. | ___ | ___ | _____ |
| 23. Used the transfer belt to transfer the person to the wheelchair. (See procedure "Transferring the Person to a Chair or Wheelchair.") | ___ | ___ | _____ |
| 24. Made sure the person's buttocks were to the back of the seat. Positioned the person in good alignment. | ___ | ___ | _____ |
| 25. Positioned the person's feet on the footplates. | ___ | ___ | _____ |
| 26. Covered the person's lap and legs with a lap blanket. Kept the blanket off the floor and wheels. | ___ | ___ | _____ |
| 27. Positioned the chair as the person preferred. Locked the wheelchair wheels according to the care plan. | ___ | ___ | _____ |

### Post-Procedure

| | S | U | Comments |
|---|---|---|---|
| 28. Provided for comfort as noted on the inside of the front book cover. | ___ | ___ | _____ |
| 29. Placed the signal light and other needed items within reach. | ___ | ___ | _____ |
| 30. Unscreened the person. | ___ | ___ | _____ |
| 31. Completed a safety check of the room as noted on the inside of the front book cover. | ___ | ___ | _____ |
| 32. Practiced hand hygiene. | ___ | ___ | _____ |
| 33. Reported and recorded observations. | ___ | ___ | _____ |

Date of Satisfactory Completion _____  Instructor's Initials_____

# Making a Closed Bed

Name: _____     Date: _____

| Quality of Life | S | U | Comments |
|---|---|---|---|
| • Knocked before entering the person's room. | ___ | ___ | _____ |
| • Addressed the person by name. | ___ | ___ | _____ |
| • Introduced yourself by name and title. | ___ | ___ | _____ |
| • Explained the procedure to the person before beginning and during the procedure. | ___ | ___ | _____ |
| • Protected the person's rights during the procedure. | ___ | ___ | _____ |
| • Handled the person gently during the procedure. | ___ | ___ | _____ |

## Pre-Procedure

| | S | U | Comments |
|---|---|---|---|
| 1. Followed "Delegation Guidelines: Making Beds." Reviewed "Promoting Safety and Comfort: Making Beds." | ___ | ___ | _____ |
| 2. Practiced hand hygiene. | ___ | ___ | _____ |
| 3. Collected clean linen: | | | |
|   • Mattress pad (if needed) | ___ | ___ | _____ |
|   • Bottom sheet (flat sheet or fitted sheet) | ___ | ___ | _____ |
|   • Plastic drawsheet or waterproof pad (if needed) | ___ | ___ | _____ |
|   • Cotton drawsheet (if needed) | ___ | ___ | _____ |
|   • Top sheet | ___ | ___ | _____ |
|   • Blanket | ___ | ___ | _____ |
|   • Bedspread | ___ | ___ | _____ |
|   • Two pillowcases | ___ | ___ | _____ |
|   • Bath towel(s) | ___ | ___ | _____ |
|   • Hand towel | ___ | ___ | _____ |
|   • Washcloth | ___ | ___ | _____ |
|   • Gown | ___ | ___ | _____ |
|   • Bath blanket | ___ | ___ | _____ |
|   • Gloves | ___ | ___ | _____ |
|   • Laundry bag | ___ | ___ | _____ |
| 4. Placed linen on a clean surface. | ___ | ___ | _____ |
| 5. Raised the bed for body mechanics. | ___ | ___ | _____ |

## Procedure

| | S | U | Comments |
|---|---|---|---|
| 6. Put on the gloves. | ___ | ___ | _____ |
| 7. Removed linen. Rolled each piece away from you. Placed each piece in a laundry bag. Discarded incontinence products or disposable bed protectors in the trash. Did not put them in the laundry bag. | ___ | ___ | _____ |
| 8. Cleaned the bed frame and mattress if this is part of your job. | ___ | ___ | _____ |

*Continued*

| Procedure—cont'd | S | U | Comments |
|---|---|---|---|
| 9. Removed and discarded the gloves. Decontaminated hands. | _____ | _____ | _____ |
| 10. Moved the mattress to the head of the bed. | _____ | _____ | _____ |
| 11. Put the mattress pad on the mattress. It was even with the top of the mattress. | _____ | _____ | _____ |
| 12. Placed the bottom sheet on the mattress pad. | | | |
|    a. Unfolded it lengthwise. | _____ | _____ | _____ |
|    b. Placed the center crease in the middle of the bed. | _____ | _____ | _____ |
|    c. Positioned the lower edge even with the bottom of the mattress. | _____ | _____ | _____ |
|    d. Placed the large hem at the top and the small hem at the bottom. | _____ | _____ | _____ |
|    e. Faced hem-stitching downward away from the person. | _____ | _____ | _____ |
| 13. Opened the sheet. Fan-folded it to the other side of the bed. | _____ | _____ | _____ |
| 14. Tucked the top of the sheet under the mattress. The sheet was tight and smooth. | _____ | _____ | _____ |
| 15. Made a mitered corner if using a flat sheet. | _____ | _____ | _____ |
| 16. Placed the plastic drawsheet on the bed (in the middle of the mattress). Or placed the waterproof pad on the bed. | _____ | _____ | _____ |
| 17. Opened the plastic drawsheet. Fan-folded it to the other side of the bed. | _____ | _____ | _____ |
| 18. Placed a cotton drawsheet over the plastic drawsheet so it covered the entire plastic drawsheet. | _____ | _____ | _____ |
| 19. Opened the cotton drawsheet. Fan-folded it to the other side of the bed. | _____ | _____ | _____ |
| 20. Tucked both drawsheets under the mattress or tucked each in separately. | _____ | _____ | _____ |
| 21. Went to the other side of the bed. | _____ | _____ | _____ |
| 22. Mitered the top corner of the flat bottom sheet. | _____ | _____ | _____ |
| 23. Pulled the bottom sheet tight so there were no wrinkles. Tucked in the sheet. | _____ | _____ | _____ |
| 24. Pulled the drawsheets tight so there were no wrinkles. Tucked both in together or separately. | _____ | _____ | _____ |
| 25. Went to the other side of the bed. | _____ | _____ | _____ |
| 26. Put the top sheet on the bed. | | | |
|    a. Unfolded it lengthwise. | _____ | _____ | _____ |
|    b. Placed the center crease in the middle. | _____ | _____ | _____ |
|    c. Placed the large hem even with the top of the mattress. | _____ | _____ | _____ |
|    d. Opened the sheet. Fan-folded it to the other side. | _____ | _____ | _____ |
|    e. Faced hem-stitching outward away from the person. | _____ | _____ | _____ |

| Procedure—cont'd | S | U | Comments |
|---|---|---|---|

     f. Did not tuck the bottom in yet. _____ _____ _____

     g. Did not tuck top linens in on the sides. _____ _____ _____

27. Placed the blanket on the bed.

     a. Unfolded it so the center crease was
       in the middle. _____ _____ _____

     b. Put the upper hem about 6 to 8 inches from
       the top of the mattress. _____ _____ _____

     c. Opened the blanket. Fan-folded it to the
       other side. _____ _____ _____

     d. If steps 33 and 34 will be done, turned the top
       sheet down over the blanket. Hem-stitching was
       down, away from the person. _____ _____ _____

28. Placed the bedspread on the bed.

     a. Unfolded it so the center crease was in
       the middle. _____ _____ _____

     b. Placed the upper hem even with the top
       of the mattress. _____ _____ _____

     c. Opened and fan-folded the spread to
       the other side. _____ _____ _____

     d. Made sure the spread facing the door was even.
       It covered all top linens. _____ _____ _____

29. Tucked in top linens together at the foot of the bed.
    They were smooth and tight. Made a mitered corner. _____ _____ _____

30. Went to the other side. _____ _____ _____

31. Straightened all top linen. Worked from the
    head of the bed to the foot. _____ _____ _____

32. Tucked in the top linens together at the foot of
    the bed. Made a mitered corner. _____ _____ _____

33. Turned the top hem of the spread under the blanket
    to make a cuff. _____ _____ _____

34. Turned the top sheet down over the spread.
    Hem-stitching was down. (If steps 33 and 34 were
    not done, the spread covered the pillow and was
    tucked under the pillow.) _____ _____ _____

35. Put the pillowcase on the pillow. Folded extra material
    under the pillow at the seam end of the pillowcase. _____ _____ _____

36. Placed the pillow on the bed. The open end was
    away from the door. The seam was toward the head
    of the bed. _____ _____ _____

## Post-Procedure

37. Provided for comfort as noted on the inside
    of the front book cover. _____ _____ _____

38. Attached the signal light to the bed or placed the signal
    light within the person's reach. _____ _____ _____

*Continued*

| Post-Procedure—cont'd | S | U | Comments |
|---|---|---|---|
| 39. Lowered the bed to its lowest position. Locked the bed wheels. | _____ | _____ | _____ |
| 40. Put towels, washcloth, gown, and bath blanket in the bedside stand. | _____ | _____ | _____ |
| 41. Completed a safety check of the room as noted on the inside of the front book cover. | _____ | _____ | _____ |
| 42. Followed agency policy for dirty linen. | _____ | _____ | _____ |
| 43. Decontaminated hands. | _____ | _____ | _____ |

Date of Satisfactory Completion _____      Instructor's Initials_____

# Making an Occupied Bed (NNAAP™)

Name: _____     Date: _____

| Quality of Life | S | U | Comments |
|---|---|---|---|

- Knocked before entering the person's room.     _____ _____ _____
- Addressed the person by name.     _____ _____ _____
- Introduced yourself by name and title.     _____ _____ _____
- Explained the procedure to the person before beginning and during the procedure.     _____ _____ _____
- Protected the person's rights during the procedure.     _____ _____ _____
- Handled the person gently during the procedure.     _____ _____ _____

## Pre-Procedure

1. Followed "Delegation Guidelines: Making Beds." Reviewed "Promoting Safety and Comfort:     _____ _____ _____
   - Making Beds"     _____ _____ _____
   - The Occupied Bed"     _____ _____ _____
2. Practiced hand hygiene.     _____ _____ _____
3. Collected the following:
   - Gloves     _____ _____ _____
   - Laundry bag     _____ _____ _____
   - Clean linen     _____ _____ _____
4. Placed linen on a clean surface.     _____ _____ _____
5. Identified the person. Checked the ID bracelet against the assignment sheet. Called the person by name.     _____ _____ _____
6. Provided for privacy.     _____ _____ _____
7. Removed the signal light.     _____ _____ _____
8. Raised the bed for body mechanics. Bed rails were up if used.     _____ _____ _____
9. Lowered the head of the bed. It was as flat as possible.     _____ _____ _____

## Procedure

10. Decontaminated hands. Put on gloves.     _____ _____ _____
11. Loosened top linens at the foot of the bed.     _____ _____ _____
12. Removed the bedspread. Then removed the blanket. Placed each over the chair.     _____ _____ _____
13. Covered the person with a bath blanket. Used the bath blanket in the bedside stand.
    a. Unfolded a bath blanket over the top sheet.     _____ _____ _____
    b. Asked the person to hold onto the bath blanket. If the person could not, tucked the top part under the person's shoulders.     _____ _____ _____
14. Lowered the bed rail near you if up.     _____ _____ _____

*Continued*

| Procedure—cont'd | S | U | Comments |
|---|---|---|---|
|    c. Grasped the top sheet under the bath blanket at the shoulders. Brought the sheet down to the foot of the bed. Removed the sheet from under the blanket. | ___ | ___ | _____ |
| 15. Positioned the person on the side of the bed away from you. Adjusted the pillow for comfort. | ___ | ___ | _____ |
| 16. Loosened bottom linens from the head to the foot of the bed. | ___ | ___ | _____ |
| 17. Fan-folded bottom linens one at a time toward the person. Started with the cotton drawsheet. (If reusing the mattress pad, did not fan-fold it.) | ___ | ___ | _____ |
| 18. Placed a clean mattress pad on the bed. Unfolded it lengthwise. The center crease was in the middle. Fan-folded the top part toward the person. (If reusing the mattress pad, straightened and smoothed any wrinkles.) | ___ | ___ | _____ |
| 19. Placed the bottom sheet on the mattress pad. Hem-stitching was away from the person. Unfolded the sheet so the crease was in the middle. The small hem was even with the bottom of the mattress. Fan-folded the top part toward the person. | ___ | ___ | _____ |
| 20. Made a mitered corner at the head of the bed. Tucked the sheet under the mattress from the head to the foot. | ___ | ___ | _____ |
| 21. Pulled the plastic drawsheet toward you over the bottom sheet. Tucked excess material under the mattress. Did the following for a clean plastic drawsheet. | ___ | ___ | _____ |
|    a. Placed the plastic drawsheet on the bed. It was in the middle of the mattress. | ___ | ___ | _____ |
|    b. Fan-folded the top part toward the person. | ___ | ___ | _____ |
|    c. Tucked in the excess fabric. | ___ | ___ | _____ |
| 22. Placed the cotton drawsheet over the plastic drawsheet so it covered the entire plastic drawsheet. Fan-folded the top part toward the person. Tucked in excess fabric. | ___ | ___ | _____ |
| 23. Raised the bed rail if used. Went to the other side and lowered the bed rail. | ___ | ___ | _____ |
| 24. Explained to the person that he or she would roll over a bump. Assured the person that he or she would not fall. | ___ | ___ | _____ |
| 25. Helped the person turn to the other side. Adjusted the pillow for comfort. | ___ | ___ | _____ |
| 26. Loosened bottom linens. Removed one piece at a time. Placed each piece in the laundry bag. Discarded disposable bed protectors and incontinence products in the trash.(Did not put them in the laundry bag.) | ___ | ___ | _____ |
| 27. Removed and discarded the gloves. Decontaminated your hands. | ___ | ___ | _____ |
| 28. Straightened and smoothed the mattress pad. | ___ | ___ | _____ |
| 29. Pulled the clean bottom sheet toward you. Made a mitered corner at the top. Tucked the sheet under the mattress from the head to the foot of the bed. | ___ | ___ | _____ |

| Procedure—cont'd | S | U | Comments |
|---|---|---|---|

30. Pulled the drawsheets tightly toward you. Tucked both under together or separately. _____ _____ _____

31. Positioned the person supine in the center of the bed. Adjusted the pillow for comfort. _____ _____ _____

32. Put the top sheet on the bed. Unfolded it lengthwise. The crease was in the middle. The large hem was even with the top of the mattress. Hem- stitching was on the outside. _____ _____ _____

33. Asked the person to hold onto the top sheet or tucked the top sheet under the person's shoulders. Removed the bath blanket. _____ _____ _____

34. Placed the blanket on the bed. Unfolded it so the crease was in the middle and it covered the person. The upper hem was 6 to 8 inches from the top of the mattress. _____ _____ _____

35. Placed the bedspread on the bed. Unfolded it so the center crease was in the middle and it covered the person. The top hem was even with the mattress top. _____ _____ _____

36. Turned the top hem of the spread under the blanket to make a cuff. _____ _____ _____

37. Brought the top sheet down over the spread to form a cuff. _____ _____ _____

38. Went to the foot of the bed. _____ _____ _____

39. Made a 2-inch toe pleat across the foot of the bed. The pleat was about 6 to 8 inches from the foot of the bed. _____ _____ _____

40. Lifted the mattress corner with one arm. Tucked all top linens under the mattress together. Made a mitered corner. _____ _____ _____

41. Raised the bed rail if used. Went to the other side and lowered the bed rail if used. _____ _____ _____

42. Straightened and smoothed top linens. _____ _____ _____

43. Tucked the top linens under bottom of the mattress. Made a mitered corner. _____ _____ _____

44. Changed the pillowcase(s). _____ _____ _____

## Post-Procedure

45. Provided for comfort as noted on the inside of the front book cover. _____ _____ _____

46. Placed the signal light within reach. _____ _____ _____

47. Lowered the bed to its lowest position. Locked the bed wheels. _____ _____ _____

48. Raised or lowered bed rails. Followed the care plan. _____ _____ _____

49. Put the towels, washcloth, gown, and bath blanket in the bedside stand. _____ _____ _____

50. Unscreened the person. _____ _____ _____

*Continued*

Post-Procedure—cont'd                          S        U              Comments

51. Completed a safety check of the room          _____  _____  _____
    as noted on the inside of the front book cover.

52. Followed agency policy for dirty linen.       _____  _____  _____

53. Decontaminated hands.                         _____  _____  _____

Date of Satisfactory Completion _____    Instructor's Initials_____

# Making a Surgical Bed

Name: _____    Date: _____

| Procedure | S | U | Comments |
|---|---|---|---|

1. Followed "Delegation Guidelines: Making Beds." Reviewed "Promoting Safety and Comfort:
   - Making Beds"
   - Surgical Beds"
2. Practiced hand hygiene.
3. Collected the following:
   - Clean linen
   - Gloves
   - Laundry bag
   - Equipment requested by the nurse
4. Placed linen on a clean surface.
5. Removed the signal light.
6. Raised the bed for body mechanics.
7. Removed all linen from the bed. Wore gloves.
8. Made a closed bed. (See procedure "Making a Closed Bed.") Did not tuck the top linens under the mattress.
9. Folded all top linens at the foot of the bed back onto the bed. The fold was even with the edge of the mattress.
10. Fan-folded linen lengthwise to the side of the bed farthest from the door.
11. Put the pillowcase(s) on the pillow(s).
12. Placed the pillow(s) on a clean surface.
13. Left the bed in its highest position.
14. Left both bed rails down.
15. Put the towels, washcloth, gown, and bath blanket in the bedside stand.
16. Moved furniture away from the bed. Allowed room for the stretcher and for the staff.
17. Did not attach the signal light to the bed.
18. Completed a safety check of the room as noted on the inside of the front book cover.
19. Followed agency policy for soiled linen.
20. Decontaminated hands.

Date of Satisfactory Completion _____    Instructor's Initials _____

# Brushing the Person's Teeth (NNAAP™)

Name: _____    Date: _____

| Quality of Life | S | U | Comments |
|---|---|---|---|

- Knocked before entering the person's room.    _____ _____ _____
- Addressed the person by name.    _____ _____ _____
- Introduced yourself by name and title.    _____ _____ _____
- Explained the procedure to the person
  before beginning and during the procedure.    _____ _____ _____
- Protected the person's rights during the procedure.    _____ _____ _____
- Handled the person gently during the procedure.    _____ _____ _____

## Pre-Procedure

1. Followed "Delegation Guidelines: Oral Hygiene."
   Reviewed "Promoting Safety and Comfort: Oral Hygiene."    _____ _____ _____
2. Practiced hand hygiene.    _____ _____ _____
3. Collected the following:
   - Toothbrush    _____ _____ _____
   - Toothpaste    _____ _____ _____
   - Mouthwash (or other solution noted on the care plan)    _____ _____ _____
   - Dental floss (if used)    _____ _____ _____
   - Water glass with cool water    _____ _____ _____
   - Straw    _____ _____ _____
   - Kidney basin    _____ _____ _____
   - Hand towel    _____ _____ _____
   - Paper towels    _____ _____ _____
   - Gloves    _____ _____ _____
4. Placed the paper towels on the overbed table.
   Arranged items on top of them.    _____ _____ _____
5. Identified the person. Checked the ID bracelet
   against the assignment sheet. Called the person by name.    _____ _____ _____
6. Provided for privacy.    _____ _____ _____
7. Raised the bed for body mechanics.
   Bed rails were up if used.    _____ _____ _____

## Procedure

8. Lowered the bed rail near you if up.    _____ _____ _____
9. Assisted the person to a sitting position or
   to a side-lying position near you.    _____ _____ _____
10. Placed the towel over the person's chest.    _____ _____ _____
11. Adjusted the overbed table so it could
    be reached with ease.    _____ _____ _____
12. Decontaminated hands. Put on the gloves.    _____ _____ _____
13. Held the toothbrush over the kidney basin.
    Poured some water over the brush.    _____ _____ _____

| Procedure—cont'd | S | U | Comments |
|---|---|---|---|

14. Applied toothpaste to the toothbrush. ___ ___ _____

15. Brushed the teeth gently. ___ ___ _____

16. Brushed the tongue gently. ___ ___ _____

17. Let the person rinse the mouth with water. Held the kidney basin under the person's chin. Repeated this step as needed. ___ ___ _____

18. Flossed the person's teeth. (optional) ___ ___ _____

  a. Broke off an 18-inch piece of floss from the dispenser. ___ ___ _____

  b. Held the floss between the middle fingers of each hand. ___ ___ _____

  c. Stretched the floss with your thumbs. ___ ___ _____

  d. Started at the upper back tooth on the right side. Worked around to the left side. ___ ___ _____

  e. Moved the floss gently up and down between the teeth. Moved floss up and down against the sides of each tooth. Worked from the top of the crown to the gum line. ___ ___ _____

  f. Moved to a new section of floss after every second tooth. ___ ___ _____

  g. Flossed the lower teeth. Used up and down motions as for the upper teeth. Started at the right side. Worked around to the left side. ___ ___ _____

19. Let the person use mouthwash or other solution. Held the kidney basin under the chin. ___ ___ _____

20. Wiped the person's mouth and removed the towel. ___ ___ _____

21. Removed and discarded the gloves. Decontaminated hands. ___ ___ _____

## Post-Procedure

22. Provided for comfort as noted on the inside of the front book cover. ___ ___ _____

23. Placed the signal light within reach. ___ ___ _____

24. Lowered the bed to its lowest position. ___ ___ _____

25. Raised or lowered bed rails. Followed the care plan. ___ ___ _____

26. Cleaned and returned equipment to its proper place. Wore gloves. ___ ___ _____

27. Wiped off the overbed table with the paper towels. Discarded the paper towels. ___ ___ _____

28. Removed the gloves. Decontaminated hands. ___ ___ _____

29. Unscreened the person. ___ ___ _____

*Continued*

| Post-Procedure—cont'd | S | U | Comments |
|---|---|---|---|
| 30. Completed a safety check of the room as noted on the inside of the front book cover. | _____ | _____ | _____ |
| 31. Followed agency policy for dirty linen. | _____ | _____ | _____ |
| 32. Decontaminated hands. | _____ | _____ | _____ |
| 33. Reported and recorded observations. | _____ | _____ | _____ |

Date of Satisfactory Completion _____    Instructor's Initials_____

## Providing Mouth Care For the Unconscious Person

Name: _____    Date: _____

| Quality of Life | S | U | Comments |
|---|---|---|---|

- Knocked before entering the person's room.    _____ _____ _____
- Addressed the person by name.    _____ _____ _____
- Introduced yourself by name and title.    _____ _____ _____
- Explained the procedure to the person
  before beginning and during the procedure.    _____ _____ _____
- Protected the person's rights during the procedure.    _____ _____ _____
- Handled the person gently during the procedure.    _____ _____ _____

### Pre-Procedure

1. Followed "Delegation Guidelines: Oral Hygiene."
   Reviewed "Promoting Safety and Comfort:    _____ _____ _____
   - Oral Hygiene"
   - Mouth Care for the Unconscious Person"
2. Practiced hand hygiene.    _____ _____ _____
3. Collected the following:
   - Cleaning agent according to the care plan    _____ _____ _____
   - Sponge swabs    _____ _____ _____
   - Padded tongue blade    _____ _____ _____
   - Water glass with cool water    _____ _____ _____
   - Hand towel    _____ _____ _____
   - Kidney basin    _____ _____ _____
   - Lip lubricant    _____ _____ _____
   - Paper towels    _____ _____ _____
   - Gloves    _____ _____ _____
4. Placed the paper towels on the overbed table.
   Arranged items on top of them.    _____ _____ _____
5. Identified the person. Checked the ID bracelet against
   the assignment sheet. Called the person by name.    _____ _____ _____
6. Provided for privacy.    _____ _____ _____
7. Raised the bed for body mechanics.
   Bed rails were up if used.    _____ _____ _____

### Procedure

8. Lowered the bed rail near you if up.    _____ _____ _____
9. Decontaminated hands. Put on the gloves.    _____ _____ _____
10. Positioned the person in a side-lying position near you.
    Turned the person's head well to the side.    _____ _____ _____
11. Placed the towel under the person's face.    _____ _____ _____
12. Placed the kidney basin under the chin.    _____ _____ _____

*Continued*

| Procedure—cont'd | S | U | Comments |
|---|---|---|---|
| 13. Separated the upper and lower teeth. Used the padded tongue blade. Was gentle. Never used force. Asked the nurse for help as needed. | | | |
| 14. Cleaned the mouth using sponge swabs moistened with the cleaning agent. | | | |
|    a. Cleaned the chewing and inner surfaces of the teeth. | | | |
|    b. Cleaned the gums and outer surfaces of the teeth. | | | |
|    c. Swabbed the roof of the mouth, inside of the cheeks, and the lips. | | | |
|    d. Swabbed the tongue. | | | |
|    e. Moistened a clean swab with water. Swabbed the mouth to rinse. | | | |
|    f. Placed used swabs in the kidney basin. | | | |
| 15. Applied lubricant to the lips. | | | |
| 16. Removed the kidney basin and supplies. | | | |
| 17. Wiped the person's mouth. Removed the towel. | | | |
| 18. Removed and discarded the gloves. Decontaminated hands. | | | |

## Post-Procedure

| | S | U | Comments |
|---|---|---|---|
| 19. Provided for comfort as noted on the inside of the front book cover. | | | |
| 20. Placed the signal light within reach. | | | |
| 21. Lowered the bed to its lowest position. | | | |
| 22. Raised or lowered the bed rails. Followed the care plan. | | | |
| 23. Cleaned and returned equipment to its proper place. Discarded disposable items. (Wore gloves.) | | | |
| 24. Wiped off the overbed table with paper towels. Discarded the paper towels. | | | |
| 25. Removed the gloves. Decontaminated hands. | | | |
| 26. Unscreened the person. | | | |
| 27. Completed a safety check of the room as noted on the inside of the front book cover. | | | |
| 28. Told the person that you were leaving the room. Told him or her when you would return. | | | |
| 29. Followed agency policy for dirty linen. | | | |
| 30. Decontaminated hands. | | | |
| 31. Reported and recorded observations. | | | |

Date of Satisfactory Completion _____      Instructor's Initials_____

## Providing Denture Care (NNAAP™)

Name: _____     Date: _____

| Quality of Life | S | U | Comments |
|---|---|---|---|

- Knocked before entering the person's room.
- Addressed the person by name.
- Introduced yourself by name and title.
- Explained the procedure to the person before beginning and during the procedure.
- Protected the person's rights during the procedure.
- Handled the person gently during the procedure.

### Pre-Procedure

1. Followed "Delegation Guidelines: Oral Hygiene." Reviewed "Promoting Safety and Comfort:
   - Oral Hygiene"
   - Denture Care"
2. Practiced hand hygiene.
3. Collected the following:
   - Denture brush or toothbrush for cleaning dentures
   - Denture cup labeled with the person's name and room number
   - Denture cleaning agent
   - Soft-bristle toothbrush or sponge swabs for oral hygiene
   - Toothpaste
   - Water glass with cool water
   - Straw
   - Mouthwash or other noted solution
   - Kidney basin
   - Two hand towels
   - Gauze squares
   - Paper towels
   - Gloves
4. Placed the paper towels on the overbed table. Arranged items on top of them.
5. Identified the person. Checked the ID bracelet against the assignment sheet. Called the person by name.
6. Provided for privacy.
7. Raised the bed for body mechanics.

### Procedure

8. Lowered the bed rail near you if used.
9. Decontaminated hands. Put on the gloves.
10. Placed a towel over the person's chest.

*Continued*

| Procedure—cont'd | S | U | Comments |
|---|---|---|---|

11. Asked the person to remove the dentures. Carefully placed them in the kidney basin. _____ _____ _____

12. Removed the dentures if the person could not do so. Used gauze squares to get a good grip on the dentures. _____ _____ _____

   a. Grasped the upper denture with the thumb and index finger. Moved it up and down slightly to break the seal. Gently removed the denture. Placed it in the kidney basin. _____ _____ _____

   b. Grasped and removed the lower denture with your thumb and index finger. Turned it slightly and lifted it out of the mouth. Placed it in the kidney basin. _____ _____ _____

13. Followed the care plan for raising bed rails. _____ _____ _____

14. Took the kidney basin, denture cup, denture brush, and cleaning agent to the sink. _____ _____ _____

15. Lined the sink with a towel. Filled the sink halfway with water. _____ _____ _____

16. Rinsed each denture under warm running water. (Some states require cool water.) _____ _____ _____

17. Returned dentures to the kidney basin. _____ _____ _____

18. Applied the denture cleaning agent to the brush. _____ _____ _____

19. Brushed the dentures. _____ _____ _____

20. Rinsed dentures under running water. Used warm or cool water as directed by the cleaning agent manufacturer (Some state competency tests require cool water.) _____ _____ _____

21. Rinsed the denture cup. Placed dentures in the denture cup. Covered the dentures with cool water. _____ _____ _____

22. Cleaned the kidney basin. _____ _____ _____

23. Took the denture cup and kidney basin to the bedside table. _____ _____ _____

24. Lowered the bed rail if up. _____ _____ _____

25. Positioned the person for oral hygiene. _____ _____ _____

26. Cleaned the person's gums and tongue. Used toothpaste and the toothbrush or sponge swab. _____ _____ _____

27. Had the person use mouthwash or noted solution. Held the kidney basin under the chin. _____ _____ _____

28. Asked the person to insert the dentures. Inserted them if the person could not. _____ _____ _____

   a. Held the upper denture firmly with your thumb and index finger. Raised the upper lip with the other hand. Inserted the denture. Gently pressed on the denture with your index fingers to make sure it was in place. _____ _____ _____

   b. Held the lower denture with your thumb and index finger. Pulled the lower lip down slightly. Inserted the denture. Gently pressed down on it to make sure it was in place. _____ _____ _____

| Procedure—cont'd | S | U | Comments |
|---|---|---|---|
| 29. Placed the denture cup in the top drawer of the bedside stand if the dentures were not worn. The dentures were in water or in a denture soaking solution. | _____ | _____ | _____ |
| 30. Wiped the person's mouth. Removed the towel. | _____ | _____ | _____ |
| 31. Removed the gloves. Decontaminated hands. | _____ | _____ | _____ |

## Post-Procedure

| | S | U | Comments |
|---|---|---|---|
| 29. Assisted with hand washing. | _____ | _____ | _____ |
| 30. Provided for comfort as noted on the inside of the front book cover. | _____ | _____ | _____ |
| 31. Placed the signal light within reach. | _____ | _____ | _____ |
| 32. Raised or lowered bed rails. Followed the care plan. | _____ | _____ | _____ |
| 33. Unscreened the person. | _____ | _____ | _____ |
| 34. Cleaned and returned equipment to its proper place. Discarded disposable items. Wore gloves for this step. | _____ | _____ | _____ |
| 35. Completed a safety check of the room as noted on the inside of the front book cover. | _____ | _____ | _____ |
| 36. Followed agency policy for dirty linen. | _____ | _____ | _____ |
| 37. Decontaminated hands. | _____ | _____ | _____ |
| 38. Reported and recorded observations. | _____ | _____ | _____ |

Date of Satisfactory Completion _____ Instructor's Initials_____

# Giving a Complete Bed Bath (NNAAP™)

Name: _____    Date: _____

| Quality of Life | S | U | Comments |
|---|---|---|---|

- Knocked before entering the person's room.          _____ _____ _____
- Addressed the person by name.          _____ _____ _____
- Introduced yourself by name and title.          _____ _____ _____
- Explained the procedure to the person before beginning and during the procedure.          _____ _____ _____
- Protected the person's rights during the procedure.          _____ _____ _____
- Handled the person gently during the procedure.          _____ _____ _____

## Pre-Procedure

1. Followed "Delegation Guidelines: Bathing." Reviewed "Promoting Safety and Comfort: Bathing."          _____ _____ _____
2. Practiced hand hygiene.          _____ _____ _____
3. Identified the person. Checked the ID bracelet against the assignment sheet. Called the person by name.          _____ _____ _____
4. Collected clean linen for a closed bed. Placed linen on a clean surface.          _____ _____ _____
5. Collected the following:
   - Wash basin          _____ _____ _____
   - Soap          _____ _____ _____
   - Bath thermometer          _____ _____ _____
   - Orange stick or nail file          _____ _____ _____
   - Washcloth          _____ _____ _____
   - Two bath towels and two hand towels          _____ _____ _____
   - Bath blanket          _____ _____ _____
   - Clothing, gown, or pajamas          _____ _____ _____
   - Lotion          _____ _____ _____
   - Powder          _____ _____ _____
   - Deodorant or antiperspirant          _____ _____ _____
   - Brush and comb          _____ _____ _____
   - Other grooming items if requested          _____ _____ _____
   - Paper towels          _____ _____ _____
   - Gloves          _____ _____ _____
6. Covered the overbed table with paper towels. Arranged items on the overbed table. Adjusted the height as needed.          _____ _____ _____
7. Provided for privacy.          _____ _____ _____
8. Raised the bed for body mechanics. Bed rails were up if used.          _____ _____ _____

| Procedure | S | U | Comments |
|---|---|---|---|
| 9. Removed the signal light. | ____ | ____ | _____ |
| 10. Decontaminated hands. Put on gloves. | ____ | ____ | _____ |
| 11. Covered the person with a bath blanket. Removed top linens. (See procedure "Making an Occupied Bed.") | ____ | ____ | _____ |
| 12. Lowered the head of the bed. It was as flat as possible. The person had at least one pillow. | ____ | ____ | _____ |
| 13. Filled the wash basin two-thirds full with water. Measured water temperature. Used a bath thermometer or tested the water by dipping your elbow or inner wrist into the basin. | ____ | ____ | _____ |
| 14. Placed the basin on the overbed table. | ____ | ____ | _____ |
| 15. Lowered the bed rail if up. | ____ | ____ | _____ |
| 16. Placed a hand towel over the person's chest. | ____ | ____ | _____ |
| 17. Made a mitt with the washcloth. Used a mitt for the entire bath. | ____ | ____ | _____ |
| 18. Washed around the person's eyes with water. Did not use soap. Gently wiped from the inner to the outer aspect of the eye with a corner of the mitt. Cleaned around the far eye first. Repeated this step for the near eye. Used a clean part of the washcloth for each stroke. | ____ | ____ | _____ |
| 19. Asked the person if you should use soap to wash the face. | ____ | ____ | _____ |
| 20. Washed the face, ears, and neck. Rinsed and patted dry with the towel on the chest. | ____ | ____ | _____ |
| 21. Helped the person move to the side of the bed near you. | ____ | ____ | _____ |
| 22. Removed the gown. Did not expose the person. | ____ | ____ | _____ |
| 23. Placed a bath towel lengthwise under the far arm. | ____ | ____ | _____ |
| 24. Supported the arm with your palm under the person's elbow. The person's forearm rested on your forearm. | ____ | ____ | _____ |
| 25. Washed the arm, shoulder, and underarm. Used long, firm strokes. Rinsed and patted dry. | ____ | ____ | _____ |
| 26. Placed the basin on the towel. Put the person's hand into the water. Washed it well. Cleaned under fingernails with an orange stick or nail file. | ____ | ____ | _____ |
| 27. Had the person exercise the hand and fingers. | ____ | ____ | _____ |
| 28. Removed the basin. Dried the hand well. Covered the arm with the bath blanket. | ____ | ____ | _____ |
| 29. Repeated steps 23 to 38 for the near arm. | ____ | ____ | _____ |
| 30. Placed a bath towel over the chest crosswise. Held the towel in place. Pulled the bath blanket from under the towel to the waist. | ____ | ____ | _____ |
| 31. Lifted the towel slightly and washed the chest. Did not expose the person. Rinsed and patted dry especially under breasts. | ____ | ____ | _____ |
| 32. Moved the towel lengthwise over the chest and abdomen. Did not expose the person. Pulled the bath blanket down to the pubic area. | ____ | ____ | _____ |

*Continued*

Procedure—cont'd                                    S        U        Comments

33. Lifted the towel slightly and washed the          _____  _____  _____
    abdomen. Rinsed and patted dry.

34. Pulled the bath blanket up to the shoulders       _____  _____  _____
    covering both arms. Removed the towel.

35. Changed soapy or cool water. Measured bath water  _____  _____  _____
    as in step 13. If bed rails were used, raised the bed rail
    near you before leaving the bedside. Lowered it when
    you returned.

36. Uncovered the far leg. Did not expose the genital area.   _____  _____  _____
    Placed a towel lengthwise under the foot and leg.

37. Bent the knee and supported the leg with your arm.   _____  _____  _____
    Washed it with long, firm strokes. Rinsed and patted dry.

38. Placed the basin on the towel near the foot.      _____  _____  _____

39. Lifted the leg slightly. Slid the basin under the foot.   _____  _____  _____

40. Placed the foot in the basin. Used an orange stick or nail   _____  _____  _____
    file to clean under toenails if necessary. If the person
    could not bend the knees:

    a. Washed the foot. Carefully separated             _____  _____  _____
       the toes. Rinsed and patted dry.

    b. Cleaned under the toenails with an               _____  _____  _____
       orange stick or nail file if necessary.

41. Removed the basin. Dried the leg and foot. Applied   _____  _____  _____
    lotion to the foot as directed by the nurse and the
    care plan. Covered the leg with the bath blanket.
    Removed the towel.

42. Repeated steps 36 to 41 for the near leg.         _____  _____  _____

43. Changed the water. Measured water temperature     _____  _____  _____
    as in step 13. If bed rails were used, raised the bed
    rail near you before leaving the bedside. Lowered it
    when you returned.

44. Turned the person onto the side away from you.    _____  _____  _____
    The person was covered with the bath blanket.

45. Uncovered the back and buttocks. Did not expose   _____  _____  _____
    the person. Placed a towel lengthwise on the bed
    along the back.

46. Washed the back. Worked from the back of the neck   _____  _____  _____
    to the lower end of the buttocks. Used long, firm,
    continuous strokes. Rinsed and dried well.

47. Gave a back massage. Unless the person wanted     _____  _____  _____
    a back massage after the bath.

48. Turned the person onto his or her back.           _____  _____  _____

49. Changed the water for perineal care. Measured water   _____  _____  _____
    temperature as in step 13. (Some state competency tests
    also require changing gloves and hand hygiene at
    this time.) If bed rails were used, raised the bed rail
    near you before leaving the bedside. Lowered it
    when you returned.

| Procedure—cont'd | S | U | Comments |
|---|---|---|---|

50. Let the person wash the genital area. Adjusted the overbed table so the person could reach the wash basin, soap, and towels with ease. Placed the signal light within reach. Asked the person to signal when finished. Made sure the person understood what to do.

51. Removed the gloves. Decontaminated hands.

52. Answered the signal light promptly. Provided perineal care if the person could not do so. Decontaminated hands and wore gloves for perineal care.

53. Gave a back massage if you had not already done so.

54. Applied deodorant or antiperspirant. Applied lotion and powder as requested.

55. Put clean garments on the person.

56. Combed and brushed the hair.

57. Made the bed.

## Post-Procedure

58. Provided for comfort as noted on the inside of the front book cover.

59. Placed the signal light within reach.

60. Lowered the bed to its lowest position.

61. Raised or lower bed rails. Followed the care plan.

62. Emptied and cleaned the wash basin. Returned it and other supplies to their proper place.

63. Wiped off the overbed table with the paper towels. Discarded the paper towels.

64. Unscreened the person.

65. Completed a safety check of the room as noted on the inside of the front book cover.

66. Followed agency policy for dirty linen.

67. Decontaminated hands.

68. Reported and recorded observations.

Date of Satisfactory Completion _____  Instructor's Initials_____

# Giving a Partial Bath

Name: _____  Date: _____

| Quality of Life | S | U | Comments |
|---|---|---|---|

- Knocked before entering the person's room.  _____ _____ _____
- Addressed the person by name.  _____ _____ _____
- Introduced yourself by name and title.  _____ _____ _____
- Explained the procedure to the person before beginning and during the procedure.  _____ _____ _____
- Protected the person's rights during the procedure.  _____ _____ _____
- Handled the person gently during the procedure.  _____ _____ _____

## Pre-Procedure

1. Followed "Delegation Guidelines: Bathing." Reviewed "Promoting Safety and Comfort: Bathing."  _____ _____ _____
2. Follow steps 2 through 7 in procedure "Giving a Complete Bed Bath."  _____ _____ _____

## Procedure

3. Made sure the bed was in the lowest position.  _____ _____ _____
4. Removed top linen. Covered the person with a bath blanket.  _____ _____ _____
5. Filled the wash basin with water. (Water was 110° to 115° F [43.3° to 46.1° C] or as directed by the nurse.) Measured water temperature with the bath thermometer or tested bath water by dipping your elbow or inner wrist into the basin.  _____ _____ _____
6. Placed the basin on the overbed table.  _____ _____ _____
7. Positioned the person in Fowler's position or assisted the person to sit at the bedside.  _____ _____ _____
8. Adjusted the overbed table so the person could reach the basin and supplies.  _____ _____ _____
9. Helped the person undress. Provided for privacy and warmth with the bath blanket.  _____ _____ _____
10. Asked the person to wash easy to reach body parts. Explained that you would wash the back and areas the person could not reach.  _____ _____ _____
11. Placed the signal light within reach. Asked the person to signal when help was needed or bathing was complete.  _____ _____ _____
12. Left the room after decontaminating hands.  _____ _____ _____
13. Returned when the signal light was on. Knocked before entering. Decontaminated hands.  _____ _____ _____
14. Changed the bath water. Measured bath water temperature as in step 5.  _____ _____ _____

Procedure—cont'd                                              S        U              Comments

15. Raised the bed for body mechanics.                    _____  _____  _____
    The far bed rail was up if used.

16. Asked what was washed. Put on gloves. Washed          _____  _____  _____
    and dried areas the person could not reach. The face,
    hands, underarms, back, buttocks, and perineal area
    were washed.

17. Removed the gloves. Decontaminated hands.             _____  _____  _____

18. Gave a back massage.                                  _____  _____  _____

19. Applied lotion, powder, and deodorant                 _____  _____  _____
    or antiperspirant as requested.

20. Helped the person put on clean garments.              _____  _____  _____

21. Assisted with hair care and other grooming needs.     _____  _____  _____

22. Assisted the person to a chair. (Lowered the bed      _____  _____  _____
    if the person transferred to a chair.) Otherwise, turned
    the person onto the side away from you.

23. Made the bed. (Raised the bed for body mechanics.)    _____  _____  _____

Post-Procedure

24. Provided for comfort as noted on the                  _____  _____  _____
    inside of the front book cover.

25. Placed the signal light within reach.                 _____  _____  _____

26. Lowered the bed to its lowest position.               _____  _____  _____

27. Raised or lowered bed rails. Followed the care plan.  _____  _____  _____

28. Emptied and cleaned the basin. Returned the           _____  _____  _____
    basin and supplies to their proper place.

29. Wiped off the overbed table with the paper            _____  _____  _____
    towels. Discarded the paper towels.

30. Unscreened the person.                                _____  _____  _____

31. Completed a safety check of the room as               _____  _____  _____
    noted on the inside of the front book cover.

32. Followed agency policy for dirty linen.               _____  _____  _____

33. Decontaminated hands.                                 _____  _____  _____

34. Reported and recorded observations.                   _____  _____  _____

Date of Satisfactory Completion _____    Instructor's Initials_____

# Assisting With a Tub Bath or Shower

Name: _____        Date: _____

| Quality of Life | S | U | Comments |
|---|---|---|---|

- Knocked before entering the person's room.    _____ _____ _____
- Addressed the person by name.    _____ _____ _____
- Introduced yourself by name and title.    _____ _____ _____
- Explained the procedure to the person before beginning and during the procedure.    _____ _____ _____
- Protected the person's rights during the procedure.    _____ _____ _____
- Handled the person gently during the procedure.    _____ _____ _____

## Pre-Procedure

1. "Followed "Delegation Guidelines:
   - "Bathing"
   - "Tub baths and showers"    _____ _____ _____
   Reviewed "Promoting Safety and Comfort:
   - "Bathing"
   - "Tub Baths and Showers"    _____ _____ _____
2. Reserved the bathtub or shower.    _____ _____ _____
3. Practiced hand hygiene.    _____ _____ _____
4. Identified the person. Checked the ID bracelet against the assignment sheet. Called the person by name.    _____ _____ _____
5. Collected the following:
   - Washcloth and two bath towels    _____ _____ _____
   - Soap    _____ _____ _____
   - Bath thermometer (for a tub bath)    _____ _____ _____
   - Clothing, gown, or pajamas    _____ _____ _____
   - Grooming items as requested    _____ _____ _____
   - Robe and non-skid footwear    _____ _____ _____
   - Rubber bath mat if needed    _____ _____ _____
   - Disposable bath mat    _____ _____ _____
   - Gloves    _____ _____ _____
   - Wheelchair or shower chair    _____ _____ _____

## Procedure

6. Placed items in the tub or shower room. Used the space provided or a chair.    _____ _____ _____
7. Cleaned and disinfected the tub or shower.    _____ _____ _____
8. Placed a rubber bath mat in the tub or on the shower floor. Did not block the drain.    _____ _____ _____
9. Placed the disposable bath mat on the floor in front of the tub or shower.    _____ _____ _____
10. Put the "Occupied" sign on the door.    _____ _____ _____

| Procedure—cont'd | S | U | Comments |
|---|---|---|---|

11. Returned to the person's room. Provided for privacy.    _____ _____ _____

12. Helped the person sit on the side of the bed.    _____ _____ _____

13. Helped the person put on a robe and non-skid footwear.    _____ _____ _____

14. Assisted or transported the person to the tub or shower room.    _____ _____ _____

15. Had the person sit on a chair. If he or she walked into the tub room or shower.    _____ _____ _____

16. Provided for privacy.    _____ _____ _____

17. For a tub bath:
    a. Filled the tub halfway with warm water (105° F; 40.5° C).    _____ _____ _____
    b. Measured water temperature with the bath thermometer or checked the digital display.    _____ _____ _____

18. For a shower:
    a. Turned on the shower.    _____ _____ _____
    b. Adjusted water temperature and pressure. Checked the digital display.    _____ _____ _____

19. Helped the person undress and remove footwear.    _____ _____ _____

20. Helped the person into the tub or shower. Positioned the shower chair, and locked the wheels.    _____ _____ _____

21. Assisted with washing if necessary. Wore gloves.    _____ _____ _____

22. Asked the person to use the signal light when done or when help was needed. Reminded the person that a tub bath lasts no longer than 20 minutes.    _____ _____ _____

23. Placed a towel across the chair.    _____ _____ _____

24. Left the room if the person could bathe alone. If not, stayed in the room or remained nearby. Removed the gloves and decontaminated hands if you left the room.    _____ _____ _____

25. Checked the person every 5 minutes.    _____ _____ _____

26. Returned when the person signaled. Knocked before entering.    _____ _____ _____

27. Turned off the shower or drained the tub. Covered the person while the tub drained.    _____ _____ _____

28. Helped the person out of the tub or shower and onto the chair.    _____ _____ _____

29. Helped the person dry off. Patted gently. Dried under breasts, between skin folds, in the perineal area, and between the toes.    _____ _____ _____

30. Assisted with lotion and other grooming items as needed.    _____ _____ _____

31. Helped the person dress and put on footwear.    _____ _____ _____

32. Helped the person return to the room. Provided for privacy.    _____ _____ _____

33. Assisted the person to a chair or into bed.    _____ _____ _____

34. Provided a back massage if the person returned to bed.    _____ _____ _____

35. Assisted with hair care and other grooming needs.    _____ _____ _____

*Continued*

| Post-Procedure | S | U | Comments |
|---|---|---|---|
| 36. Provided for comfort as noted on the inside of the front book cover. | _____ | _____ | _____ |
| 37. Placed the signal light within reach. | _____ | _____ | _____ |
| 38. Raised or lowered bed rails. Followed the care plan. | _____ | _____ | _____ |
| 39. Unscreened the person. | _____ | _____ | _____ |
| 40. Completed safety check of the room as noted on the inside of the front book cover. | _____ | _____ | _____ |
| 41. Cleaned and disinfected the tub or shower. Removed soiled linen. Wore gloves for this step. | _____ | _____ | _____ |
| 42. Discarded disposable items. Put the "UNOCCUPIED" sign on the door. Returned supplies to their proper place. | _____ | _____ | _____ |
| 43. Followed agency policy for dirty linen. | _____ | _____ | _____ |
| 44. Decontaminated hands. | _____ | _____ | _____ |
| 45. Reported and recorded observations. | _____ | _____ | _____ |

Date of Satisfactory Completion _____    Instructor's Initials_____

# Giving a Back Massage

Name: _____    Date: _____

| Quality of Life | S | U | Comments |
|---|---|---|---|

- Knocked before entering the person's room.
- Addressed the person by name.
- Introduced yourself by name and title.
- Explained the procedure to the person before beginning and during the procedure.
- Protected the person's rights during the procedure.
- Handled the person gently during the procedure.

## Pre-Procedure

1. Followed "Delegation Guidelines: Back Massage." Reviewed "Promoting Safety and Comfort: Back Massage."
2. Practiced hand hygiene.
3. Identified the person. Checked the ID bracelet against the assignment sheet. Called the person by name.
4. Collected the following:
   - Bath blanket
   - Bath towel
   - Lotion
5. Provided for privacy.
6. Raised the bed for body mechanics. Bed rails were up if used.

## Procedure

7. Lowered the bed rail near you if up.
8. Positioned the person in the prone or side-lying position with the back toward you.
9. Exposed the back, shoulders, upper arms, and buttocks. Covered the rest of the body with the bath blanket.
10. Laid the towel on the bed along the back. (If the person was in the side-lying position.)
11. Warmed the lotion.
12. Explained that the lotion may feel cool and wet.
13. Applied lotion to the lower back area.
14. Stroked up from the buttocks to the shoulders. Then stroked down over the upper arms. Stroked up the upper arms, across the shoulders, and down the back to the buttocks. Used firm strokes. Kept hands in contact with the person's skin.

*Continued*

| Procedure—cont'd | S | U | Comments |
|---|---|---|---|
| 15. Repeated Step 14 for at least 3 minutes. | _____ | _____ | _____ |
| 16. Kneaded by grasping skin between your thumb and fingers. Kneaded half of the back. Started at the buttocks and move up to the shoulder. Then kneaded down from the shoulder to the buttocks. Repeated on the other half of the back. | _____ | _____ | _____ |
| 17. Applied lotion to bony areas. Used circular motions with the tips of your index and middle fingers. (Did not massage reddened bony areas.) | _____ | _____ | _____ |
| 18. Used fast movements to stimulate. Used slow movements to relax the person. | _____ | _____ | _____ |
| 19. Stroked with long, firm movements to end the massage. Told the person you were finishing. | _____ | _____ | _____ |
| 20. Covered the person. Removed the towel and bath blanket. | _____ | _____ | _____ |

## Post-Procedure

| | S | U | Comments |
|---|---|---|---|
| 21. Provided for comfort as noted on the inside of the front book cover. | _____ | _____ | _____ |
| 22. Placed the signal light within reach. | _____ | _____ | _____ |
| 23. Lowered the bed to its lowest position. | _____ | _____ | _____ |
| 24. Raised or lowered bed rails. Followed the care plan. | _____ | _____ | _____ |
| 25. Returned lotion to its proper place. | _____ | _____ | _____ |
| 26. Unscreened the person. | _____ | _____ | _____ |
| 27. Completed a safety check of the room as noted on the inside of the front book cover. | _____ | _____ | _____ |
| 28. Followed agency policy for dirty linen. | _____ | _____ | _____ |
| 29. Decontaminated hands. | _____ | _____ | _____ |
| 30. Reported and recorded observations. | _____ | _____ | _____ |

Date of Satisfactory Completion _____    Instructor's Initials_____

# Giving Female Perineal Care (NNAAP™)

Name: _____    Date: _____

| Quality of Life | S | U | Comments |
|---|---|---|---|

- Knocked before entering the person's room.  _____ _____ _____
- Addressed the person by name.  _____ _____ _____
- Introduced yourself by name and title.  _____ _____ _____
- Explained the procedure to the person before beginning and during the procedure.  _____ _____ _____
- Protected the person's rights during the procedure.  _____ _____ _____
- Handled the person gently during the procedure.  _____ _____ _____

## Pre-Procedure

1. Followed "Delegation Guidelines: Perineal Care." Reviewed "Promoting Safety and Comfort: Perineal Care."  _____ _____ _____
2. Practiced hand hygiene.  _____ _____ _____
3. Collected the following:
   - Soap or other cleaning agent as directed.  _____ _____ _____
   - At least 4 washcloths  _____ _____ _____
   - Bath towel  _____ _____ _____
   - Bath blanket  _____ _____ _____
   - Bath thermometer  _____ _____ _____
   - Wash basin  _____ _____ _____
   - Waterproof pad  _____ _____ _____
   - Gloves  _____ _____ _____
   - Paper towels  _____ _____ _____
4. Covered the overbed table with paper towels. Arranged items on top of them.  _____ _____ _____
5. Identified the person. Checked the ID bracelet against the assignment sheet. Called her by name.  _____ _____ _____
6. Provided for privacy.  _____ _____ _____
7. Raised the bed for body mechanics. Bed rails were up if used.  _____ _____ _____

## Procedure

8. Lowered the bed rail near you if up.  _____ _____ _____
9. Decontaminated hands. Put on gloves.  _____ _____ _____
10. Covered the person with a bath blanket. Moved top linens to the foot of the bed.  _____ _____ _____
11. Positioned the person on her back.  _____ _____ _____
12. Draped her.  _____ _____ _____
13. Raised the bed rail if used.  _____ _____ _____
14. Filled the wash basin. (Water was about 105° to 109° F [40.5° to 42.7° C]). Measured water temperature according to agency policy.  _____ _____ _____

*Continued*

| Procedure—cont'd | S | U | Comments |
|---|---|---|---|

15. Placed the basin on the overbed table.

16. Lowered the bed rail if up.

17. Helped the person flex her knees and spread her legs, or helped her spread her legs as much as possible with her knees straight.

18. Placed a waterproof pad under her buttocks.

19. Folded the corner of the bath blanket between her legs onto her abdomen.

20. Wet the washcloths.

21. Squeezed out excess water from a washcloth. Made a mitted washcloth. Applied soap.

22. Separated the labia. Cleaned downward from front to back with one stroke.

23. Repeated steps 21 and 22 until the area was clean. Used a clean part of the washcloth for each stroke. Used more than one washcloth if needed.

24. Rinsed the perineum with a clean washcloth. Separated the labia. Stroked downward from front to back. Repeated as necessary. Used a clean part of the washcloth for each stroke. Used more than one washcloth if needed.

25. Patted the area dry with the towel. Dried from front to back.

26. Folded the blanket back between her legs.

27. Helped the person lower her legs and turn onto her side away from you.

28. Applied soap to a mitted washcloth.

29. Cleaned the rectal area. Cleaned from the vagina to the anus with one stroke.

30. Repeated steps 28 and 29 until the area was clean. Used a clean part of the washcloth for each stroke. Used more than one washcloth if needed.

31. Rinsed the rectal area with a washcloth. Stroked from the vagina to the anus. Repeated as necessary. Used a clean part of the washcloth for each stroke. Used more than one washcloth if needed.

32. Patted the area dry with the towel. Dried from front to back.

33. Removed the waterproof pad.

34. Provided clean and dry linens and incontinence products as needed.

35. Removed and discarded the gloves. Decontaminated hands.

## Post-Procedure

36. Covered the person. Removed the bath blanket.

37. Provided for comfort as noted on the inside of the front book cover.

38. Placed the signal light within reach.          \_\_\_\_\_  \_\_\_\_\_  _____

39. Lowered the bed to its lowest position.        \_\_\_\_\_  \_\_\_\_\_  _____

40. Raised or lowered bed rails. Followed the care plan.   \_\_\_\_\_  \_\_\_\_\_  _____

41. Emptied and cleaned the wash basin. Wore gloves.   \_\_\_\_\_  \_\_\_\_\_  _____

42. Returned the basin and supplies to their proper place.   \_\_\_\_\_  \_\_\_\_\_  _____

43. Wiped off the overbed table with the paper towels. Discarded the paper towels.   \_\_\_\_\_  \_\_\_\_\_  _____

44. Removed the gloves. Decontaminated hands.      \_\_\_\_\_  \_\_\_\_\_  _____

45. Unscreened the person.                          \_\_\_\_\_  \_\_\_\_\_  _____

46. Completed a safety check of the room as noted on the inside of the front book cover.   \_\_\_\_\_  \_\_\_\_\_  _____

47. Followed agency policy for dirty linen.        \_\_\_\_\_  \_\_\_\_\_  _____

48. Decontaminated hands.                           \_\_\_\_\_  \_\_\_\_\_  _____

49. Reported and recorded observations.            \_\_\_\_\_  \_\_\_\_\_  _____

Date of Satisfactory Completion _____     Instructor's Initials_____

# Giving Male Perineal Care (NNAAP™)

Name: _____    Date: _____

| Quality of Life | S | U | Comments |
|---|---|---|---|

- Knocked before entering the person's room.     _____ _____ _____
- Addressed the person by name.     _____ _____ _____
- Introduced yourself by name and title.     _____ _____ _____
- Explained the procedure to the person before beginning and during the procedure.     _____ _____ _____
- Protected the person's rights during the procedure.     _____ _____ _____
- Handled the person gently during the procedure.     _____ _____ _____

## Procedure

1. Followed steps 1 through 16 in procedure "Giving Female Perineal Care." Draped the person for male perineal care.     _____ _____ _____

2. Retracted the foreskin if the person was uncircumcised.     _____ _____ _____

3. Grasped the penis.     _____ _____ _____

4. Cleaned the tip. Used a circular motion. Started at the meatus of the urethra, and worked outward. Repeated as needed. Used a clean part of the washcloth each time.     _____ _____ _____

5. Rinsed the area with another washcloth.     _____ _____ _____

6. Returned the foreskin to its natural position.     _____ _____ _____

7. Cleaned the shaft of the penis. Used firm downward strokes. Rinsed the area.     _____ _____ _____

8. Helped the person flex his knees and his legs, or helped him spread his legs as much as possible with his knees straight.     _____ _____ _____

9. Cleaned the scrotum. Rinsed well. Observed for redness and irritation in the skin folds.     _____ _____ _____

10. Patted dry the penis and scrotum. Used the towel.     _____ _____ _____

11. Folded the bath blanket back between his legs.     _____ _____ _____

12. Helped him lower his legs and turn onto his side away from you.     _____ _____ _____

13. Cleaned the rectal area. (See procedure "Giving Female Perineal Care.") Rinsed and dried well.     _____ _____ _____

| Procedure—cont'd | S | U | Comments |
|---|---|---|---|
| 14. Removed the waterproof pad. | _____ | _____ | _____ |
| 15. Provided clean and dry linens and incontinence products as needed. | _____ | _____ | _____ |
| 16. Removed and discarded the gloves. Decontaminated hands. | _____ | _____ | _____ |

## Post-Procedure

| | | | |
|---|---|---|---|
| 17. Followed steps 37 through 49 in procedure "Giving Female Perineal Care." | _____ | _____ | _____ |

Date of Satisfactory Completion _____  Instructor's Initials_____

# Brushing and Combing the Person's Hair

Name: _____    Date: _____

| Quality of Life | S | U | Comments |
|---|---|---|---|

- Knocked before entering the person's room.
- Addressed the person by name.
- Introduced yourself by name and title.
- Explained the procedure to the person before beginning and during the procedure.
- Protected the person's rights during the procedure.
- Handled the person gently during the procedure.

## Pre-Procedure

1. Followed "Delegation Guidelines: Brushing and Combing Hair."Reviewed "Promoting Safety and Comfort: Brushing and Combing Hair."
2. Practiced hand hygiene.
3. Identified the person. Checked the ID bracelet the assignment sheet. Called the person by name.
4. Asked the person how to style hair.
5. Collected the following:
   - Comb and brush
   - Bath towel
   - Hair care items as requested
6. Arranged items on the bedside stand.
7. Provided for privacy.

## Procedure

8. Lowered the bed rail if used.
9. Helped the person to the chair. The person put on a robe and non-skid footwear. (If the person was in bed, raised the bed for body mechanics. Bed rails were up if used. Lowered the near bed rail. Assisted the person to semi-Fowler's position if allowed.)
10. Placed a towel across the back and shoulders or across the pillow.
11. Asked the person to remove eyeglasses. Put them in the eyeglass case. Put the case inside the bedside stand.
12. Used the comb to part the hair.
    a. Parted hair down the middle into 2 sides.
    b. Divided one side into 2 smaller sections using comb.
13. Brushed one of the small sections of hair. Started at the scalp and brushed toward the hair ends. Did the same for the other small section of hair.

| Procedure—cont'd | S | U | Comments |
|---|---|---|---|
| 14. Repeated steps 12b and 13 for the other side. | _____ | _____ | _____ |
| 15. Styled the hair as the person preferred. | _____ | _____ | _____ |
| 16. Removed the towel. | _____ | _____ | _____ |
| 17. Let the person put on the eyeglasses. | _____ | _____ | _____ |

## Post-Procedure

| | S | U | Comments |
|---|---|---|---|
| 18. Provided for comfort as noted on the inside of the front book cover. | _____ | _____ | _____ |
| 19. Placed the signal light within reach. | _____ | _____ | _____ |
| 20. Lowered the bed to its lowest position. | _____ | _____ | _____ |
| 21. Raised or lowered bed rails. Followed the care plan. | _____ | _____ | _____ |
| 22. Cleaned and returned items to their proper place. | _____ | _____ | _____ |
| 23. Unscreened the person. | _____ | _____ | _____ |
| 24. Completed a safety check of the room as noted on the inside of the front book cover. | _____ | _____ | _____ |
| 25. Followed agency policy for dirty linen. | _____ | _____ | _____ |
| 26. Decontaminated hands. | _____ | _____ | _____ |

Date of Satisfactory Completion _____ Instructor's Initials_____

# Shampooing the Person's Hair (NNAAP™)

Name: _____  Date: _____

| Quality of Life | S | U | Comments |
|---|---|---|---|

- Knocked before entering the person's room.  _____ _____ _____
- Addressed the person by name.  _____ _____ _____
- Introduced yourself by name and title.  _____ _____ _____
- Explained the procedure to the person before beginning and during the procedure.  _____ _____ _____
- Protected the person's rights during the procedure.  _____ _____ _____
- Handled the person gently during the procedure.  _____ _____ _____

## Pre-Procedure

1. Followed "Delegation Guidelines: Shampooing." Reviewed "Promoting Safety and Comfort: Shampooing."  _____ _____ _____
2. Practiced hand hygiene.  _____ _____ _____
3. Collected the following:
   - Two bath towels  _____ _____ _____
   - Washcloth  _____ _____ _____
   - Shampoo  _____ _____ _____
   - Hair conditioner (if requested)  _____ _____ _____
   - Bath thermometer  _____ _____ _____
   - Pitcher or nozzle (if needed)  _____ _____ _____
   - Shampoo tray (if needed)  _____ _____ _____
   - Basin or pan (if needed)  _____ _____ _____
   - Waterproof pad (if needed)  _____ _____ _____
   - Gloves (if needed)  _____ _____ _____
   - Comb and brush  _____ _____ _____
   - Hair dryer  _____ _____ _____
4. Arranged items nearby.  _____ _____ _____
5. Identified the person. Checked the ID bracelet against the assignment sheet. Called the person by name.  _____ _____ _____
6. Provided for privacy.  _____ _____ _____
7. Raised the bed for body mechanics for a shampoo in bed. Bed rails were up if used.  _____ _____ _____
8. Decontaminated hands.  _____ _____ _____
9. Lowered the bed rail near you if up.  _____ _____ _____

## Procedure

10. Covered the person's chest with a towel.  _____ _____ _____
11. Brushed and combed the hair to remove snarls and tangles.  _____ _____ _____

| Procedure—cont'd | S | U | Comments |
|---|---|---|---|

12. Positioned the person for the method used to shampoo the person in bed.  _____  _____  _____

   a. Lowered the head of the bed and removed the pillow.  _____  _____  _____

   b. Placed the waterproof pad and shampoo tray under the head and shoulders.  _____  _____  _____

   c. Supported the head and neck with a folded towel if necessary.  _____  _____  _____

13. Raised the bed rail if used.  _____  _____  _____

14. Obtained water. Temperature was about 105° F [40.5° C]. Tested water temperature according to agency policy.  _____  _____  _____

15. Lowered the bed rail near you if up.  _____  _____  _____

16. Put on gloves (if needed).  _____  _____  _____

17. Asked the person to hold a dampened hand towel or washcloth over the eyes. (Some state competency tests require a washcloth.) It did not cover the nose and mouth.  _____  _____  _____

18. Used the pitcher or nozzle to wet the hair.  _____  _____  _____

19. Applied a small amount of shampoo.  _____  _____  _____

20. Worked up a lather with both hands. Started at the hairline. Worked toward the back of the head.  _____  _____  _____

21. Massaged the scalp with the fingertips. Did not scratch the scalp.  _____  _____  _____

22. Rinsed the hair.  _____  _____  _____

23. Repeat steps 19 through 22 until the water runs clear.  _____  _____  _____

24. Applied conditioner. Followed directions on the container.  _____  _____  _____

25. Squeezed water from the person's hair.  _____  _____  _____

26. Covered hair with a bath towel. Used the towel on the person's chest.  _____  _____  _____

27. Removed the shampoo tray and waterproof pad.  _____  _____  _____

28. Dried the person's face with the towel.  _____  _____  _____

29. Helped the person raise the head if appropriate. For the person in bed, raised the head of the bed.  _____  _____  _____

30. Rubbed the hair and scalp with the towel. Used the second towel if the first was wet.  _____  _____  _____

31. Combed the hair to remove snarls and tangles.  _____  _____  _____

32. Dried and styled hair as quickly as possible.  _____  _____  _____

33. Removed and discarded the gloves (if used). Decontaminated hands.  _____  _____  _____

## Post-Procedure

34. Provided for comfort as noted on the inside of the front book cover.  _____  _____  _____

35. Placed the signal light within reach.  _____  _____  _____

36. Lowered the bed to its lowest position.  _____  _____  _____

37. Raised or lowered bed rails. Followed the care plan.  _____  _____  _____

*Continued*

| Post-Procedure—cont'd | S | U | Comments |
|---|---|---|---|
| 38. Unscreened the person. | _____ | _____ | _____ |
| 39. Completed a safety check of the room as noted on the inside of the front book cover. | _____ | _____ | _____ |
| 40. Cleaned and returned equipment to its proper place. Cleaned brush and comb. Discarded disposable items. | _____ | _____ | _____ |
| 41. Followed agency policy for dirty linen. | _____ | _____ | _____ |
| 42. Decontaminated hands. | _____ | _____ | _____ |
| 43. Reported and recorded observations. | _____ | _____ | _____ |

Date of Satisfactory Completion _____    Instructor's Initials_____

# Shaving the Person

Name: _____     Date: _____

| Quality of Life | S | U | Comments |
|---|---|---|---|

- Knocked before entering the person's room.  _____ _____ _____
- Addressed the person by name.  _____ _____ _____
- Introduced yourself by name and title.  _____ _____ _____
- Explained the procedure to the person before beginning and during the procedure.  _____ _____ _____
- Protected the person's rights during the procedure.  _____ _____ _____
- Handled the person gently during the procedure.  _____ _____ _____

## Pre-Procedure

1. Followed "Delegation Guidelines: Shaving." Reviewed "Promoting Safety and Comfort: Shaving."  _____ _____ _____
2. Practiced hand hygiene.  _____ _____ _____
3. Collected the following:
   - Wash basin  _____ _____ _____
   - Bath towel  _____ _____ _____
   - Hand towel  _____ _____ _____
   - Washcloth  _____ _____ _____
   - Safety razor  _____ _____ _____
   - Mirror  _____ _____ _____
   - Shaving cream, soap, or lotion  _____ _____ _____
   - Shaving brush  _____ _____ _____
   - After-shave or lotion  _____ _____ _____
   - Tissues or paper towels  _____ _____ _____
   - Paper towels  _____ _____ _____
   - Gloves  _____ _____ _____
4. Arranged paper towels and supplies on the overbed table.  _____ _____ _____
5. Identified the person. Checked the ID bracelet against the assignment sheet. Called the person by name.  _____ _____ _____
6. Provided for privacy.  _____ _____ _____
7. Raised the bed for body mechanics. Bed rails were up if used.  _____ _____ _____

## Procedure

8. Filled the basin with warm water.  _____ _____ _____
9. Placed the basin on the overbed table.  _____ _____ _____
10. Lowered the bed rail near you if up.  _____ _____ _____
11. Decontaminated hands. Put on gloves.  _____ _____ _____
12. Assisted the person to semi-Fowler's position if allowed or to the supine position.  _____ _____ _____
13. Adjusted lighting to clearly see the person's face.  _____ _____ _____

*Continued*

| Procedure—cont'd | S | U | Comments |
|---|---|---|---|
| 14. Placed the bath towel over the chest. | _____ | _____ | _____ |
| 15. Adjusted the overbed table for easy reach. | _____ | _____ | _____ |
| 16. Tightened the razor blade to the shaver. | _____ | _____ | _____ |
| 17. Washed the person's face. Did not dry. | _____ | _____ | _____ |
| 18. Wet the washcloth or hand towel. Wrung it out. | _____ | _____ | _____ |
| 19. Applied the washcloth or hand towel to the face for a few minutes. | _____ | _____ | _____ |
| 20. Applied shaving cream with hands, or used a shaving brush to apply lather. | _____ | _____ | _____ |
| 21. Held the skin taut with one hand. | _____ | _____ | _____ |
| 22. Shaved in the direction of hair growth. Used shorter strokes around the chin and lips. | _____ | _____ | _____ |
| 23. Rinsed the razor often. Wiped it with tissues or paper towels. | _____ | _____ | _____ |
| 24. Applied direct pressure to any bleeding areas. | _____ | _____ | _____ |
| 25. Washed off any remaining shaving cream or soap. Patted with a towel. | _____ | _____ | _____ |
| 26. Applied after-shave lotion if requested. | _____ | _____ | _____ |
| 27. Removed the towel and gloves. Decontaminated hands. | _____ | _____ | _____ |

### Post-Procedure

| | S | U | Comments |
|---|---|---|---|
| 28. Provided for comfort as noted on the inside of the front book cover. | _____ | _____ | _____ |
| 29. Placed the signal light within reach. | _____ | _____ | _____ |
| 30. Lowered the bed to its lowest position. | _____ | _____ | _____ |
| 31. Raised or lowered bed rails. Followed the care plan. | _____ | _____ | _____ |
| 32. Cleaned and return equipment and supplies to their proper place. Discarded disposable items. Wore gloves. | _____ | _____ | _____ |
| 33. Wiped off the overbed table with the paper towels. Discarded the paper towels. | _____ | _____ | _____ |
| 34. Removed the gloves. Decontaminated hands. | _____ | _____ | _____ |
| 35. Unscreened the person. | _____ | _____ | _____ |
| 36. Completed a safety check of the room as noted on the inside of the front book cover. | _____ | _____ | _____ |
| 37. Followed agency policy for dirty linen. | _____ | _____ | _____ |
| 38. Decontaminated hands. | _____ | _____ | _____ |
| 39. Reported nicks, cuts, irritation, or bleeding to the nurse. Reported and recorded other observations. | _____ | _____ | _____ |

Date of Satisfactory Completion _____     Instructor's Initials_____

# Giving Nail and Foot Care (NNAAP™)

Name: _____    Date: _____

| Quality of Life | S | U | Comments |
|---|---|---|---|

- Knocked before entering the person's room.    _____ _____ _____
- Addressed the person by name.    _____ _____ _____
- Introduced yourself by name and title.    _____ _____ _____
- Explained the procedure to the person before beginning and during the procedure.    _____ _____ _____
- Protected the person's rights during the procedure.    _____ _____ _____
- Handled the person gently during the procedure.    _____ _____ _____

## Pre-Procedure

1. Followed "Delegation Guidelines: Nail and Foot Care." Reviewed "Promoting Safety and Comfort: Nail and Foot Care."    _____ _____ _____
2. Practiced hand hygiene.    _____ _____ _____
3. Collected the following:
   - Wash basin or whirlpool foot bath    _____ _____ _____
   - Soap    _____ _____ _____
   - Bath thermometer    _____ _____ _____
   - Bath towel    _____ _____ _____
   - Hand towel    _____ _____ _____
   - Washcloth    _____ _____ _____
   - Kidney basin    _____ _____ _____
   - Nail clippers    _____ _____ _____
   - Orange stick    _____ _____ _____
   - Emery board or nail file    _____ _____ _____
   - Lotion for hands    _____ _____ _____
   - Lotion or petrolatum jelly for feet    _____ _____ _____
   - Paper towels    _____ _____ _____
   - Bath mat    _____ _____ _____
   - Gloves    _____ _____ _____
4. Arranged paper towels and other items on the overbed table.    _____ _____ _____
5. Identified the person. Checked the ID bracelet against the assignment sheet. Called the person by name.    _____ _____ _____
6. Provided for privacy.    _____ _____ _____
7. Assisted the person to the bedside chair. Placed the signal light within reach.    _____ _____ _____

*Continued*

| Procedure | S | U | Comments |
|-----------|---|---|----------|
| 8. Placed the bath mat under the feet. | _____ | _____ | _____ |
| 9. Filled the wash basin or whirlpool foot bath ⅔ (two-thirds) full with water. Followed the nurse's directions for water temperature. (Measured water temperature with a bath thermometer or tested it by dipping your elbow or inner wrist into the basin. Followed agency policy.) | _____ | _____ | _____ |
| 10. Placed the basin or foot bath on the bath mat. | _____ | _____ | _____ |
| 11. Helped the person put the feet into the basin or foot bath. Both feet were completely covered with water. | _____ | _____ | _____ |
| 12. Adjusted the overbed table in front of the person. | _____ | _____ | _____ |
| 13. Filled the kidney basin ⅔ (two-thirds) full with water. Measured water temperature (See step 9). | _____ | _____ | _____ |
| 14. Placed the kidney basin on the overbed table. | _____ | _____ | _____ |
| 15. Placed the person's fingers into the basin. Positioned the arms for comfort. | _____ | _____ | _____ |
| 16. Let the fingers soak for 5 to 10 minutes. Let the feet soak for 15 to 20 minutes. Rewarmed water as needed. | _____ | _____ | _____ |
| 17. Decontaminated hands. Put on gloves. | _____ | _____ | _____ |
| 18. Removed the kidney basin. | _____ | _____ | _____ |
| 19. Cleaned under the fingernails with the orange stick. Used a towel to wipe the orange stick after each nail. | _____ | _____ | _____ |
| 20. Dried the hands and between the fingers. | | | |
| 21. Clipped fingernails straight across with the nail clippers. | _____ | _____ | _____ |
| 22. Shaped nails with an emery board or nail file. Nails were smooth with no rough edges. | _____ | _____ | _____ |
| 23. Pushed cuticles back with the orange stick or a washcloth. | _____ | _____ | _____ |
| 24. Applied lotion to the hands. Warmed lotion before applying it. | _____ | _____ | _____ |
| 25. Moved the overbed table to the side. | _____ | _____ | _____ |
| 26. Washed the feet and between the toes with soap and a washcloth. Rinsed the feet and between the toes. | _____ | _____ | _____ |
| 27. Removed the feet from the basin or foot bath. Dried thoroughly, especially between the toes. | _____ | _____ | _____ |
| 28. Applied lotion or petrolatum jelly to the tops and soles of the feet. Did not apply between the toes. Warmed lotion before applying it. Removed excess lotion with a towel. | _____ | _____ | _____ |
| 29. Removed and discarded the gloves. Decontaminated hands. | _____ | _____ | _____ |
| 30. Helped the person put on non-skid footwear. | _____ | _____ | _____ |

## Post-Procedure

| | | | |
|-----------|---|---|----------|
| 31. Provided for comfort as noted on the inside of the front book cover. | _____ | _____ | _____ |
| 32. Placed the signal light within reach. | _____ | _____ | _____ |

| Post-Procedure—cont'd | S | U | Comments |
|---|---|---|---|
| 33. Raised or lowered bed rails. Followed the care plan. | _____ | _____ | _____ |
| 34. Cleaned and returned equipment and supplies to their proper place. Discarded disposable items. Wore gloves for this step. | _____ | _____ | _____ |
| 35. Removed the gloves. Decontaminated hands. | _____ | _____ | _____ |
| 36. Unscreened the person. | _____ | _____ | _____ |
| 37. Completed a safety check of the room as noted on the inside of the front book cover. | _____ | _____ | _____ |
| 38. Followed agency policy for dirty linen. | _____ | _____ | _____ |
| 39. Decontaminated hands. | _____ | _____ | _____ |
| 40. Reported and recorded observations. | _____ | _____ | _____ |

Date of Satisfactory Completion _____     Instructor's Initials_____

# Changing the Gown of the Person With an IV

Name: _____     Date: _____

| Quality of Life | S | U | Comments |
|---|---|---|---|
| • Knocked before entering the person's room. | _____ | _____ | _____ |
| • Addressed the person by name. | _____ | _____ | _____ |
| • Introduced yourself by name and title. | _____ | _____ | _____ |
| • Explained the procedure to the person before beginning and during the procedure. | _____ | _____ | _____ |
| • Protected the person's rights during the procedure. | _____ | _____ | _____ |
| • Handled the person gently during the procedure. | _____ | _____ | _____ |

## Pre-Procedure

| | | | |
|---|---|---|---|
| 1. Followed "Delegation Guidelines: Changing Gowns." Reviewed "Promoting Safety and Comfort: Changing Gowns." | _____ | _____ | _____ |
| 2. Practiced hand hygiene. | _____ | _____ | _____ |
| 3. Got a clean gown and a bath blanket. | _____ | _____ | _____ |
| 4. Identified the person. Checked the ID bracelet against the assignment sheet. Called the person by name. | _____ | _____ | _____ |
| 5. Provided for privacy. | _____ | _____ | _____ |
| 6. Raised the bed for body mechanics. Bed rails were up if used. | _____ | _____ | _____ |

## Procedure

| | | | |
|---|---|---|---|
| 7. Lowered the bed rail near you if up. | _____ | _____ | _____ |
| 8. Covered the person with a bath blanket. Fan-folded linens to the foot of the bed. | _____ | _____ | _____ |
| 9. Untied the gown. Freed parts that the person was lying on. | _____ | _____ | _____ |
| 10. Removed the gown from the arm with no IV. | _____ | _____ | _____ |
| 11. Gathered up the sleeve of the arm with the IV. Slid it over the IV site and tubing. Removed the arm and hand from the sleeve. | _____ | _____ | _____ |
| 12. Kept the sleeve gathered. Slid your arm along the tubing to the bag. | _____ | _____ | _____ |
| 13. Removed the bag from the pole. Slid the bag and tubing through the sleeve. Did not pull on the tubing. Kept the bag above the person. | _____ | _____ | _____ |
| 14. Hung the IV bag on the pole. | _____ | _____ | _____ |
| 15. Gathered the sleeve of the clean gown that would go on the arm with the IV infusion. | _____ | _____ | _____ |
| 16. Removed the bag from the pole. Slipped the sleeve over the bag at the shoulder part of the gown. Hung the bag. | _____ | _____ | _____ |

| Procedure—cont'd | S | U | Comments |
|---|---|---|---|

17. Slid the gathered sleeve over the tubing, hand, arm, and IV site. Then slid it onto the shoulder. _____ _____ _____

18. Put the other side of the gown on the person. Fastened the gown. _____ _____ _____

19. Covered the person. Removed the bath blanket. _____ _____ _____

## Post-Procedure

20. Provided for comfort as noted on the inside of the front book cover. _____ _____ _____

21. Placed the signal light within reach. _____ _____ _____

22. Lowered the bed to its lowest position. _____ _____ _____

23. Raised or lowered bed rails. Followed the care plan. _____ _____ _____

24. Unscreened the person. _____ _____ _____

25. Completed a safety check of the room as noted on the inside of the front book cover. _____ _____ _____

26. Followed agency policy for dirty linen. _____ _____ _____

27. Decontaminated hands. _____ _____ _____

28. Asked the nurse to check the flow rate. _____ _____ _____

29. Reported and recorded observations. _____ _____ _____

Date of Satisfactory Completion _____    Instructor's Initials_____

# Undressing the Person

Name: _____    Date: _____

| Quality of Life | S | U | Comments |
|---|---|---|---|

- Knocked before entering the person's room.
- Addressed the person by name.
- Introduced yourself by name and title.
- Explained the procedure to the person before beginning and during the procedure.
- Protected the person's rights during the procedure.
- Handled the person gently during the procedure.

## Pre-Procedure

1. Followed "Delegation Guidelines: Dressing and Undressing."
2. Practiced hand hygiene.
3. Collected a bath blanket and clothing requested by the person.
4. Identified the person. Checked the ID bracelet against the assignment sheet. Called the person by name.
5. Provided for privacy.
6. Raised the bed for body mechanics. Bed rails were up if used.
7. Lowered the bed rail on the person's weak side.
8. Positioned the person supine.
9. Covered the person with the bath blanket. Fanfolded linens to the foot of the bed.

## Procedure

10. To remove garments that opened in the back:
    a. Raised the head and shoulders, or turned the person onto the side away from you.
    b. Undid buttons, zippers, ties, or snaps.
    c. Brought the sides of the garment to the sides of the person. If the person was in a side-lying position, tucked the far side under the person. Folded the near side onto the chest.
    d. Positioned the person supine.
    e. Slid the garment off the shoulder on the strong side. Removed it from the arm.
    f. Repeated step 10e for the weak side.
11. To remove garments that opened in the front:
    a. Undid buttons, zippers, ties, or snaps.

| Procedure—cont'd | S | U | Comments |
|---|---|---|---|

b. Slid the garment off the shoulder and arm on the strong side.

c. Assisted the person to sit up or raised the head and shoulders. Brought the garment over to the weak side.

d. Lowered the head and shoulders. Removed the garment from the weak side.

e. If you could not raise the head and shoulders:

   (1) Turned the person toward you. Tucked the removed part under the person.

   (2) Turned the person onto the side away from you.

   (3) Pulled the side of the garment out from under the person. Made sure the person would not lie on it when supine.

   (4) Returned the person to the supine position.

   (5) Removed the garment from the weak side.

12. To remove pullover garments:

  a. Undid any buttons, zippers, ties, or snaps.

  b. Removed the garment from the strong side.

  c. Raised the head and shoulders, or turned the person onto the side away from you. Brought the garment up to the person's neck.

  d. Removed the garment from the weak side.

  e. Brought the garment over the person's head.

  f. Positioned the person in the supine position.

13. To remove pants or slacks:

  a. Removed footwear.

  b. Positioned the person supine.

  c. Undid buttons, zippers, ties, snaps, or buckles.

  d. Removed the belt.

  e. Asked the person to lift the buttocks off the bed. Slid the pants down over the hips and buttocks. Had the person lower the hips and buttocks.

  f. If the person could not raise the hips off the bed:

   (1) Turned the person toward you.

   (2) Slid the pants off the hip and buttock on the strong side.

   (3) Turned the person away from you.

   (4) Slid the pants off the hip and buttock on the weak side.

  g. Slid the pants down the legs and over the feet.

14. Dressed the person. See procedure "Dressing the Person."

*Continued*

| Post-Procedure | S | U | Comments |
|---|---|---|---|
| 15. Provided for comfort as noted on the inside of the front book cover. | _____ | _____ | _____ |
| 16. Placed the signal light within reach. | _____ | _____ | _____ |
| 17. Lowered the bed to its lowest level. | _____ | _____ | _____ |
| 18. Raised or lowered bed rails. Followed the care plan. | _____ | _____ | _____ |
| 19. Unscreened the person. | _____ | _____ | _____ |
| 20. Completed a safety check of the room as noted on the inside of the front book cover. | _____ | _____ | _____ |
| 21. Followed agency policy for soiled clothing. | _____ | _____ | _____ |
| 22. Decontaminated hands. | _____ | _____ | _____ |
| 23. Reported and recorded observations. | _____ | _____ | _____ |

Date of Satisfactory Completion _____    Instructor's Initials_____

# Dressing the Person (NNAAP™)

Name: _____     Date: _____

| Quality of Life | S | U | Comments |
|---|---|---|---|

- Knocked before entering the person's room.
- Addressed the person by name.
- Introduced yourself by name and title.
- Explained the procedure to the person before beginning and during the procedure.
- Protected the person's rights during the procedure.
- Handled the person gently during the procedure.

### Pre-Procedure

1. Followed "Delegation Guidelines: Dressing and Undressing."
2. Practiced hand hygiene.
3. Asked the person what he or she would like to wear.
4. Got a bath blanket and clothing requested by the person.
5. Identified the person. Checked the ID bracelet against the assignment sheet. Called the person by name.
6. Provided for privacy.
7. Raised the bed for body mechanics. Bed rails were up if used.
8. Lowered the bed rail (if up) on the person's strong side.
9. Positioned the person supine.
10. Covered the person with the bath blanket. Fan-folded linens to the foot of the bed.
11. Undressed the person (See procedure "Undressing the Person.")

### Procedure

12. To put on garments that opened in the back:
    a. Slid the garment onto the arm and shoulder of the weak side.
    b. Slid the garment onto the arm and shoulder of the strong side.
    c. Raised the person's head and shoulders.
    d. Brought the sides to the back.
    e. If the person could not raise the head and shoulders:
       (1) Turned the person toward you.
       (2) Brought one side of the garment to the person's back.

*Continued*

| Procedure—cont'd | S | U | Comments |
|---|---|---|---|

    (3) Turned the person away from you. _____ _____ _____

    (4) Brought the other side to the person's back. _____ _____ _____

  f. Fastened buttons, ties, snaps, or zippers. _____ _____ _____

  g. Positioned the person supine. _____ _____ _____

13. To put on garments that opened in the front:

  a. Slid the garment onto the arm and shoulder on the weak side. _____ _____ _____

  b. Raised the head and shoulders. Brought the side of the garment around to the back. Lowered the person down. Slid the garment onto the arm and shoulder of the strong arm. _____ _____ _____

  c. If the person could not raise the head and shoulders:

    (1) Turned the person away from you. _____ _____ _____

    (2) Tuck the garment under the person. _____ _____ _____

    (3) Turned the person toward you. _____ _____ _____

    (4) Pulled the garment out from under the person. _____ _____ _____

    (5) Turned the person back to the supine position. _____ _____ _____

    (6) Slid the garment over the arm and shoulder of the strong arm. _____ _____ _____

  d. Fastened buttons, ties, snaps, or zippers. _____ _____ _____

14. To put on pullover garments:

  a. Positioned the person supine. _____ _____ _____

  b. Brought the neck of the garment over the head. _____ _____ _____

  c. Slid the arm and shoulder of the garment onto the weak side. _____ _____ _____

  d. Raised the person's head and shoulders. _____ _____ _____

  e. Brought the garment down. _____ _____ _____

  f. Slid the arm and shoulder of the garment onto the strong side. _____ _____ _____

  g. If the person could not assume a semi-sitting position:

    (1) Turned the person away from you. _____ _____ _____

    (2) Tucked the garment under the person. _____ _____ _____

    (3) Turned the person toward you. _____ _____ _____

    (4) Pulled the garment out from under the person. _____ _____ _____

    (5) Positioned the person supine. _____ _____ _____

    (6) Slid the arm and shoulder of the garment onto the strong side. _____ _____ _____

  h. Fastened buttons, ties, snaps, or zippers. _____ _____ _____

15. To put on pants or slacks:

  a. Slid the pants over the feet and up the legs. _____ _____ _____

  b. Asked the person to raise the hips and buttocks off the bed. _____ _____ _____

| Procedure—cont'd | S | U | Comments |
|---|---|---|---|

   c. Brought the pants up over the hips and buttocks. \_\_\_\_ \_\_\_\_ _____

   d. Asked the person to lower the hips and buttocks. \_\_\_\_ \_\_\_\_ _____

   e. If the person could not raise the hips and buttocks:

     (1) Turned the person onto strong side away from you. \_\_\_\_ \_\_\_\_ _____

     (2) Pulled the pants over the hip and buttock on the weak side. \_\_\_\_ \_\_\_\_ _____

     (3) Turned the person onto the weak side toward you. \_\_\_\_ \_\_\_\_ _____

     (4) Pulled the pants over the hip and buttock on the strong side. \_\_\_\_ \_\_\_\_ _____

     (5) Positioned the person supine. \_\_\_\_ \_\_\_\_ _____

   f. Fastened buttons, ties, snaps, the zipper, and the belt buckle. \_\_\_\_ \_\_\_\_ _____

16. Put socks and non-skid footwear on the person. \_\_\_\_ \_\_\_\_ _____

17. Helped the person get out of bed. If the person stayed in bed, covered the person and removed the bath blanket. \_\_\_\_ \_\_\_\_ _____

## Post-Procedure

18. Provided for comfort as noted on the inside of the front book cover. \_\_\_\_ \_\_\_\_ _____

19. Placed the signal light within reach. \_\_\_\_ \_\_\_\_ _____

20. Lowered the bed to its lowest position. \_\_\_\_ \_\_\_\_ _____

21. Raised or lowered bed rails. Followed the care plan. \_\_\_\_ \_\_\_\_ _____

22. Unscreened the person. \_\_\_\_ \_\_\_\_ _____

23. Completed a safety check of the room as noted on the inside of the front book cover. \_\_\_\_ \_\_\_\_ _____

24. Followed agency policy for soiled clothing. \_\_\_\_ \_\_\_\_ _____

25. Decontaminated hands. \_\_\_\_ \_\_\_\_ _____

26. Reported and recorded observations. \_\_\_\_ \_\_\_\_ _____

Date of Satisfactory Completion _____     Instructor's Initials_____

# Giving the Bedpan (NNAAP™)

Name: _____     Date: _____

| Quality of Life | S | U | Comments |
|---|---|---|---|

- Knocked before entering the person's room.    _____ _____ _____
- Addressed the person by name.    _____ _____ _____
- Introduced yourself by name and title.    _____ _____ _____
- Explained the procedure to the person before beginning and during the procedure.    _____ _____ _____
- Protected the person's rights during the procedure.    _____ _____ _____
- Handled the person gently during the procedure.    _____ _____ _____

## Pre-Procedure

1. Followed "Delegation Guidelines: Bedpans." Reviewed "Promoting Safety and Comfort: Bedpans."    _____ _____ _____
2. Provided for privacy.    _____ _____ _____
3. Practiced hand hygiene.    _____ _____ _____
4. Put on gloves.    _____ _____ _____
5. Collected the following:
   - Bedpan    _____ _____ _____
   - Bedpan cover    _____ _____ _____
   - Toilet tissue    _____ _____ _____
   - Waterproof pad if required by agency    _____ _____ _____
6. Arranged equipment on the chair or bed.    _____ _____ _____

## Procedure

7. Warmed and dried the bedpan if necessary.    _____ _____ _____
8. Lowered the bed rail near you if up.    _____ _____ _____
9. Positioned the person supine. Raised the head of the bed slightly.    _____ _____ _____
10. Folded the top linens and gown out of the way. Kept the lower body covered.    _____ _____ _____
11. Asked the person to flex the knees and raise the buttocks by pushing against the mattress with the feet.    _____ _____ _____
12. Slid your hand under the lower back. Helped raise the buttocks. If using a waterproof pad, placed it under the buttocks.    _____ _____ _____
13. Slid the bedpan under the person.    _____ _____ _____
14. If the person could not assist in getting on the bedpan:
    a. Placed the waterproof pad under the buttocks, if using one.    _____ _____ _____
    b. Turned the person onto the side away from you.    _____ _____ _____
    c. Placed the bedpan firmly against the buttocks.    _____ _____ _____
    d. Pushed the bedpan down and toward the person.    _____ _____ _____

| Procedure—cont'd | S | U | Comments |
|---|---|---|---|

    e. Held the bedpan securely.Turned the person onto the back.
    f. Made sure the bedpan was centered under the person.
15. Covered the person.
16. Raised the head of the bed so the person was in a sitting position.
17. Made sure the person was correctly positioned on the bedpan.
18. Raised the bed rail if used.
19. Placed the toilet tissue and signal light within reach.
20. Asked the person to signal when done or when help was needed.
21. Removed the gloves. Decontaminated hands.
22. Left the room and closed the door.
23. Returned when the person signaled. Or checked on the person every 5 minutes. Knocked before entering.
24. Decontaminated hands. Put on gloves.
25. Raised the bed for body mechanics. Lowered the bed rail (if used) and the head of the bed.
26. Asked the person to raise the buttocks. Removed the bedpan, or held the bedpan and turned the person onto the side away from you.
27. Cleaned the genital area if the person could not do so. Cleaned from front (urethra) to back (anus) with toilet tissue. Used fresh tissue for each wipe. Provided perineal care if needed. Removed and discarded the waterproof pad if using one.
28. Covered the bedpan. Took it to the bathroom. Raised the bed rail (if used) before leaving the bedside.
29. Noted the color, amount, and character of urine or feces.
30. Emptied the bedpan contents into the toilet and flushed.
31. Rinsed the bedpan. Poured the rinse into the toilet and flushed.
32. Cleaned the bedpan with a disinfectant.
33. Removed soiled gloves. Practiced hand hygiene and put on clean gloves.
34. Returned the bedpan and clean cover to the bedside stand.
35. Helped the person with hand washing.
36. Removed the gloves. Decontaminated hands.

## Post-Procedure

37. Provided for comfort as noted on the inside of the front book cover.
38. Placed the signal light within reach.
39. Lowered the bed to its lowest position.

*Continued*

| Post-Procedure—cont'd | S | U | Comments |
|---|---|---|---|
| 40. Raised or lowered bed rails. Followed the care plan. | _____ | _____ | _____ |
| 41. Unscreened the person. | _____ | _____ | _____ |
| 42. Completed a safety check of the room as noted on the inside of the front book cover. | _____ | _____ | _____ |
| 43. Followed agency policy for soiled linen. | _____ | _____ | _____ |
| 44. Decontaminated hands. | _____ | _____ | _____ |
| 45. Reported and recorded observations. | _____ | _____ | _____ |

Date of Satisfactory Completion _____    Instructor's Initials_____

Giving the Urinal (NNAAP™)

Name: _____     Date: _____

| Quality of Life | S | U | Comments |
|---|---|---|---|

- Knocked before entering the person's room.
- Addressed the person by name.
- Introduced yourself by name and title.
- Explained the procedure to the person before beginning and during the procedure.
- Protected the person's rights during the procedure.
- Handled the person gently during the procedure.

### Pre-Procedure

1. Followed "Delegation Guidelines: Urinals." Reviewed "Promoting Safety and Comfort: Urinals."
2. Provided for privacy.
3. Determined if the man would stand, sit, or lie in bed.
4. Practiced hand hygiene.
5. Put on gloves.

### Procedure

6. Gave him the urinal if he was in bed. Reminded him to tilt the bottom down to prevent spills.
7. If he was going to stand:
   a. Helped him sit on the side of the bed.
   b. Put non-skid footwear on him.
   c. Helped him stand. Provided support if he was unsteady.
   d. Gave him the urinal.
8. Positioned the urinal if necessary. Positioned his penis in the urinal if he could not do so.
9. Placed the signal light within reach. Asked him to signal when done or if he needed help. Checked on him every 5 minutes.
10. Provided for privacy.
11. Removed the gloves. Decontaminated hands.
12. Left the room and closed the door.
13. Returned when he signaled. Or checked on him every 5 minutes. Knocked before entering.
14. Decontaminated hands. Put on gloves.
15. Closed the cap on the urinal. Took it to the bathroom.
16. Noted the color, amount, and character of the urine.
17. Emptied the urinal into the toilet and flushed.
18. Rinsed the urinal with cold water. Poured the rinse into the toilet and flushed.

*Continued*

| Procedure—cont'd | S | U | Comments |
|---|---|---|---|
| 19. Cleaned the urinal with a disinfectant. | _____ | _____ | _____ |
| 20. Returned the urinal to its proper place. | _____ | _____ | _____ |
| 21. Removed soiled gloves. Practiced hand hygiene and put on clean gloves. | _____ | _____ | _____ |
| 22. Assisted him with hand washing. | _____ | _____ | _____ |
| 23. Removed the gloves. Decontaminated hands. | _____ | _____ | _____ |

### Post-Procedure

| | S | U | Comments |
|---|---|---|---|
| 24. Provided for comfort as noted on the inside of the front book cover. | _____ | _____ | _____ |
| 25. Placed the signal light within reach. | _____ | _____ | _____ |
| 26. Raised or lower bed rails. Followed the care plan. | _____ | _____ | _____ |
| 27. Unscreened him. | _____ | _____ | _____ |
| 28. Completed a safety check of the room as noted on the inside of the front book cover. | _____ | _____ | _____ |
| 29. Followed agency policy for soiled linen. | _____ | _____ | _____ |
| 30. Decontaminated hands. | _____ | _____ | _____ |
| 31. Reported and recorded observations. | _____ | _____ | _____ |

Date of Satisfactory Completion _____    Instructor's Initials_____

## Helping the Person to the Commode

Name: _____    Date: _____

|  | S | U | Comments |
|---|---|---|---|

### Quality of Life

- Knocked before entering the person's room.
- Addressed the person by name.
- Introduced yourself by name and title.
- Explained the procedure to the person before beginning and during the procedure.
- Protected the person's rights during the procedure.
- Handled the person gently during the procedure.

### Pre-Procedure

1. Followed "Delegation Guidelines: Commodes." Reviewed "Promoting Safety and Comfort: Commodes."
2. Provided for privacy.
3. Practiced hand hygiene.
4. Put on gloves.
5. Collected the following:
   - Commode
   - Toilet tissue
   - Bath blanket
   - Transfer belt

### Procedure

6. Brought the commode next to the bed. Removed the chair seat and container lid.
7. Helped the person sit on the side of the bed. Lowered the bed rail if used.
8. Helped the person put on a robe and non-skid footwear.
9. Assisted the person to the commode. Used the transfer belt.
10. Covered the person with a bath blanket for warmth.
11. Placed the toilet tissue and signal light within reach.
12. Asked the person to signal when done or when help was needed. (Stayed with the person if necessary. Was respectful and provided as much privacy as possible.)
13. Removed the gloves. Decontaminated hands.
14. Left the room. Closed the door.
15. Returned when the person signaled. Or checked on the person every 5 minutes. Knocked before entering.
16. Decontaminated hands. Put on the gloves.
17. Helped the person clean the genital area as needed. Removed the gloves, and practiced hand hygiene.

*Continued*

| Procedure—cont'd | S | U | Comments |
|---|---|---|---|

18. Helped the person back to bed using the transfer belt. Removed the robe, transfer belt, and footwear. Raised the bed rail if used.   _____ _____ _____

19. Put on clean gloves. Removed and covered the commode container. Cleaned the commode.   _____ _____ _____

20. Took the container to the bathroom.   _____ _____ _____

21. Observed urine and feces for color, amount, and character.   _____ _____ _____

22. Emptied the container contents into the toilet and flushed.   _____ _____ _____

23. Rinsed the container. Poured the rinse into the toilet and flushed.   _____ _____ _____

24. Cleaned and disinfected the container.   _____ _____ _____

25. Returned the container to the commode. Returned other supplies to their proper place.   _____ _____ _____

26. Returned the commode to its proper place.   _____ _____ _____

27. Removed soiled gloves. Practiced hand hygiene and put on clean gloves.   _____ _____ _____

28. Assisted the person with hand washing.   _____ _____ _____

29. Removed the gloves. Decontaminated hands.   _____ _____ _____

## Post-Procedure

30. Provided for comfort as noted on the inside of the front book cover.   _____ _____ _____

31. Placed the signal light within reach.   _____ _____ _____

32. Raised or lowered bed rails. Followed the care plan.   _____ _____ _____

33. Unscreened the person.   _____ _____ _____

34. Completed a safety check of the room as noted on the inside of the front book cover.   _____ _____ _____

35. Followed agency policy for soiled linen.   _____ _____ _____

36. Decontaminated hands.   _____ _____ _____

37. Reported and recorded observations.   _____ _____ _____

Date of Satisfactory Completion _____   Instructor's Initials_____

# Giving Catheter Care

Name: _____          Date: _____

| Quality of Life | S | U | Comments |
|---|---|---|---|

- Knocked before entering the person's room.  _____ _____ _____
- Addressed the person by name.  _____ _____ _____
- Introduced yourself by name and title.  _____ _____ _____
- Explained the procedure to the person before beginning and during the procedure.  _____ _____ _____
- Protected the person's rights during the procedure.  _____ _____ _____
- Handled the person gently during the procedure.  _____ _____ _____

## Pre-Procedure

1. Followed "Delegation Guidelines: Catheters." Reviewed "Promoting Safety and Comfort: Catheters."  _____ _____ _____
2. Practiced hand hygiene.  _____ _____ _____
3. Collected the following:
   - Items for perineal care (Chapter13)  _____ _____ _____
   - Gloves  _____ _____ _____
   - Waterproof pad  _____ _____ _____
   - Bath blanket  _____ _____ _____
4. Identified the person. Checked the ID bracelet against the assignment sheet. Called the person by name.  _____ _____ _____
5. Provided for privacy.  _____ _____ _____
6. Raised the bed for body mechanics. Bed rails were up if used.  _____ _____ _____

## Procedure

7. Lowered the bed rail near you if up.  _____ _____ _____
8. Decontaminated hands. Put on the gloves.  _____ _____ _____
9. Covered the person with a bath blanket. Fan-folded top linens to the foot of the bed.  _____ _____ _____
10. Draped the person for perineal care. (See procedure "Giving Female Perineal Care" in Chapter 13.)  _____ _____ _____
11. Folded back the bath blanket to expose the genital area.  _____ _____ _____
12. Placed the waterproof pad under the buttocks. Asked the person to flex the knees and raise the buttocks off the bed.  _____ _____ _____
13. Separated the labia (female). In an uncircumcised male, retracted the foreskin. Checked for crusts, abnormal drainage, or secretions.  _____ _____ _____
14. Gave perineal care. (See procedure "Giving Female Perineal Care" or "Giving Male Perineal Care" in Chapter 13.)  _____ _____ _____
15. Applied soap to a clean, wet washcloth.  _____ _____ _____

*Continued*

| Procedure—cont'd | S | U | Comments |
|---|---|---|---|

16. Held the catheter near the meatus. _____ _____ _____

17. Cleaned the catheter from the meatus down the catheter about 4 inches. Cleaned downward, away from the meatus with 1 stroke. Did not tug or pull on the catheter. Repeated as needed with a clean area of the washcloth. Used a clean washcloth if needed. _____ _____ _____

18. Rinsed the catheter with a clean washcloth. Rinsed from the meatus down the catheter about 4 inches. Rinsed downward, away from the meatus with 1 stroke. Did not tug or pull on the catheter. Repeated as needed with a clean area of the washcloth. Used a clean washcloth if needed. _____ _____ _____

19. Patted dry the perineal area. Dried from front to back. _____ _____ _____

20. Returned the foreskin to its natural position. _____ _____ _____

21. Secured the catheter. Coiled and secured tubing. _____ _____ _____

22. Removed the waterproof pad. _____ _____ _____

23. Covered the person. Removed the bath blanket. _____ _____ _____

24. Removed the gloves. Decontaminated hands. _____ _____ _____

## Post-Procedure

25. Provided for comfort as noted on the inside of the front book cover. _____ _____ _____

26. Placed the signal light within reach. _____ _____ _____

27. Lowered the bed to its lowest position. _____ _____ _____

28. Raised or lowered bed rails. Followed the care plan. _____ _____ _____

29. Cleaned and returned equipment to its proper place. Discarded disposable items. Wore gloves for this step. _____ _____ _____

30. Removed the gloves. Decontaminated hands. _____ _____ _____

31. Unscreened the person. _____ _____ _____

32. Completed a safety check of the room as noted on the inside of the front book cover. _____ _____ _____

33. Followed agency policy for soiled linen. _____ _____ _____

34. Decontaminated hands. _____ _____ _____

35. Reported and recorded observations. _____ _____ _____

Date of Satisfactory Completion _____ Instructor's Initials _____

## Emptying a Urinary Drinage Bag

Name: _____      Date: _____

| Quality of Life | S | U | Comments |
|---|---|---|---|
| • Knocked before entering the person's room. | _____ | _____ | _____ |
| • Addressed the person by name. | _____ | _____ | _____ |
| • Introduced yourself by name and title. | _____ | _____ | _____ |
| • Explained the procedure to the person before beginning and during the procedure. | _____ | _____ | _____ |
| • Protected the person's rights during the procedure. | _____ | _____ | _____ |
| • Handled the person gently during the procedure. | _____ | _____ | _____ |

**Pre-Procedure**

| | S | U | Comments |
|---|---|---|---|
| 1. Followed "Delegation Guidelines: Drainage Systems." Reviewed "Promoting Safety and Comfort: Drainage Systems." | _____ | _____ | _____ |
| 2. Collected equipment: | | | |
| • Graduate | _____ | _____ | _____ |
| • Gloves | _____ | _____ | _____ |
| • Paper towels | _____ | _____ | _____ |
| 3. Practiced hand hygiene. | _____ | _____ | _____ |
| 4. Identified the person. Checked the ID bracelet against the assignment sheet. Called the person by name. | _____ | _____ | _____ |
| 5. Provided for privacy. | _____ | _____ | _____ |

**Procedure**

| | S | U | Comments |
|---|---|---|---|
| 6. Put on the gloves. | _____ | _____ | _____ |
| 7. Placed a paper towel on the floor. Placed the graduate on top of it. | _____ | _____ | _____ |
| 8. Positioned the graduate under the collection bag. | _____ | _____ | _____ |
| 9. Opened the clamp on the drain. | _____ | _____ | _____ |
| 10. Let all urine drain into the graduate. Did not let the drain touch the graduate. | _____ | _____ | _____ |
| 11. Closed and positioned the clamp. | _____ | _____ | _____ |
| 12. Measured urine. | _____ | _____ | _____ |
| 13. Removed and discarded the paper towel. | _____ | _____ | _____ |
| 14. Emptied the contents of the graduate into the toilet and flushed. | _____ | _____ | _____ |
| 15. Rinsed the graduate. Emptied the rinse into the toilet and flushed. | _____ | _____ | _____ |
| 16. Cleaned and disinfected the graduate. | _____ | _____ | _____ |
| 17. Returned the graduate to its proper place. | _____ | _____ | _____ |

*Continued*

| Procedure—cont'd | S | U | Comments |
|---|---|---|---|

18. Removed the gloves. Practiced hand hygiene.  _____ _____ _____
19. Recorded the time and amount on the
    intake and output (I&O) record.  _____ _____ _____

## Post-Procedure

20. Provided for comfort as noted on the inside of the
    front book cover.  _____ _____ _____
21. Placed the signal light within reach.  _____ _____ _____
22. Unscreened the person.  _____ _____ _____
23. Completed a safety check of the room as noted
    on the inside of the front book cover.  _____ _____ _____
24. Reported and recorded the amount and
    other observations.  _____ _____ _____

Date of Satisfactory Completion _____  Instructor's Initials_____

## Applying a Condom Catheter

Name: _____    Date: _____

|  | S | U | Comments |
|---|---|---|---|
| **Quality of Life** | | | |
| • Knocked before entering the person's room. | ___ | ___ | _____ |
| • Addressed the person by name. | ___ | ___ | _____ |
| • Introduced yourself by name and title. | ___ | ___ | _____ |
| • Explained the procedure to the person before beginning and during the procedure. | ___ | ___ | _____ |
| • Protected the person's rights during the procedure. | ___ | ___ | _____ |
| • Handled the person gently during the procedure. | ___ | ___ | _____ |

**Pre-Procedure**

| | | | |
|---|---|---|---|
| 1. Followed "Delegation Guidelines: Condom Catheters." Reviewed "Promoting Safety and Comfort: Condom Catheters." | ___ | ___ | _____ |
| 2. Practiced hand hygiene. | ___ | ___ | _____ |
| 3. Collected the following: | | | |
|   • Condom catheter | ___ | ___ | _____ |
|   • Elastic tape | ___ | ___ | _____ |
|   • Drainage bag or leg bag | ___ | ___ | _____ |
|   • Cap for the drainage bag | ___ | ___ | _____ |
|   • Basin of warm water | ___ | ___ | _____ |
|   • Soap | ___ | ___ | _____ |
|   • Towel and washcloths | ___ | ___ | _____ |
|   • Bath blanket | ___ | ___ | _____ |
|   • Gloves | ___ | ___ | _____ |
|   • Waterproof pad | ___ | ___ | _____ |
|   • Paper towels | ___ | ___ | _____ |
| 4. Arranged paper towels and equipment on the overbed table. | ___ | ___ | _____ |
| 5. Identified the person. Checked the ID bracelet against the assignment sheet. Called the person by name. | ___ | ___ | _____ |
| 6. Provided for privacy. | ___ | ___ | _____ |
| 7. Raised the bed for body mechanics. Bed rails were up if used. | ___ | ___ | _____ |

**Procedure**

| | | | |
|---|---|---|---|
| 8. Lowered the bed rail near you if up. | ___ | ___ | _____ |
| 9. Decontaminated hands. Put on the gloves. | ___ | ___ | _____ |
| 10. Covered the person with a bath blanket. Lowered top linens to the knees. | ___ | ___ | _____ |
| 11. Asked the person to raise his buttocks off the bed or turned him onto his side away from you. | ___ | ___ | _____ |
| 12. Slid the waterproof pad under his buttocks. | ___ | ___ | _____ |

*Continued*

| Procedure—cont'd | S | U | Comments |
|---|---|---|---|

13. Had the person lower his buttocks or turned him onto his back.    _____ _____ _____

14. Secured the drainage bag to the bed frame or had a leg bag ready. Closed the drain.    _____ _____ _____

15. Exposed the genital area.    _____ _____ _____

16. Removed the condom catheter.

   a. Removed the tape. Rolled the sheath off the penis.    _____ _____ _____

   b. Disconnected the drainage tubing from the condom. Capped the drainage tube.    _____ _____ _____

   c. Discarded the tape and condom.    _____ _____ _____

17. Provided perineal care. (See procedure "Giving Male Perineal Care" in Chapter 13.) Observed the penis for reddened areas and skin breakdown or irritation.    _____ _____ _____

18. Removed the protective backing from the condom.    _____ _____ _____

19. Held the penis firmly. Rolled the condom onto the penis. Left a 1-inch space between the penis and the end of the catheter.    _____ _____ _____

20. Secured the condom.    _____ _____ _____

   a. For a self-adhering condom: pressed the condom to the penis.    _____ _____ _____

   b. For a condom secured with elastic tape: applied elastic tape in a spiral. Did not apply the tape completely around the penis.    _____ _____ _____

21. Made sure the penis tip did not touch the condom. Made sure the condom was not twisted.    _____ _____ _____

22. Connected the condom to the drainage tubing. Coiled excess tubing on the bed or attached a leg bag.    _____ _____ _____

23. Removed the waterproof pad and gloves. Discarded them. Practiced hand hygiene.    _____ _____ _____

24. Covered the person. Removed the bath blanket.    _____ _____ _____

## Post-Procedure

25. Provided for comfort as noted on the inside of the front book cover.    _____ _____ _____

26. Placed the signal light within reach.    _____ _____ _____

27. Lowered the bed to its lowest position.    _____ _____ _____

28. Raised or lowered bed rails. Followed the care plan.    _____ _____ _____

29. Unscreened the person.    _____ _____ _____

30. Decontaminated hands. Put on clean gloves.    _____ _____ _____

31. Measured and recorded the amount of urine in the bag. Cleaned or discarded the collection bag.    _____ _____ _____

32. Cleaned and returned the wash basin and other equipment. Returned items to their proper place.    _____ _____ _____

| Post-Procedure—cont'd | S | U | Comments |
|---|---|---|---|
| 33. Removed the gloves. Decontaminated hands. | _____ | _____ | _____ |
| 34. Completed a safety check of the room as noted on the inside of the front book cover. | _____ | _____ | _____ |
| 35. Reported and recorded observations. | _____ | _____ | _____ |

Date of Satisfactory Completion _____   Instructor's Initials_____

# Giving a Cleansing Enema

Name: _____        Date: _____

| Quality of Life | S | U | Comments |
|---|---|---|---|

- Knocked before entering the person's room.
- Addressed the person by name.
- Introduced yourself by name and title.
- Explained the procedure to the person before beginning and during the procedure.
- Protected the person's rights during the procedure.
- Handled the person gently during the procedure.

## Pre-Procedure

1. Followed "Delegation Guidelines: Enemas." Reviewed "Promoting Safety and Comfort: Enemas."
2. Practiced hand hygiene.
3. Collected the following:
   - Bedpan or commode
   - Disposable enema kit as directed by the nurse (enema bag, tube, clamp, and waterproof pad)
   - Bath thermometer
   - Waterproof pad (if not in the enema kit)
   - Water-soluble lubricant
   - Gloves
   - 3 to 5 ml (1 teaspoon) castile soap or 1 to 2 teaspoons of salt
   - Toilet tissue
   - Bath blanket
   - IV pole
   - Robe and non-skid footwear
   - Paper towels
4. Identified the person. Checked the ID bracelet with the assignment sheet. Called the person by name.
5. Provided for privacy.
6. Raised the bed for body mechanics. Bed rails were up if used.

## Procedure

7. Lowered the bed rail near you if up.
8. Decontaminated hands. Put on gloves.
9. Covered the person with a bath blanket. Fan-folded top linens to the foot of the bed.
10. Positioned the IV pole so the enema bag was 12 inches above the anus, or it was at a height directed by the nurse.

| Procedure—cont'd | S | U | Comments |
|---|---|---|---|

11. Raised the bed rail if used. \_\_\_\_ \_\_\_\_ _____

12. Prepared the enema:

    a. Closed the clamp on the tube. \_\_\_\_ \_\_\_\_ _____

    b. Adjusted water flow until it was lukewarm. \_\_\_\_ \_\_\_\_ _____

    c. Filled the enema bag for the amount ordered. \_\_\_\_ \_\_\_\_ _____

    d. Measured water temperature with the bath thermometer (Usually 105°F [40.5° C] for adults) \_\_\_\_ \_\_\_\_ _____

    e. Prepared the enema solution as directed by the nurse:

       (1) Saline enema: added salt as directed \_\_\_\_ \_\_\_\_ _____

       (2) Soapsuds enema: added castile soap as directed \_\_\_\_ \_\_\_\_ _____

       (3) Tap-water enema: added nothing \_\_\_\_ \_\_\_\_ _____

    f. Stirred the solution with the bath thermometer. Scooped off any suds. (SSE) \_\_\_\_ \_\_\_\_ _____

    g. Sealed the bag. \_\_\_\_ \_\_\_\_ _____

    h. Hung the bag on the IV pole. \_\_\_\_ \_\_\_\_ _____

13. Lowered the bed rail near you if up. \_\_\_\_ \_\_\_\_ _____

14. Positioned the person in Sims' position or in a left side-lying position. \_\_\_\_ \_\_\_\_ _____

15. Placed a waterproof pad under the buttocks. \_\_\_\_ \_\_\_\_ _____

16. Exposed the anal area. \_\_\_\_ \_\_\_\_ _____

17. Placed the bedpan behind the person. \_\_\_\_ \_\_\_\_ _____

18. Positioned the enema tube in the bedpan. Removed the cap from the tubing. \_\_\_\_ \_\_\_\_ _____

19. Opened the clamp. Let solution flow through the tube to remove air. Clamped the tube. \_\_\_\_ \_\_\_\_ _____

20. Lubricated the tube 3 to 4 inches from the tip. \_\_\_\_ \_\_\_\_ _____

21. Separated the buttocks to see the anus. \_\_\_\_ \_\_\_\_ _____

22. Asked the person to take a deep breath through the mouth. \_\_\_\_ \_\_\_\_ _____

23. Inserted the tube gently 3 to 4 inches into the adult's rectum. Did this when the person was exhaling. Stopped if the person complained of pain, resistance was felt, or bleeding occurred. \_\_\_\_ \_\_\_\_ _____

24. Checked the amount of solution in the bag. \_\_\_\_ \_\_\_\_ _____

25. Unclamped the tube. Gave the solution slowly. \_\_\_\_ \_\_\_\_ _____

26. Asked the person to take slow deep breaths. \_\_\_\_ \_\_\_\_ _____

27. Clamped the tube if the person needed to defecate, had cramping, or started to expel solution. Unclamped when symptoms subsided. \_\_\_\_ \_\_\_\_ _____

28. Gave the amount of solution ordered. Stopped if the person could not tolerate the procedure. \_\_\_\_ \_\_\_\_ _____

29. Clamped the tube before it was empty. \_\_\_\_ \_\_\_\_ _____

30. Held toilet tissue around the tube and against the anus. Removed the tube. \_\_\_\_ \_\_\_\_ _____

*Continued*

| Procedure—cont'd | S | U | Comments |
|---|---|---|---|

31. Discarded the toilet tissue into the bedpan. _____ _____ _____

32. Wrapped the tubing tip with paper towels. Placed it inside the enema bag. _____ _____ _____

33. Helped the person onto the bedpan.Raised the head of the bed, and raised the bed rail if used. Or assisted the person to the bathroom or commode. The person wore a robe and non-skid footwear when up. The bed was in the lowest position. _____ _____ _____

34. Placed the signal light and toilet tissue within reach. Reminded the person not to flush the toilet. _____ _____ _____

35. Discarded disposable items. _____ _____ _____

36. Removed the gloves. Decontaminated hands. _____ _____ _____

37. Left the room if the person could be left alone. _____ _____ _____

38. Returned when the person signaled. Or checked on the person every 5 minutes. Knocked before entering. _____ _____ _____

39. Decontaminated hands and put on gloves. Lowered the bed rail if up. _____ _____ _____

40. Observed enema results for amount, color, consistency, and odor. Called for the nurse to observe the results. _____ _____ _____

41. Provided perineal care as needed. _____ _____ _____

42. Removed the waterproof pad. _____ _____ _____

43. Emptied, cleaned, and disinfected the bedpan or commode. Flushed the toilet after the nurse observed the results. Returned items to their proper place. _____ _____ _____

44. Removed the gloves. Practiced hand hygiene. _____ _____ _____

45. Assisted with hand washing. Wore gloves if needed. _____ _____ _____

46. Covered the person. Removed the bath blanket. _____ _____ _____

## Post-Procedure

47. Provided for comfort as noted on the inside of the front book cover. _____ _____ _____

48. Placed the signal light within reach. _____ _____ _____

49. Lowered the bed to its lowest position. _____ _____ _____

50. Raised or lowered bed rails. Followed the care plan. _____ _____ _____

51. Unscreened the person. _____ _____ _____

52. Completed a safety check of the room as noted on the inside of the front book cover. _____ _____ _____

53. Followed agency policy for soiled linen and used supplies. _____ _____ _____

54. Decontaminated hands. _____ _____ _____

55. Reported and recorded observations. _____ _____ _____

Date of Satisfactory Completion _____    Instructor's Initials_____

## Giving a Small-Volume Enema

Name: _____     Date: _____

| Quality of Life | S | U | Comments |
|---|---|---|---|

- Knocked before entering the person's room.   _____ _____ _____
- Addressed the person by name.   _____ _____ _____
- Introduced yourself by name and title.   _____ _____ _____
- Explained the procedure to the person before beginning and during the procedure.   _____ _____ _____
- Protected the person's rights during the procedure.   _____ _____ _____
- Handled the person gently during the procedure.   _____ _____ _____

### Pre-Procedure

1. Followed "Delegation Guidelines: Enemas." Reviewed "Promoting Safety and Comfort: Enemas."   _____ _____ _____
2. Practiced hand hygiene.   _____ _____ _____
3. Collected the following:
   - Small volume enema   _____ _____ _____
   - Bedpan or commode   _____ _____ _____
   - Waterproof pad   _____ _____ _____
   - Toilet tissue   _____ _____ _____
   - Gloves   _____ _____ _____
   - Robe and non-skid footwear   _____ _____ _____
   - Bath blanket   _____ _____ _____
4. Identified the person. Checked the ID bracelet with the assignment sheet. Called the person by name.   _____ _____ _____
5. Provided for privacy.   _____ _____ _____
6. Raised the bed for body mechanics. Bed rails were up if used.   _____ _____ _____

### Procedure

7. Lowered the bed rail near you if up.   _____ _____ _____
8. Decontaminated hands. Put on the gloves.   _____ _____ _____
9. Covered the person with a bath blanket. Fan-folded top linens to the foot of the bed.   _____ _____ _____
10. Positioned the person in Sims' or a left side-lying position.   _____ _____ _____
11. Placed the waterproof pad under the buttocks.   _____ _____ _____
12. Exposed the anal area.   _____ _____ _____
13. Positioned the bedpan near the person.   _____ _____ _____
14. Removed the cap from the enema tip.   _____ _____ _____
15. Separated the buttocks to see the anus.   _____ _____ _____

*Continued*

| Procedure—cont'd | S | U | Comments |
|---|---|---|---|
| 16. Asked the person to take a deep breath through the mouth. | _____ | _____ | _____ |
| 17. Inserted the enema tip 2 inches into the rectum. Did this when the person was exhaling. Inserted the tip gently. Stopped if the person complained of pain, resistance was felt, or bleeding occurred. | _____ | _____ | _____ |
| 18. Squeezed and rolled the bottle gently. Released pressure on the bottle after the tip was removed from the rectum. | _____ | _____ | _____ |
| 19. Put the bottle into the box, tip first. | _____ | _____ | _____ |
| 20. Helped the person onto the bedpan; raised the head of the bed. Raised or lowered bed rails according to the care plan. Or assisted the person to the bathroom or commode. The person wore a robe and non-skid footwear when up. The bed was in the lowest position. | _____ | _____ | _____ |
| 21. Placed the signal light and toilet tissue within reach. Reminded the person not to flush the toilet. | _____ | _____ | _____ |
| 22. Discarded disposable items. | _____ | _____ | _____ |
| 23. Removed the gloves. Decontaminated hands. | _____ | _____ | _____ |
| 24. Left the room if the person could be left alone. | _____ | _____ | _____ |
| 25. Returned when the person signaled. Or checked on the person every 5 minutes. Knocked before entering. | _____ | _____ | _____ |
| 26. Decontaminated hands. Put on gloves. | _____ | _____ | _____ |
| 27. Lowered the bed rail if up. | _____ | _____ | _____ |
| 28. Observed enema results for amount, color, consistency, shape, and odor. | _____ | _____ | _____ |
| 29. Helped the person with perineal care. | _____ | _____ | _____ |
| 30. Removed the waterproof pad. | _____ | _____ | _____ |
| 31. Emptied, cleaned, and disinfected the bedpan or commode. Flushed the toilet after the nurse observed the results. | _____ | _____ | _____ |
| 32. Returned equipment to its proper place. | _____ | _____ | _____ |
| 33. Removed the gloves. Practiced hand hygiene. | _____ | _____ | _____ |
| 34. Assisted the person with hand washing. Wore gloves if necessary. | _____ | _____ | _____ |
| 35. Returned top linens. Removed the bath blanket. | _____ | _____ | _____ |

## Post-Procedure

| | S | U | Comments |
|---|---|---|---|
| 36. Followed steps 47 through 55 in procedure "Giving a Cleansing Enema." | _____ | _____ | _____ |

Date of Satisfactory Completion _____     Instructor's Initials_____

## Preparing the Person For a Meal

Name: _____          Date: _____

| Quality of Life | S | U | Comments |
|---|---|---|---|

- Knocked before entering the person's room.
- Addressed the person by name.
- Introduced yourself by name and title.
- Explained the procedure to the person before beginning and during the procedure.
- Protected the person's rights during the procedure.
- Handled the person gently during the procedure.

### Pre-Procedure

1. Followed "Delegation Guidelines: Preparing for Meals." Reviewed "Promoting Safety and Comfort: Preparing for Meals."
2. Practiced hand hygiene.
3. Collected the following:
   - Equipment for oral hygiene
   - Bedpan, urinal, commode, or specimen pan and toilet tissue
   - Wash basin
   - Soap
   - Washcloth
   - Towel
   - Gloves
4. Provided for privacy.

### Procedure

5. Made sure eyeglasses and hearing aids were in place.
6. Assisted with oral hygiene. Made sure dentures were in place. Wore gloves and practiced hand hygiene after removing them.
7. Assisted with elimination. Made sure the incontinent person was clean and dry. Wore gloves and practiced hand hygiene after removing them.
8. Assisted the person with hand washing. Wore gloves and practiced hand hygiene after removing them.
9. Did the following if the person would eat in bed:
   a. Raised the head of the bed to a comfortable position.
   b. Cleaned the overbed table. Adjusted it in front of the person.

*Continued*

| Procedure—cont'd | S | U | Comments |
|---|---|---|---|
| c. Placed the signal light within reach. | _____ | _____ | _____ |
| d. Unscreened the person. | _____ | _____ | _____ |
| 10. Did the following if the person would sit in a chair: | | | |
| a. Positioned the person in a chair or wheelchair. | _____ | _____ | _____ |
| b. Removed items from the overbed table. Cleaned the table. | _____ | _____ | _____ |
| c. Adjusted the overbed table in front of the person. | _____ | _____ | _____ |
| d. Placed the signal light within reach. | _____ | _____ | _____ |
| e. Unscreened the person. | _____ | _____ | _____ |
| 11. Assisted the person to the dining area (if the person would eat in the dining area). | _____ | _____ | _____ |

## Post-Procedure

| | S | U | Comments |
|---|---|---|---|
| 12. Provided for comfort as noted on the inside of the front book cover. | _____ | _____ | _____ |
| 13. Cleaned and returned equipment to its proper place. Wore gloves for this step. | _____ | _____ | _____ |
| 14. Straightened the room. Eliminated unpleasant noise, odors, or equipment. | _____ | _____ | _____ |
| 15. Completed a safety check of the room as noted on the inside of the front book cover. | _____ | _____ | _____ |
| 16. Removed the gloves. Decontaminated hands. | _____ | _____ | _____ |

Date of Satisfactory Completion _____   Instructor's Initials_____

## Serving Meal Trays

Name: _____     Date: _____

| Quality of Life | S | U | Comments |
|---|---|---|---|
| • Knocked before entering the person's room. | _____ | _____ | _____ |
| • Addressed the person by name. | _____ | _____ | _____ |
| • Introduced yourself by name and title. | _____ | _____ | _____ |
| • Explained the procedure to the person before beginning and during the procedure. | _____ | _____ | _____ |
| • Protected the person's rights during the procedure. | _____ | _____ | _____ |
| • Handled the person gently during the procedure. | _____ | _____ | _____ |

### Pre-Procedure

| | S | U | Comments |
|---|---|---|---|
| 1. Followed "Delegation Guidelines: Serving Meal Trays." Reviewed "Promoting Safety and Comfort: Serving Meal Trays." | _____ | _____ | _____ |
| 2. Practiced hand hygiene. | _____ | _____ | _____ |

### Procedure

| | S | U | Comments |
|---|---|---|---|
| 3. Made sure the tray was complete. Checked items on the tray with the dietary card. Made sure adaptive equipment was included. | _____ | _____ | _____ |
| 4. Identified the person. Checked the ID bracelet with the dietary card. Called the person by name. | _____ | _____ | _____ |
| 5. Placed the tray within the person's reach. Adjusted the overbed table as needed. | _____ | _____ | _____ |
| 6. Removed food covers. Opened cartons, cut meat, and buttered bread as needed. | _____ | _____ | _____ |
| 7. Placed the napkin, clothes protector, adaptive equipment, and eating utensils within reach. | _____ | _____ | _____ |
| 8. Measured and recorded intake if ordered (Chapter 18). Noted the amount and type of foods eaten. | _____ | _____ | _____ |
| 9. Checked for and removed any food in the mouth. Wore gloves. Decontaminated hands after removing the gloves. | _____ | _____ | _____ |
| 10. Removed the tray. | _____ | _____ | _____ |
| 11. Cleaned spills. Changed soiled linen and clothing. | _____ | _____ | _____ |
| 12. Helped the person return to bed if needed. | _____ | _____ | _____ |

### Post-Procedure

| | S | U | Comments |
|---|---|---|---|
| 13. Assisted the person with oral hygiene and hand washing. Wore gloves. | _____ | _____ | _____ |
| 14. Removed the gloves. Decontaminated hands. | _____ | _____ | _____ |

*Continued*

| Post-Procedure—cont'd | S | U | Comments |
|---|---|---|---|
| 15. Provided for comfort as noted on inside of the front book cover. | _____ | _____ | _____ |
| 16. Placed the signal light within reach. | _____ | _____ | _____ |
| 17. Raised or lowered bed rails. Followed the care plan. | _____ | _____ | _____ |
| 18. Completed a safety check of the room as noted on the inside of the front book cover. | _____ | _____ | _____ |
| 19. Followed agency policy for soiled linen. | _____ | _____ | _____ |
| 20. Decontaminated hands. | _____ | _____ | _____ |
| 21. Reported and recorded observations. | _____ | _____ | _____ |

Date of Satisfactory Completion _____    Instructor's Initials_____

# Feeding the Person

Name: _____          Date: _____

| Quality of Life | S | U | Comments |
|---|---|---|---|

**Quality of Life**

- Knocked before entering the person's room.
- Addressed the person by name.
- Introduced yourself by name and title.
- Explained the procedure to the person before beginning and during the procedure.
- Protected the person's rights during the procedure.
- Handled the person gently during the procedure.

**Pre-Procedure**

1. Followed "Delegation Guidelines: Feeding the Person." Reviewed "Promoting Safety and Comfort:Feeding the Person."
2. Practiced hand hygiene.
3. Positioned the person in a comfortable position for eating (usually sitting or Fowler's).
4. Got the tray. Placed it on the overbed table or dining table.

**Procedure**

5. Identified the person. Checked the ID bracelet with the dietary card. Called the person by name.
6. Draped a napkin across the person's chest and underneath the chin.
7. Told the person what foods and fluids were on the tray.
8. Prepared food for eating. Seasoned food as the person preferred and was allowed on the care plan.
9. Served foods in the order the person preferred. Identified foods as you served them. Alternated between solid and liquid foods. Used a spoon for safety. Allowed enough time for chewing and swallowing. Did not rush the person.
10. Checked the person's mouth before offering more food. Made sure the person's mouth was empty between bites and swallows.
11. Used straws for liquids if the person could not drink out of a glass or cup. Had one straw for each liquid. Provided short straws for weak persons.
12. Wiped the person's hands, face, and mouth as needed during the meal. Used the napkin.
13. Followed the care plan if the person had dysphagia. Gave thickened liquid with a spoon.
14. Conversed with the person in a pleasant manner.
15. Encouraged the person to eat as much as possible.

*Continued*

| Procedure—cont'd | S | U | Comments |
|---|---|---|---|
| 16. Wiped the person's mouth with a napkin. Discarded the napkin. | _____ | _____ | _____ |
| 17. Noted how much and which foods were eaten. | _____ | _____ | _____ |
| 18. Measured and recorded intake if ordered (Chapter 18). | _____ | _____ | _____ |
| 19. Removed the tray. | _____ | _____ | _____ |
| 20. Took the person back to his or her room (if in the dining room). | _____ | _____ | _____ |
| 21. Assisted the person with oral hygiene and hand washing. Provided for privacy, and put on gloves. Decontaminated hands after removing the gloves. | _____ | _____ | _____ |

**Post-Procedure**

| | S | U | Comments |
|---|---|---|---|
| 22. Provided for comfort as noted on the inside of the front book cover. | _____ | _____ | _____ |
| 23. Placed the signal light within reach. | _____ | _____ | _____ |
| 24. Raised or lowered bed rails. Followed the care plan. | _____ | _____ | _____ |
| 25. Completed a safety check of the room as noted on the inside of the front book cover. | _____ | _____ | _____ |
| 26. Returned the food tray to the food cart. | _____ | _____ | _____ |
| 27. Decontaminated hands. | _____ | _____ | _____ |
| 28. Reported and recorded observations. | _____ | _____ | _____ |

Date of Satisfactory Completion _____    Instructor's Initials_____

## Taking a Temprature With a Glass Thermometer

Name: _____     Date: _____

| Quality of Life | S | U | Comments |
|---|---|---|---|

- Knocked before entering the person's room.
- Addressed the person by name.
- Introduced yourself by name and title.
- Explained the procedure to the person before beginning and during the procedure.
- Protected the person's rights during the procedure.
- Handled the person gently during the procedure.

### Pre-Procedure

1. Followed "Delegation Guidelines: Taking Temperatures." Reviewed "Promoting Safety and Comfort:
   - Glass Thermometers"
   - Taking Temperatures"
2. For an oral temperature, asked the person not to eat, drink, smoke, or chew gum for at least 15 to 20 minutes or as required by agency policy.
3. Practiced hand hygiene.
4. Collected the following:
   - Oral or rectal thermometer and holder
   - Tissues
   - Plastic covers if used
   - Gloves
   - Toilet tissue (rectal temperature)
   - Water-soluble lubricant (rectal temperature)
   - Towel (axillary temperature)
5. Identified the person. Checked the ID bracelet against the assignment sheet. Called the person by name.
6. Provided for privacy.

### Procedure

7. Put on the gloves.
8. Rinsed the thermometer in cold water if it was soaking in a disinfectant. Dried it with tissues.
9. Checked for breaks, cracks, or chips.
10. Shook down the thermometer below the lowest number. Held the thermometer by the stem.
11. Inserted it into a plastic cover if used.
12. For an oral temperature:
    a. Asked the person to moisten the lips.
    b. Placed the bulb end of the thermometer under the tongue and to one side.

*Continued*

| Procedure—cont'd | S | U | Comments |
|---|---|---|---|

   c. Asked the person to close the lips around the thermometer to hold it in place. \_\_\_\_ \_\_\_\_ _____

   d. Asked the person not to talk. Reminded the person not to bite down on the thermometer. \_\_\_\_ \_\_\_\_ _____

   e. Left it in place for 2 to 3 minutes or as required by agency policy. (Some state competency tests require leaving the thermometer in place for 3 minutes.) \_\_\_\_ \_\_\_\_ _____

13. For a rectal temperature:

   a. Positioned the person in Sims' position. \_\_\_\_ \_\_\_\_ _____

   b. Put a small amount of lubricant on a tissue. Lubricated the bulb end of the thermometer. \_\_\_\_ \_\_\_\_ _____

   c. Folded back top linens to expose the anal area. \_\_\_\_ \_\_\_\_ _____

   d. Raised the upper buttock to expose the anus. \_\_\_\_ \_\_\_\_ _____

   e. Inserted the thermometer 1 inch into the rectum. Did not force the thermometer. \_\_\_\_ \_\_\_\_ _____

   f. Held the thermometer in place for 2 minutes or as required by agency policy. Did not let go of it while it was in the rectum. \_\_\_\_ \_\_\_\_ _____

14. For an axillary temperature:

   a. Helped the person remove an arm from the gown. Did not expose the person. \_\_\_\_ \_\_\_\_ _____

   b. Dried the axilla with the towel. \_\_\_\_ \_\_\_\_ _____

   c. Placed the bulb end of the thermometer in the center of the axilla. \_\_\_\_ \_\_\_\_ _____

   d. Asked the person to place the arm over the chest to hold the thermometer in place. Held it and the arm in place if he or she could not help. \_\_\_\_ \_\_\_\_ _____

   e. Left the thermometer in place for 5 to 10 minutes or as required by agency policy. \_\_\_\_ \_\_\_\_ _____

15. Removed the thermometer. \_\_\_\_ \_\_\_\_ _____

16. Used tissues to remove the plastic cover. Discarded the cover and tissue. Wiped the thermometer with a tissue if no cover was used. Wiped from the stem to the bulb end. Discarded the tissue. \_\_\_\_ \_\_\_\_ _____

17. Read the thermometer. \_\_\_\_ \_\_\_\_ _____

18. Noted the person's name and temperature on the notepad or assignment sheet. Wrote R for a rectal temperature. Wrote A for an axillary temperature. \_\_\_\_ \_\_\_\_ _____

19. For a rectal temperature:

   a. Placed used toilet tissue on several thicknesses of toilet tissue. \_\_\_\_ \_\_\_\_ _____

   b. Placed the thermometer on clean toilet tissue. \_\_\_\_ \_\_\_\_ _____

   c. Wiped the anal area to remove excess lubricant and any feces. \_\_\_\_ \_\_\_\_ _____

   d. Covered the person. \_\_\_\_ \_\_\_\_ _____

| Procedure—cont'd | S | U | Comments |
|---|---|---|---|
| 20. For an axillary temperature: Helped the person put the gown back on. | ____ | ____ | _____ |
| 21. Shook down the thermometer. | ____ | ____ | _____ |
| 22. Cleaned the thermometer according to agency policy. Returned it to the holder. | ____ | ____ | _____ |
| 23. Discarded tissue and disposed of toilet tissue. | ____ | ____ | _____ |
| 24. Removed the gloves. Decontaminated hands. | ____ | ____ | _____ |

## Post-Procedure

| | S | U | Comments |
|---|---|---|---|
| 25. Provided for comfort as noted on the inside of the front book cover. | ____ | ____ | _____ |
| 26. Placed the signal light within reach. | ____ | ____ | _____ |
| 27. Unscreened the person. | ____ | ____ | _____ |
| 28. Completed a safety check of the room as noted on the inside of the front book cover. | ____ | ____ | _____ |
| 29. Decontaminated hands. | ____ | ____ | _____ |
| 30. Reported and recorded the temperature. Noted the temperature site. Reported any abnormal temperature at once. | ____ | ____ | _____ |

Date of Satisfactory Completion _____    Instructor's Initials_____

# Taking a Temperature With an Electronic Thermometer

Name: _____        Date: _____

| Quality of Life | S | U | Comments |
|---|---|---|---|

- Knocked before entering the person's room.    _____ _____ _____
- Addressed the person by name.    _____ _____ _____
- Introduced yourself by name and title.    _____ _____ _____
- Explained the procedure to the person before beginning and during the procedure.    _____ _____ _____
- Protected the person's rights during the procedure.    _____ _____ _____
- Handled the person gently during the procedure.    _____ _____ _____

**Pre-Procedure**

1. Followed "Delegation Guidelines: Taking Temperatures." Reviewed "Promoting Safety and Comfort: Taking Temperatures."    _____ _____ _____
2. For an oral temperature, asked the person not to eat, drink, smoke, or chew gum for at least 15 to 20 minutes.    _____ _____ _____
3. Collected the following:
   - Thermometer—electronic or tympanic membrane    _____ _____ _____
   - Probe (Blue for an oral or axillary temperature. Red for a rectal temperature)    _____ _____ _____
   - Probe covers    _____ _____ _____
   - Toilet tissue (rectal temperature)    _____ _____ _____
   - Water-soluble lubricant (rectal temperature)    _____ _____ _____
   - Gloves    _____ _____ _____
   - Towel (axillary temperature)    _____ _____ _____
4. Plugged the probe into the thermometer. (This was not done for a tympanic membrane thermometer.)    _____ _____ _____
5. Practiced hand hygiene.    _____ _____ _____
6. Identified the person. Checked the ID bracelet against the assignment sheet. Called the person by name.    _____ _____ _____

**Procedure**

7. Provided for privacy. Positioned the person for an oral, rectal, axillary, or tympanic membrane temperature.    _____ _____ _____
8. Put on gloves if contact with blood, body fluids, secretions, or excretions was likely.    _____ _____ _____
9. Inserted the probe into a probe cover.    _____ _____ _____
10. For an oral temperature:
    a. Asked the person to open the mouth and raise the tongue.    _____ _____ _____

| Procedure—cont'd | S | U | Comments |
|---|---|---|---|

b. Placed the covered probe at the base of the tongue and to one side. \_\_\_\_\_ \_\_\_\_\_ _____

c. Asked the person to lower the tongue and close the mouth. \_\_\_\_\_ \_\_\_\_\_ _____

11. For a rectal temperature:

   a. Placed some lubricant on toilet tissue. \_\_\_\_\_ \_\_\_\_\_ _____

   b. Lubricated the end of the covered probe. \_\_\_\_\_ \_\_\_\_\_ _____

   c. Exposed the anal area. \_\_\_\_\_ \_\_\_\_\_ _____

   d. Raised the upper buttock. \_\_\_\_\_ \_\_\_\_\_ _____

   e. Inserted the probe ½ inch into the rectum. \_\_\_\_\_ \_\_\_\_\_ _____

   f. Held the probe in place. \_\_\_\_\_ \_\_\_\_\_ _____

12. For an axillary temperature:

   a. Helped the person remove an arm from the gown. Did not expose the person. \_\_\_\_\_ \_\_\_\_\_ _____

   b. Dried the axilla with the towel. \_\_\_\_\_ \_\_\_\_\_ _____

   c. Placed the covered probe in the axilla. \_\_\_\_\_ \_\_\_\_\_ _____

   d. Placed the person's arm over the chest. \_\_\_\_\_ \_\_\_\_\_ _____

   e. Held the probe in place. \_\_\_\_\_ \_\_\_\_\_ _____

13. For a tympanic membrane temperature:

   a. Asked the person to turn the head so the ear was in front of you. \_\_\_\_\_ \_\_\_\_\_ _____

   b. Pulled up and back on the ear to straighten the ear canal. \_\_\_\_\_ \_\_\_\_\_ _____

   c. Inserted the covered probe gently. \_\_\_\_\_ \_\_\_\_\_ _____

14. Started the thermometer. \_\_\_\_\_ \_\_\_\_\_ _____

15. Held the probe in place until a tone was heard or a flashing or steady light was seen. \_\_\_\_\_ \_\_\_\_\_ _____

16. Read the temperature on the display. \_\_\_\_\_ \_\_\_\_\_ _____

17. Removed the probe. Pressed the eject button to discard the cover. \_\_\_\_\_ \_\_\_\_\_ _____

18. Noted the person's name and temperature on the notepad or assignment sheet. Noted the temperature site. \_\_\_\_\_ \_\_\_\_\_ _____

19. Returned the probe to the holder. \_\_\_\_\_ \_\_\_\_\_ _____

20. Helped the person put the gown back on (axillary temperature). For a rectal temperature: \_\_\_\_\_ \_\_\_\_\_ _____

   a. Wiped the anal area with toilet tissue to remove lubricant. \_\_\_\_\_ \_\_\_\_\_ _____

   b. Covered the person. \_\_\_\_\_ \_\_\_\_\_ _____

   c. Disposed of used toilet tissue. \_\_\_\_\_ \_\_\_\_\_ _____

   d. Removed the gloves. Decontaminated hands. \_\_\_\_\_ \_\_\_\_\_ _____

*Continued*

Post-Procedure                                         S        U              Comments

21. Provided for comfort as noted on          _____  _____  _____
    the inside of the front book cover.

22. Placed the signal light within reach.      _____  _____  _____

23. Unscreened the person.                     _____  _____  _____

24. Completed a safety check of the room as noted   _____  _____  _____
    on the inside of the front book cover.

25. Returned the thermometer to the charging unit.   _____  _____  _____

26. Decontaminated hands.                      _____  _____  _____

27. Reported and recorded the temperature. Noted   _____  _____  _____
    the temperature site. Reported any abnormal
    temperature at once.

Date of Satisfactory Completion _____    Instructor's Initials_____

Taking a Radial Pulse (NNAAP™)

Name: _____    Date: _____

| Quality of Life | S | U | Comments |
|---|---|---|---|

- Knocked before entering the person's room.      _____ _____ _____
- Addressed the person by name.      _____ _____ _____
- Introduced yourself by name and title.      _____ _____ _____
- Explained the procedure to the person
  before beginning and during the procedure.      _____ _____ _____
- Protected the person's rights during the procedure.      _____ _____ _____
- Handled the person gently during the procedure.      _____ _____ _____

## Pre-Procedure

1. Followed "Delegation Guidelines: Taking Pulses."
   Reviewed "Promoting Safety and Comfort:
   Taking Pulses."      _____ _____ _____
2. Practiced hand hygiene.      _____ _____ _____
3. Identified the person. Checked the ID bracelet against
   the assignment sheet. Called the person by name.      _____ _____ _____
4. Provided for privacy.      _____ _____ _____

## Procedure

5. Had the person sit or lie down.      _____ _____ _____
6. Located the radial pulse. Used the
   first 2 or 3 middle fingers.      _____ _____ _____
7. Noted if the pulse was strong or
   weak, and regular or irregular.      _____ _____ _____
8. Counted the pulse for 30 seconds. Multiplied      _____ _____ _____
   the number of beats by 2. Or counted the pulse for
   1 minute as directed by the nurse or if required
   by agency policy. (Some state competency tests require
   counting the pulse for 1 minute.)
9. Counted the pulse for 1 minute if it was irregular.      _____ _____ _____
10. Noted the person's name and pulse on the note      _____ _____ _____
    pad or assignment sheet. Noted the strength of
    the pulse. Noted if it was regular or irregular.

## Post-Procedure

11. Provided for comfort as noted on the inside      _____ _____ _____
    of the front book cover.
12. Placed the signal light within reach.      _____ _____ _____
13. Unscreened the person.      _____ _____ _____

*Continued*

Post-Procedure—cont'd                              S         U              Comments

14. Completed a safety check of the room          _____   _____   _____
    as noted on the inside of the front book cover.

15. Decontaminated hands.                         _____   _____   _____

16. Reported and recorded the pulse rate and      _____   _____   _____
    observations. Reported an abnormal pulse at once.

Date of Satisfactory Completion _____    Instructor's Initials_____

## Taking an Apical Pulse

Name: _____     Date: _____

| Quality of Life | S | U | Comments |
|---|---|---|---|

- Knocked before entering the person's room.     _____ _____ _____
- Addressed the person by name.     _____ _____ _____
- Introduced yourself by name and title.     _____ _____ _____
- Explained the procedure to the person before beginning and during the procedure.     _____ _____ _____
- Protected the person's rights during the procedure.     _____ _____ _____
- Handled the person gently during the procedure.     _____ _____ _____

### Pre-Procedure

1. Followed "Delegation Guidelines: Taking Pulses." Reviewed "Promoting Safety and Comfort: Using a Stethoscope."     _____ _____ _____
2. Collected a stethoscope and antiseptic wipes.     _____ _____ _____
3. Practiced hand hygiene.     _____ _____ _____
4. Identified the person. Checked the ID bracelet against the assignment sheet. Called the person by name.     _____ _____ _____
5. Provided for privacy.     _____ _____ _____

### Procedure

6. Cleaned the earpieces and diaphragm with the wipes.     _____ _____ _____
7. Had the person sit or lie down.     _____ _____ _____
8. Exposed the nipple area of the left chest. Did not expose a woman's breasts.     _____ _____ _____
9. Warmed the diaphragm in your palm.     _____ _____ _____
10. Placed the earpieces in your ears.     _____ _____ _____
11. Found the apical pulse. Placed the diaphragm 2 to 3 inches to the left of the breastbone and below the left nipple.     _____ _____ _____
12. Counted the pulse for 1 minute. Noted if it was regular or irregular.     _____ _____ _____
13. Covered the person. Removed the earpieces.     _____ _____ _____
14. Noted the person's name and pulse on the notepad or assignment sheet. Noted if the pulse was regular or irregular.     _____ _____ _____

### Post-Procedure

15. Provided for comfort as noted on the inside of the front book cover.     _____ _____ _____
16. Placed the signal light within reach.     _____ _____ _____

*Continued*

| Post-Procedure—cont'd | S | U | Comments |
|---|---|---|---|
| 17. Returned the stethoscope to its proper place. | _____ | _____ | _____ |
| 18. Unscreened the person. | _____ | _____ | _____ |
| 19. Cleaned the earpieces and diaphragm with the wipes. | _____ | _____ | _____ |
| 20. Completed a safety check of the room as noted on the inside of the front book cover. | _____ | _____ | _____ |
| 21. Decontaminated hands. | _____ | _____ | _____ |
| 22. Reported and recorded observations. Recorded the pulse rate with *Ap* for apical pulse. Reported an abnormal pulse at once. | _____ | _____ | _____ |

Date of Satisfactory Completion _____     Instructor's Initials_____

# Counting Respirations (NNAAP™)

Name: _____          Date: _____

| Procedure | S | U | Comments |
|---|---|---|---|

1. Followed "Delegation Guidelines: Respirations."     _____ _____ _____
2. Kept your fingers or the stethoscope over
   the pulse site.                                     _____ _____ _____
3. Did not tell the person you were
   counting respirations.                              _____ _____ _____
4. Began counting when the chest rose. Counted each    _____ _____ _____
   rise and fall of the chest as 1 respiration.
5. Noted the following:
   - If respirations were regular                      _____ _____ _____
   - If both sides of the chest rose equally           _____ _____ _____
   - The depth of respirations                         _____ _____ _____
   - If the person had any pain or difficulty breathing _____ _____ _____
6. Counted respirations for 30 seconds. Multiplied     _____ _____ _____
   the number by 2. (Some state competency tests require
   counting respirations for 1 minute.)
7. Counted respirations for 1 minute if they were abnormal _____ _____ _____
   or irregular.
8. Noted the person's name, respiratory rate, and      _____ _____ _____
   other observations on the notepad or assignment sheet.

## Post-Procedure

9. Provided for comfort as noted                       _____ _____ _____
   on the inside of the front book cover.
10. Placed the signal light within reach.              _____ _____ _____
11. Unscreened the person.                             _____ _____ _____
12. Completed a safety check of the room as noted      _____ _____ _____
    on the inside of the front book cover.
13. Decontaminated hands.                              _____ _____ _____
14. Reported and recorded the respiratory rate and     _____ _____ _____
    observations. Reported abnormal respirations at once.

Date of Satisfactory Completion _____          Instructor's Initials_____

# Measuring Blood Pressure (NNAAP™)

Name: _____    Date: _____

| | S | U | Comments |
|---|---|---|---|

## Quality of Life

- Knocked before entering the person's room.    _____ _____ _____
- Addressed the person by name.    _____ _____ _____
- Introduced yourself by name and title.    _____ _____ _____
- Explained the procedure to the person
  before beginning and during the procedure.    _____ _____ _____
- Protected the person's rights during the procedure.    _____ _____ _____
- Handled the person gently during the procedure.    _____ _____ _____

## Pre-Procedure

1. Followed "Delegation Guidelines: Measuring
   Blood Pressures." Reviewed "Promoting
   Safety and Comfort:    _____ _____ _____
   - "Using a Stethoscope"
   - "Equipment"
2. Collected the following:
   - Sphygmomanometer    _____ _____ _____
   - Stethoscope    _____ _____ _____
   - Antiseptic wipes    _____ _____ _____
3. Practiced hand hygiene.    _____ _____ _____
4. Identified the person. Checked the ID bracelet against
   the assignment sheet. Called the person by name.    _____ _____ _____
5. Provided for privacy.    _____ _____ _____

## Procedure

6. Wiped the stethoscope earpieces and
   diaphragm with the wipes.    _____ _____ _____
7. Had the person sit or lie down.    _____ _____ _____
8. Positioned the person's arm level
   with the heart. The palm was up.    _____ _____ _____
9. Stood no more than 3 feet away from the
   manometer. The mercury model was vertical, on a
   flat surface, and at eye level. The aneroid type was
   directly in front of you.    _____ _____ _____
10. Exposed the upper arm.    _____ _____ _____
11. Squeezed the cuff to expel any remaining air.
    Closed the valve on the bulb.    _____ _____ _____
12. Found the brachial artery at the inner aspect of the elbow.    _____ _____ _____
    Used your fingertips.
13. Placed the arrow on the cuff over the brachial artery.    _____ _____ _____
    Wrapped the cuff around the upper arm at least
    1 inch above the elbow. It was even and snug.

| Procedure—cont'd | S | U | Comments |
|---|---|---|---|

14. One-step method:
   a. Placed the stethoscope earpieces in your ears. ___ ___ _____
   b. Found the radial or brachial artery. ___ ___ _____
   c. Inflated the cuff until the pulse could no longer be felt. Noted this point. ___ ___ _____
   d. Inflated the cuff 30 mm Hg beyond the point where you last felt the pulse. ___ ___ _____

15. Two-step method:
   a. Found the radial or brachial artery. ___ ___ _____
   b. Inflated the cuff until you could no longer feel the pulse. Noted this point. ___ ___ _____
   c. Inflated the cuff 30 mm Hg beyond the point where you last felt the pulse. ___ ___ _____
   d. Deflated the cuff slowly. Noted the point when you felt the pulse. ___ ___ _____
   e. Waited 30 seconds. ___ ___ _____
   f. Placed the stethoscope earpieces in your ears. ___ ___ _____
   g. Inflated the cuff 30 mm Hg beyond the point where you felt the pulse return. ___ ___ _____

16. Placed the diaphragm over the brachial artery. Did not place it under the cuff. ___ ___ _____

17. Deflated the cuff at an even rate of 2 to 4 millimeters per second. Turned the valve counterclockwise to deflate the cuff. ___ ___ _____

18. Noted the point where you heard the first sound. ___ ___ _____

19. Continued to deflate the cuff. Noted the point where the sound disappeared. ___ ___ _____

20. Deflated the cuff completely. Removed it from the person's arm. Removed the stethoscope earpieces from your ears. ___ ___ _____

21. Noted the person's name and blood pressure on the notepad or assignment sheet. ___ ___ _____

22. Returned the cuff to the case or wall holder. ___ ___ _____

## Post-Procedure

23. Provided for comfort as noted on the inside of the front book cover. ___ ___ _____

24. Placed the signal light within reach. ___ ___ _____

25. Unscreened the person. ___ ___ _____

26. Completed a safety check of the room as noted on the inside of the front book cover. ___ ___ _____

27. Cleaned the earpieces and diaphragm with the wipes. ___ ___ _____

*Continued*

| Post-Procedure—cont'd | S | U | Comments |
|---|---|---|---|
| 28. Returned the equipment to its proper place. | _____ | _____ | _____ |
| 29. Decontaminated hands. | _____ | _____ | _____ |
| 30. Reported and recorded the blood pressure. Reported an abnormal blood pressure at once. | _____ | _____ | _____ |

Date of Satisfactory Completion _____     Instructor's Initials _____

# Measuring Intake and Output (NNAAP™)

Name: _____    Date: _____

| Quality of Life | S | U | Comments |
|---|---|---|---|

- Knocked before entering the person's room.
- Addressed the person by name.
- Introduced yourself by name and title.
- Explained the procedure to the person before beginning and during the procedure.
- Protected the person's rights during the procedure.
- Handled the person gently during the procedure.

### Pre-Procedure

1. Followed "Delegation Guidelines: Intake and Output." Reviewed "Promoting Safety and Comfort: Intake and Output."
2. Practiced hand hygiene.
3. Collected the following:
   - Intake and output (I&O) record
   - Graduates
   - Gloves

### Procedure

4. Put on gloves.
5. Measured intake as follows:
   a. Poured liquid remaining in a container into the graduate.
   b. Measured the amount at eye level. Kept the container level.
   c. Checked the serving amount on the I&O record.
   d. Subtracted the remaining amount from the full serving amount. Recorded the amount.
   e. Poured the fluid in the graduate back into the container.
   f. Repeated steps 5a through 5e for each liquid.
   g. Added the amounts from each liquid together.
   h. Recorded the time and amount on the I&O record.
6. Measured output as follows:
   a. Poured the fluid into the graduate used to measure output.
   b. Measured the amount at eye level. Kept the container level.

*Continued*

| Procedure—cont'd | S | U | Comments |
|---|---|---|---|
| 7. Disposed of fluid in the toilet. Avoided splashes. | _____ | _____ | _____ |
| 8. Cleaned and rinsed the graduates. Disposed of rinse into the toilet. Returned the graduates to their proper place. | _____ | _____ | _____ |
| 9. Cleaned and rinsed the bedpan, urinal, kidney basin, or other drainage container. Discarded the rinse into the toilet. Returned the item to its proper place. | _____ | _____ | _____ |
| 10. Removed the gloves. Decontaminated hands. | _____ | _____ | _____ |
| 11. Recorded the amount on the I&O record. | _____ | _____ | _____ |

## Post-Procedure

| | S | U | Comments |
|---|---|---|---|
| 12. Provided for comfort as noted on the inside of the front book cover. | _____ | _____ | _____ |
| 13. Made sure the signal light was within reach. | _____ | _____ | _____ |
| 14. Completed a safety check of the room as noted on the inside of the front book cover. | _____ | _____ | _____ |
| 15. Reported and recorded observations. | _____ | _____ | _____ |

Date of Satisfactory Completion _____    Instructor's Initials_____

# Measuring Weight and Height (NNAAP™)

Name: _____    Date: _____

| Quality of Life | S | U | Comments |
|---|---|---|---|

- Knocked before entering the person's room.
- Addressed the person by name.
- Introduced yourself by name and title.
- Explained the procedure to the person before beginning and during the procedure.
- Protected the person's rights during the procedure.
- Handled the person gently during the procedure.

## Pre-Procedure

1. Followed "Delegation Guidelines: Measuring Weight and Height." Reviewed "Promoting Safety and Comfort: Measuring Weight and Height."
2. Asked the person to void.
3. Practiced hand hygiene.
4. Brought the scale and paper towels to the person's room.
5. Decontaminated hands.
6. Identified the person. Checked the ID bracelet against the assignment sheet. Called the person by name.
7. Provided for privacy.

## Procedure

8. Placed the paper towels on the scale platform.
9. Raised the height rod.
10. Moved the weights to zero (0). The pointer was in the middle.
11. Had the person remove the robe and footwear. Assisted as needed.
12. Helped the person stand on the scale. The person stood in the center of the scale. Arms were at the side.
13. Moved the weights until the balance pointer was in the middle.
14. Noted the weight on the notepad or assignment sheet.
15. Asked the person to stand very straight.
16. Lowered the height rod until it rested on the person's head.

*Continued*

| Procedure—cont'd | S | U | Comments |
|---|---|---|---|
| 17. Noted the height on the notepad or assignment sheet. | _____ | _____ | _____ |
| 18. Helped the person step off the scale. | _____ | _____ | _____ |
| 19. Helped the person put on a robe and non-skid footwear if he or she would be up. Or helped the person back to bed. | _____ | _____ | _____ |
| 20. Lowered the height rod. Adjusted the weight to zero (0) if agency policy. | _____ | _____ | _____ |

### Post-Procedure

| | S | U | Comments |
|---|---|---|---|
| 21. Provided for comfort as noted on the inside of the front book cover. | _____ | _____ | _____ |
| 22. Placed the signal light within reach. | _____ | _____ | _____ |
| 23. Raised or lowered bed rails. Followed the care plan. | _____ | _____ | _____ |
| 24. Unscreened the person. | _____ | _____ | _____ |
| 25. Discarded the paper towels. | _____ | _____ | _____ |
| 26. Completed a safety check of the room as noted on the inside of the front book cover. | _____ | _____ | _____ |
| 27. Returned the scale to its proper place. | _____ | _____ | _____ |
| 28. Decontaminated hands. | _____ | _____ | _____ |
| 29. Reported and recorded the measurements. | _____ | _____ | _____ |

Date of Satisfactory Completion _____  Instructor's Initials_____

## Collecting a Random Urine Specimen

Name: _____   Date: _____

| | S | U | Comments |
|---|---|---|---|

### Quality of Life

- Knocked before entering the person's room.   _____ _____ _____
- Addressed the person by name.   _____ _____ _____
- Introduced yourself by name and title.   _____ _____ _____
- Explained the procedure to the person
  before beginning and during the procedure.   _____ _____ _____
- Protected the person's rights during the procedure.   _____ _____ _____
- Handled the person gently during the procedure.   _____ _____ _____

### Pre-Procedure

1. Followed "Delegation Guidelines: Urine Specimens."
   Reviewed "Promoting Safety and Comfort: Urine
   Specimens."   _____ _____ _____
2. Practiced hand hygiene. Put on gloves.   _____ _____ _____
3. Collected the following:
   - Voiding receptacle—bedpan and cover, urinal,
     or specimen pan   _____ _____ _____
   - Specimen container and lid   _____ _____ _____
   - Label   _____ _____ _____
   - Gloves   _____ _____ _____
   - Plastic bag   _____ _____ _____

### Procedure

4. Labeled the container.   _____ _____ _____
5. Put the container and lid in the bathroom.   _____ _____ _____
6. Removed the gloves. Decontaminated hands.   _____ _____ _____
7. Identified the person. Checked the ID bracelet against
   the requisition slip. Called the person by name.   _____ _____ _____
8. Provided for privacy.   _____ _____ _____
9. Put on the gloves.   _____ _____ _____
10. Asked the person to void into the receptacle.
    Reminded the person to put toilet tissue into
    the wastebasket or toilet (not in the bedpan or
    specimen pan).   _____ _____ _____
11. Took the receptacle to the bathroom.   _____ _____ _____
12. Poured about 120 ml (4 oz) of urine into
    the specimen container. Disposed of excess urine.   _____ _____ _____
13. Placed the lid on the specimen container.
    Put the container in the plastic bag.   _____ _____ _____
14. Cleaned and returned the receptacle
    to its proper place.   _____ _____ _____

*Continued*

| Procedure—cont'd | S | U | Comments |
|---|---|---|---|
| 15. Removed the gloves and practiced hand hygiene. Put on clean gloves. | _____ | _____ | _____ |
| 16. Assisted the person with hand washing. | _____ | _____ | _____ |
| 17. Removed the gloves. Decontaminated hands. | _____ | _____ | _____ |

**Post-Procedure**

| | | | |
|---|---|---|---|
| 18. Provided for comfort as noted on the inside of the front book cover. | _____ | _____ | _____ |
| 19. Placed the signal light within reach. | _____ | _____ | _____ |
| 20. Raised or lowered bed rails. Followed the care plan. | _____ | _____ | _____ |
| 21. Unscreened the person. | _____ | _____ | _____ |
| 22. Completed a safety check of the room as noted on the inside of the front book cover. | _____ | _____ | _____ |
| 23. Decontaminated hands. | _____ | _____ | _____ |
| 24. Reported and recorded observations. | _____ | _____ | _____ |
| 25. Took the specimen and the requisition slip to the storage area or laboratory. | _____ | _____ | _____ |

Date of Satisfactory Completion _____   Instructor's Initials _____

## Collecting a Midstream Specimen

Name: _____           Date: _____

| Quality of Life | S | U | Comments |
|---|---|---|---|

- Knocked before entering the person's room.                 _____ _____ _____
- Addressed the person by name.                              _____ _____ _____
- Introduced yourself by name and title.                     _____ _____ _____
- Explained the procedure to the person
  before beginning and during the procedure.                 _____ _____ _____
- Protected the person's rights during the procedure.        _____ _____ _____
- Handled the person gently during the procedure.            _____ _____ _____

### Pre-Procedure

1. Followed "Delegation Guidelines: Urine Specimens."        _____ _____ _____
   Reviewed "Promoting Safety and Comfort:
   Urine Specimens."
2. Practiced hand hygiene. Put on gloves.                    _____ _____ _____
3. Collected the following:
   - Midstream specimen kit (with antiseptic solution)       _____ _____ _____
   - Label                                                   _____ _____ _____
   - Disposable gloves                                       _____ _____ _____
   - Sterile gloves (if not part of the kit)                 _____ _____ _____
   - Voiding receptacle—bedpan, urinal,                      _____ _____ _____
     or commode if needed
   - Plastic bag                                             _____ _____ _____
   - Supplies for perineal care                              _____ _____ _____
4. Labeled the container.                                    _____ _____ _____
5. Removed the gloves. Decontaminated hands.                 _____ _____ _____
6. Identified the person. Checked the ID bracelet against    _____ _____ _____
   the requisition slip. Called the person by name.
7. Provided for privacy.                                     _____ _____ _____

### Procedure

8. Provided perineal care. Wore gloves for this step.        _____ _____ _____
   Decontaminated hands after removing them.
9. Opened the sterile kit.                                   _____ _____ _____
10. Put on the sterile gloves.                               _____ _____ _____
11. Poured the antiseptic solution over the cotton balls.    _____ _____ _____
12. Opened the sterile specimen container. Did not touch     _____ _____ _____
    the inside of the container or lid. Set the lid down
    so the inside was up.
13. For a female: cleaned the perineum with cotton balls.    _____ _____ _____
    a. Spread the labia with your thumb and index finger.    _____ _____ _____
       Used your non-dominant hand. (The hand did not
       touch anything sterile after this step.)

*Continued*

Procedure—cont'd                                           S          U              Comments

   b. Cleaned down the urethral area from front
      to back. Used a clean cotton ball for each stroke.    _____  _____  _____

   c. Kept the labia separated to collect the
      urine specimen (steps 15 through 18).                 _____  _____  _____

14. For a male: cleaned the penis with cotton balls.        _____  _____  _____

   a. Held the penis with the non-dominant hand.            _____  _____  _____

   b. Cleaned the penis starting at the meatus. Used a
      cotton ball and cleaned in a circular motion.         _____  _____  _____
      Started at the center and work outward.

   c. Kept holding the penis until the
      specimen was collected (steps 15 through 18).          _____  _____

15. Asked the person to void into the receptacle.           _____  _____  _____

16. Passed the specimen container into the stream
    of urine. Kept the labia separated.                     _____  _____  _____

17. Collected about 30 to 60 ml of urine (1 to 2 oz).       _____  _____  _____

18. Removed the specimen container
    before the person stopped voiding.                      _____  _____  _____

19. Released the labia or penis.                            _____  _____  _____

20. Let the person finish voiding into the receptacle.      _____  _____  _____

21. Put the lid on the specimen container.
    Touched only the outside of the container or lid.       _____  _____  _____

22. Wiped the outside of the container.                     _____  _____  _____

23. Placed the container in a plastic bag.                  _____  _____  _____

24. Provided toilet tissue after
    the person was done voiding.                            _____  _____  _____

25. Took the receptacle to the bathroom.                    _____  _____  _____

26. Measured urine if intake and output was ordered.
    Included the amount in the specimen container.          _____  _____  _____

27. Cleaned the receptacle and other items.
    Returned equipment to its proper place.                 _____  _____  _____

28. Removed soiled gloves. Practiced hygiene.               _____  _____  _____

29. Put on clean gloves.                                    _____  _____  _____

30. Assisted the person with hand washing.                  _____  _____  _____

31. Removed the gloves. Decontaminated hands.               _____  _____  _____

Post-Procedure

32. Follow steps 18 through 25 in procedure
    "Collecting a Random Urine Specimen."                   _____  _____  _____

Date of Satisfactory Completion _____    Instructor's Initials_____

## Collecting a Double-Voided Specimen

Name: _____     Date: _____

| Quality of Life | S | U | Comments |
|---|---|---|---|

- Knocked before entering the person's room.
- Addressed the person by name.
- Introduced yourself by name and title.
- Explained the procedure to the person before beginning and during the procedure.
- Protected the person's rights during the procedure.
- Handled the person gently during the procedure.

### Pre-Procedure

1. Followed "Delegation Guidelines: Urine Specimens." Reviewed "Promoting Safety and Comfort: Urine Specimens."
2. Practiced hand hygiene. Put on gloves.
3. Collected the following:
   - Voiding receptacle—bedpan, urinal, commode, or specimen pan
   - Two specimen containers
   - Urine testing equipment
   - Gloves
4. Removed the gloves. Decontaminated hands.
5. Identified the person. Checked the ID bracelet against the assignment sheet. Called the person by name.
6. Provided for privacy.

### Procedure

7. Put on the gloves.
8. Asked the person to void into the receptacle. Reminded the person not to put toilet tissue in the receptacle.
9. Took the receptacle to the bathroom.
10. Poured some urine into the specimen container.
11. Tested the specimen in case a second specimen could not be obtained. Discarded the urine. Noted the result on the assignment sheet.
12. Cleaned the receptacle and returned the receptacle to its proper place.
13. Removed the gloves and practiced hand hygiene. Put on clean gloves.
14. Assisted the person with hand washing.
15. Removed the gloves. Decontaminated your hands.
16. Asked the person to drink an 8-ounce glass of water.

*Continued*

| Procedure—cont'd | S | U | Comments |
|---|---|---|---|
| 17. Provided for comfort as noted on the inside of the front book cover. Raised the bed rails if needed. Placed the signal light within reach. | _____ | _____ | _____ |
| 18. Unscreened the person. | _____ | _____ | _____ |
| 19. Decontaminated hands. | _____ | _____ | _____ |
| 20. Completed a safety check of the room as noted on the inside of the front book cover. | _____ | _____ | _____ |
| 21. Returned to the room in 20 to 30 minutes. | _____ | _____ | _____ |
| 22. Repeated steps 6 through 15. | _____ | _____ | _____ |

**Post-Procedure**

| | S | U | Comments |
|---|---|---|---|
| 23. Provided for comfort as noted on the inside of the front book cover. | _____ | _____ | _____ |
| 24. Raised the bed rails if needed. Followed the care plan. | _____ | _____ | _____ |
| 25. Placed the signal light within reach. | _____ | _____ | _____ |
| 26. Unscreened the person. | _____ | _____ | _____ |
| 27. Completed a safety check of the room as noted on the inside of the front book cover. | _____ | _____ | _____ |
| 28. Decontaminated hands. | _____ | _____ | _____ |
| 29. Reported the results of the second test and any other observations. | _____ | _____ | _____ |

Date of Satisfactory Completion _____    Instructor's Initials_____

## Testing Urine With Reagent Strips

Name: _____     Date: _____

| Quality of Life | S | U | Comments |
|---|---|---|---|

Quality of Life                                    S        U        Comments

- Knocked before entering the person's room.         _____  _____  _____
- Addressed the person by name.                      _____  _____  _____
- Introduced yourself by name and title.             _____  _____  _____
- Explained the procedure to the person
  before beginning and during the procedure.         _____  _____  _____
- Protected the person's rights during the procedure. _____  _____  _____
- Handled the person gently during the procedure.    _____  _____  _____

### Pre-Procedure

1. Followed "Delegation Guidelines: Testing Urine."
   Reviewed "Promoting Safety and Comfort:
   Testing Urine."                                    _____  _____  _____
2. Practiced hand hygiene.                            _____  _____  _____
3. Identified the person. Checked the ID bracelet against
   the assignment sheet. Called the person by name.   _____  _____  _____

### Procedure

4. Put on the gloves.                                 _____  _____  _____
5. Collected the following:
   - Urine specimen (routine specimen for pH and
     occult blood; double-voided specimen for sugar
     and ketones)                                     _____  _____  _____
   - Reagent strip as ordered                         _____  _____  _____
   - Gloves                                           _____  _____  _____
6. Removed a strip from the bottle. Put the cap
   on the bottle at once. The cap was tight.          _____  _____  _____
7. Dipped the strip test areas into the urine.        _____  _____  _____
8. Removed the strip after the correct amount of time.
   Followed the manufacturer's instructions.          _____  _____  _____
9. Tapped the strip gently against the container to
   remove excess urine.                               _____  _____  _____
10. Waited the required amount of time. Followed the
    manufacturer's instructions.                      _____  _____  _____
11. Compared the strip with the color chart on the bottle.
    Read the results.                                 _____  _____  _____
12. Discarded disposable items and the specimen.      _____  _____  _____
13. Removed the gloves. Decontaminated hands.         _____  _____  _____

### Post-Procedure

14. Provided for comfort as noted on the inside of the
    front book cover.                                 _____  _____  _____
15. Placed the signal light within reach.             _____  _____  _____

*Continued*

| Post-Procedure—cont'd | S | U | Comments |
|---|---|---|---|
| 16. Cleaned and returned equipment to its proper place. Wore gloves for this step. | _____ | _____ | _____ |
| 17. Completed a safety check of the room as noted on the inside of the front book cover. | _____ | _____ | _____ |
| 18. Removed the gloves. Practiced hand hygiene. | _____ | _____ | _____ |
| 19. Reported and recorded the results and other observations. | _____ | _____ | _____ |

Date of Satisfactory Completion _____    Instructor's Initials_____

## Collecting a Stool Specimen

Name: _____    Date: _____

| Quality of Life | S | U | Comments |
|---|---|---|---|
| • Knocked before entering the person's room. | _____ | _____ | _____ |
| • Addressed the person by name. | _____ | _____ | _____ |
| • Introduced yourself by name and title. | _____ | _____ | _____ |
| • Explained the procedure to the person before beginning and during the procedure. | _____ | _____ | _____ |
| • Protected the person's rights during the procedure. | _____ | _____ | _____ |
| • Handled the person gently during the procedure. | _____ | _____ | _____ |

### Pre-Procedure

| | S | U | Comments |
|---|---|---|---|
| 1. Followed "Delegation Guidelines: Stool Specimens." Reviewed "Promoting Safety and Comfort: Stool Specimens." | _____ | _____ | _____ |
| 2. Practiced hand hygiene. Put on gloves. | _____ | _____ | _____ |
| 3. Collected the following: | | | |
| • Bedpan and cover or commode | _____ | _____ | _____ |
| • Urinal for voiding | _____ | _____ | _____ |
| • Specimen pan for the toilet or commode | _____ | _____ | _____ |
| • Specimen container and lid | _____ | _____ | _____ |
| • Tongue blade | _____ | _____ | _____ |
| • Disposable bag | _____ | _____ | _____ |
| • Gloves | _____ | _____ | _____ |
| • Toilet tissue | _____ | _____ | _____ |
| • Laboratory requisition slip | _____ | _____ | _____ |
| • Plastic bag | _____ | _____ | _____ |

### Procedure

| | S | U | Comments |
|---|---|---|---|
| 4. Labeled the container. | _____ | _____ | _____ |
| 5. Removed the gloves. Decontaminated hands. | _____ | _____ | _____ |
| 6. Identified the person. Checked the ID bracelet against the requisition slip. Called the person by name. | _____ | _____ | _____ |
| 7. Provided for privacy. | _____ | _____ | _____ |
| 8. Put on gloves. | _____ | _____ | _____ |
| 9. Asked the person to void. Provided the bedpan, commode, or urinal for voiding if the person did not use the bathroom. Emptied and cleaned the device. | _____ | _____ | _____ |
| 10. Put the specimen pan on the toilet if the person would use the bathroom. Placed it at the back of the toilet. | _____ | _____ | _____ |
| 11. Assisted the person onto the bedpan or to the toilet or commode. The person wore a robe and non-skid footwear when up. | _____ | _____ | _____ |

*Continued*

| Procedure—cont'd | S | U | Comments |
|---|---|---|---|
| 12. Asked the person not to put toilet tissue in the bedpan, commode, or specimen pan. Provided a bag for toilet tissue. | _____ | _____ | _____ |
| 13. Placed the signal light and toilet tissue within reach. Raised or lowered bed rails. Followed the care plan. | _____ | _____ | _____ |
| 14. Removed the gloves and decontaminated hands. Left the room. | _____ | _____ | _____ |
| 15. Returned when the person signaled. Or checked on the person every 5 minutes. Knocked before entering. Decontaminated hands. | _____ | _____ | _____ |
| 16. Lowered the bed rail near you if up. | _____ | _____ | _____ |
| 17. Put on the gloves. Provided perineal care if needed. | _____ | _____ | _____ |
| 18. Used a tongue blade to take about 2 tablespoons of stool to the specimen container. Took the sample from the middle of a formed stool. If required by agency policy, took stool from 2 different places on the specimen. | _____ | _____ | _____ |
| 19. Put the lid on the specimen container. Did not touch the inside of the lid or container. Placed the container in the plastic bag. | _____ | _____ | _____ |
| 20. Wrapped the tongue blade in toilet tissue. | _____ | _____ | _____ |
| 21. Discarded the tongue blade into the bag. | _____ | _____ | _____ |
| 22. Emptied, cleaned, and disinfected equipment. | _____ | _____ | _____ |
| 23. Removed the gloves. Decontaminated hands. | _____ | _____ | _____ |
| 24. Returned equipment to its proper place. | _____ | _____ | _____ |
| 25. Put on clean gloves. | _____ | _____ | _____ |
| 26. Assisted the person with hand washing. | _____ | _____ | _____ |
| 27. Removed the gloves. Decontaminated hands. | _____ | _____ | _____ |

## Post-Procedure

| | S | U | Comments |
|---|---|---|---|
| 28. Provided for comfort as noted on the inside of the front book cover. | _____ | _____ | _____ |
| 29. Placed the signal light within reach. | _____ | _____ | _____ |
| 30. Raised or lowered bed rails. Followed the care plan. | _____ | _____ | _____ |
| 31. Unscreened the person. | _____ | _____ | _____ |
| 32. Completed a safety check of the room as noted on the inside of the front book cover. | _____ | _____ | _____ |
| 33. Took the specimen and requisition slip to the storage area or laboratory. | _____ | _____ | _____ |
| 34. Decontaminated hands. | _____ | _____ | _____ |
| 35. Reported and recorded observations. | _____ | _____ | _____ |

Date of Satisfactory Completion _____     Instructor's Initials_____

## Collecting a Sputum Specimen

Name: _____        Date: _____

| Quality of Life | S | U | Comments |
|---|---|---|---|

- Knocked before entering the person's room.
- Addressed the person by name.
- Introduced yourself by name and title.
- Explained the procedure to the person before beginning and during the procedure.
- Protected the person's rights during the procedure.
- Handled the person gently during the procedure.

### Pre-Procedure

1. Followed "Delegation Guidelines: Sputum Specimens." Reviewed "Promoting Safety and Comfort: Sputum Specimens."
2. Practiced hand hygiene.
3. Collected the following:
   - Sputum specimen container and label
   - Laboratory requisition slip
   - Disposable bag
   - Gloves
   - Tissues
4. Labeled the container.
5. Identified the person. Checked the ID bracelet against the requisition slip. Called the person by name.
6. Provided for privacy. If able the person used the bathroom for the procedure.

### Procedure

7. Put on the gloves.
8. Asked the person to rinse the mouth out with clear water.
9. Had the person hold the container. Only the outside was touched.
10. Asked the person to cover the mouth and nose with tissues when coughing.
11. Asked the person to take 2 or 3 deep breaths and cough up the sputum.
12. Had the person expectorate directly into the container. Sputum did not touch the outside.
13. Collected 1 to 2 tablespoons of sputum unless told to collect more.
14. Put the lid on the container.

*Continued*

| Procedure—cont'd | S | U | Comments |
|---|---|---|---|
| 15. Placed the container in the bag. Attached the requisition slip to the bag. | _____ | _____ | _____ |
| 16. Removed the gloves and decontaminated your hands. Put on clean gloves. | _____ | _____ | _____ |
| 17. Assisted the person with hand washing. | _____ | _____ | _____ |
| 18. Removed the gloves. Decontaminated hands. | _____ | _____ | _____ |

## Post-Procedure

| | S | U | Comments |
|---|---|---|---|
| 19. Provided for comfort as noted on the inside of the front book cover. | _____ | _____ | _____ |
| 20. Placed the signal light within reach. | _____ | _____ | _____ |
| 21. Unscreened the person. | _____ | _____ | _____ |
| 22. Completed a safety check of the room as noted on the inside of the front book cover. | _____ | _____ | _____ |
| 23. Decontaminated hands. | _____ | _____ | _____ |
| 24. Took the bag to the laboratory or storage area. | _____ | _____ | _____ |
| 25. Decontaminated hands. | _____ | _____ | _____ |
| 26. Reported and recorded observations. | _____ | _____ | _____ |

Date of Satisfactory Completion _____     Instructor's Initials_____

# Performing Range-of-Motion Excercises

Name: _____     Date: _____

| Quality of Life | S | U | Comments |
|---|---|---|---|

- Knocked before entering the person's room.
- Addressed the person by name.
- Introduced yourself by name and title.
- Explained the procedure to the person before beginning and during the procedure.
- Protected the person's rights during the procedure.
- Handled the person gently during the procedure.

## Pre-Procedure

1. Followed "Delegation Guidelines: Range-of-Motion Exercises." Reviewed "Promoting Safety and Comfort: Range-of-Motion Exercises."
2. Practiced hand hygiene.
3. Identified the person. Checked the ID bracelet against the assignment sheet. Called the person by name.
4. Obtained a bath blanket.
5. Provided for privacy.
6. Raised the bed for body mechanics. Bed rails were up if used.

## Procedure

7. Lowered the bed rail near you if up.
8. Positioned the person supine.
9. Covered the person with a bath blanket. Fan-folded top linens to the foot of the bed.
10. Exercised the neck if allowed by the agency and if the RN instructed you to do so:
    a. Placed your hands over the person's ears to support the head. Supported the jaws with your fingers.
    b. Flexion—brought the head forward. The chin touched the chest.
    c. Extension—straightened the head.
    d. Hyperextension—brought the head backward until the chin pointed up.
    e. Rotation—turned the head from side to side.
    f. Lateral flexion—moved the head to the right and to the left.

*Continued*

| Procedure—cont'd | S | U | Comments |
|---|---|---|---|

g. Repeated flexion, extension, hyperextension, rotation, and lateral flexion 5 times—or the number of times stated on the care plan.    \_\_\_\_\_  \_\_\_\_\_  _____

11. Exercised the shoulder:

   a. Grasped the wrist with one hand. Grasped the elbow with the other hand.    \_\_\_\_\_  \_\_\_\_\_  _____

   b. Flexion—raised the arm straight in front and over the head.    \_\_\_\_\_  \_\_\_\_\_  _____

   c. Extension—brought the arm down to the side.    \_\_\_\_\_  \_\_\_\_\_  _____

   d. Hyperextension—moved the arm behind the body. (Did this if the person was sitting in a straight-backed chair or was standing.)    \_\_\_\_\_  \_\_\_\_\_  _____

   e. Abduction—moved the straight arm away from the side of the body.    \_\_\_\_\_  \_\_\_\_\_  _____

   f. Adduction—moved the straight arm to the side of the body.    \_\_\_\_\_  \_\_\_\_\_  _____

   g. Internal rotation—bent the elbow. Placed it at the same level as the shoulder. Moved the forearm down toward the body.    \_\_\_\_\_  \_\_\_\_\_  _____

   h. External rotation—moved the forearm toward the head.    \_\_\_\_\_  \_\_\_\_\_  _____

   i. Repeated flexion, extension, hyperextension, abduction, adduction, and internal and external rotation 5 times—or the number of times stated on the care plan.    \_\_\_\_\_  \_\_\_\_\_  _____

12. Exercised the elbow:

   a. Grasped the person's wrist with one hand. Grasped the elbow with the other hand.    \_\_\_\_\_  \_\_\_\_\_  _____

   b. Flexion—bent the arm so the same-side shoulder was touched.    \_\_\_\_\_  \_\_\_\_\_  _____

   c. Extension—straightened the arm.    \_\_\_\_\_  \_\_\_\_\_  _____

   d. Repeated flexion and extension 5 times—or the number of times stated on the care plan.    \_\_\_\_\_  \_\_\_\_\_  _____

13. Exercised the forearm:

   a. Pronation—turned the hand so the palm was down.    \_\_\_\_\_  \_\_\_\_\_  _____

   b. Supination—turned the hand so the palm was up.    \_\_\_\_\_  \_\_\_\_\_  _____

   c. Repeated pronation and supination 5 times—or the number of times stated on the care plan.    \_\_\_\_\_  \_\_\_\_\_  _____

14. Exercised the wrist:

   a. Held the wrist with both of your hands.    \_\_\_\_\_  \_\_\_\_\_  _____

   b. Flexion—bent the hand down.    \_\_\_\_\_  \_\_\_\_\_  _____

   c. Extension—straightened the hand.    \_\_\_\_\_  \_\_\_\_\_  _____

   d. Hyperextension—bent the hand back.    \_\_\_\_\_  \_\_\_\_\_  _____

   e. Radial flexion—turned the hand toward the thumb.    \_\_\_\_\_  \_\_\_\_\_  _____

   f. Ulnar flexion—turned the hand toward the little finger.

| Procedure—cont'd | S | U | Comments |
|---|---|---|---|

g. Repeated flexion, extension, hyperextension, and radial flexion and ulnar flexion 5 times—or the number of times stated on the care plan. _____ _____ _____

15. Exercised the thumb:

    a. Held the person's hand with one hand. Held the thumb with your other hand. _____ _____ _____

    b. Abduction—moved the thumb out from the inner part of the index finger. _____ _____ _____

    c. Adduction—moved the thumb back next to the index finger. _____ _____ _____

    d. Opposition—touched each fingertip with the thumb. _____ _____ _____

    e. Flexion—bent the thumb into the hand. _____ _____ _____

    f. Extension—moved the thumb out to the side of the fingers. _____ _____ _____

    g. Repeated abduction, adduction, opposition, flexion, and extension 5 times—or the number of times stated on the care plan. _____ _____ _____

16. Exercised the fingers:

    a. Abduction—spread the fingers and the thumb apart. _____ _____ _____

    b. Adduction—brought the fingers and thumb together. _____ _____ _____

    c. Extension—straightened the fingers so the fingers, hand, and arm were straight. _____ _____ _____

    d. Flexion—made a fist. _____ _____ _____

    e. Repeated abduction, adduction, extension, and flexion 5 times—or the number of times stated on the care plan. _____ _____ _____

17. Exercised the hip:

    a. Supported the leg. Placed one hand under the knee. Placed your other hand under the ankle. _____ _____ _____

    b. Flexion—raised the leg. _____ _____ _____

    c. Extension—straightened the leg. _____ _____ _____

    d. Abduction—moved the leg away from the body. _____ _____ _____

    e. Adduction—moved the leg toward the other leg. _____ _____ _____

    f. Internal rotation—turned the leg inward. _____ _____ _____

    g. External rotation—turned the leg outward. _____ _____ _____

    h. Repeated flexion, extension, abduction, adduction, and internal and external rotation 5 times—or the number of times stated on the care plan. _____ _____ _____

18. Exercised the knee:

    a. Supported the knee. Placed one hand under the knee. Placed your other hand under the ankle. _____ _____ _____

    b. Flexion—bent the leg. _____ _____ _____

    c. Extension—straightened the leg. _____ _____ _____

*Continued*

| Procedure—cont'd | S | U | Comments |
|---|---|---|---|

d. Repeated flexion and extension of the knee 5 times— or the number of times stated on the care plan.  \_\_\_\_\_ \_\_\_\_\_ _____

19. Exercised the ankle:

   a. Supported the foot and ankle. Placed one hand under the foot. Placed your other hand under the ankle.  \_\_\_\_\_ \_\_\_\_\_ _____

   b. Dorsiflexion—pulled the foot forward. Pushed down on the heel at the same time.  \_\_\_\_\_ \_\_\_\_\_ _____

   c. Plantar flexion—turned the foot down, or pointed the toes.  \_\_\_\_\_ \_\_\_\_\_ _____

   d. Repeated dorsiflexion and plantar flexion 5 times—or the number of times stated on the care plan.  \_\_\_\_\_ \_\_\_\_\_ _____

20. Exercised the foot:

   a. Continued to support the foot and ankle.  \_\_\_\_\_ \_\_\_\_\_ _____

   b. Pronation—turned the outside of the foot up and the inside down.  \_\_\_\_\_ \_\_\_\_\_ _____

   c. Supination—turned the inside of the foot up and the outside down.  \_\_\_\_\_ \_\_\_\_\_ _____

   d. Repeated pronation and supination 5 times—or the number of times stated on the care plan.  \_\_\_\_\_ \_\_\_\_\_ _____

21. Exercised the toes:

   a. Flexion—curled the toes.  \_\_\_\_\_ \_\_\_\_\_ _____

   b. Extension—straightened the toes.  \_\_\_\_\_ \_\_\_\_\_ _____

   c. Abduction—spread the toes apart.  \_\_\_\_\_ \_\_\_\_\_ _____

   d. Adduction—pulled the toes together.  \_\_\_\_\_ \_\_\_\_\_ _____

   e. Repeated flexion, extension, abduction, and adduction 5 times—or the number of times stated on the care plan.  \_\_\_\_\_ \_\_\_\_\_ _____

22. Covered the leg. Raised the bed rail if used.  \_\_\_\_\_ \_\_\_\_\_ _____

23. Went to the other side. Lowered the bed rail near you if up.  \_\_\_\_\_ \_\_\_\_\_ _____

24. Repeated steps 11 through 21.  \_\_\_\_\_ \_\_\_\_\_ _____

## Post-Procedure

25. Provided for comfort as noted on the inside of the front book cover.  \_\_\_\_\_ \_\_\_\_\_ _____

26. Removed the bath blanket.  \_\_\_\_\_ \_\_\_\_\_ _____

27. Placed the signal light within reach.  \_\_\_\_\_ \_\_\_\_\_ _____

28. Lowered the bed to its lowest level.  \_\_\_\_\_ \_\_\_\_\_ _____

29. Raised or lowered bed rails. Followed the care plan.  \_\_\_\_\_ \_\_\_\_\_ _____

30. Returned the bath blanket to its proper place.  \_\_\_\_\_ \_\_\_\_\_ _____

31. Unscreened the person.  \_\_\_\_\_ \_\_\_\_\_ _____

| Post-Procedure—cont'd | S | U | Comments |
|---|---|---|---|
| 32. Completed a safety check of the room as noted on the inside of the front book cover. | _____ | _____ | _____ |
| 33. Decontaminated hands. | _____ | _____ | _____ |
| 34. Reported and recorded observations. | _____ | _____ | _____ |

Date of Satisfactory Completion _____  Instructor's Initials_____

# Helping the Person to Walk (NNAAP™)

Name: _____     Date: _____

| Quality of Life | S | U | Comments |
|---|---|---|---|

- Knocked before entering the person's room.     _____ _____ _____
- Addressed the person by name.     _____ _____ _____
- Introduced yourself by name and title.     _____ _____ _____
- Explained the procedure to the person
  before beginning and during the procedure.     _____ _____ _____
- Protected the person's rights during the procedure.     _____ _____ _____
- Handled the person gently during the procedure.     _____ _____ _____

## Pre-Procedure

1. Followed "Delegation Guidelines: Ambulation."
   Reviewed "Promoting Safety and Comfort: Ambulation."     _____ _____ _____
2. Practiced hand hygiene.     _____ _____ _____
3. Collected the following:
   - Robe and non-skid shoes     _____ _____ _____
   - Paper or sheet to protect bottom linen     _____ _____ _____
   - Gait (transfer) belt     _____ _____ _____
4. Identified the person. Checked the ID bracelet against
   the assignment sheet. Called the person by name.     _____ _____ _____
5. Provided for privacy.     _____ _____ _____

## Procedure

6. Lowered the bed to its lowest position. Locked the
   bed wheels. Lowered the bed rail if up.     _____ _____ _____
7. Fan-folded top linens to the foot of the bed.     _____ _____ _____
8. Placed the paper or sheet under the person's feet.
   Put the shoes on the person. Fastened the shoes.     _____ _____ _____
9. Helped the person to dangle. (See procedure "Helping
   the Person Sit on the Side of the Bed[Dangle]")     _____ _____ _____
10. Helped the person put on the robe.     _____ _____ _____
11. Applied the gait belt. (See procedure "Applying a
    Transfer Belt" in Chapter 11)     _____ _____ _____
12. Helped the person stand. (See procedure
    "Transferring the Person to a Chair or Wheelchair"
    in Chapter 11) Grasped the belt at each side.
    If not using a gait belt, placed your arms under the
    person's arms around to the shoulder blades.     _____ _____ _____
13. Stood at the person's weak side while the person
    gained balance. Held the belt at the side and back.
    If not using a gait belt, had one arm around the back
    and the other at the elbow to support the person.     _____ _____ _____

## Procedure—cont'd                                    S        U        Comments

14. Encouraged the person to stand erect (in Chapter 11)   _____ _____ _____
    with the head up and back straight.

15. Helped the person walk. Walked to the side and         _____ _____ _____
    slightly behind the person on the person's weak side.
    Provided support with the gait belt. If not using a
    gait belt, had one arm around the back and the
    other at the elbow to support the person. Encouraged
    the person to use the hand rail on his or her strong side.

16. Encouraged the person to walk normally.                _____ _____ _____
    (The heel should strike the floor first.) Discouraged
    shuffling, sliding, or walking on tiptoes.

17. Walked the required distance if the person             _____ _____ _____
    tolerated the activity. Did not rush the person.

18. Helped the person return to bed. Removed the gait belt.  _____ _____ _____
    (See procedure "Transferring the Person From a Chair or
    Wheelchair to Bed" in Chapter 11.)

19. Lowered the head of the bed. Helped the                _____ _____ _____
    person to the center of the bed.

20. Removed the shoes. Removed the paper or                _____ _____ _____
    sheet over the bottom sheet.

## Post-Procedure

21. Provided for comfort as noted on the inside of the     _____ _____ _____
    front book cover.

22. Placed the signal light within reach.                  _____ _____ _____

23. Raised or lowered bed rails. Followed the care plan.   _____ _____ _____

24. Returned the robe and shoes to their proper place.     _____ _____ _____

25. Unscreened the person.                                 _____ _____ _____

26. Completed a safety check of the room as noted on the   _____ _____ _____
    inside of the front book cover.

27. Decontaminated hands.                                  _____ _____ _____

28. Reported and recorded observations.                    _____ _____ _____

Date of Satisfactory Completion _____  Instructor's Initials_____

# Helping the Falling Person

Name: _____   Date: _____

| Procedure | S | U | Comments |
|---|---|---|---|

**Procedure**

1. Stood with your feet apart. Kept your back straight.    _____ _____ _____

2. Brought the person close to your body as fast as possible. Used the gait belt. Or wrapped your arms around the person's waist. The person could also be held under the arms if necessary.    _____ _____ _____

3. Moved your leg so the person's buttocks rested on it. Moved the leg near the person.    _____ _____ _____

4. Lowered the person to the floor. The person slid down your leg to the floor. Bent at your hips and knees as you lowered the person.    _____ _____ _____

5. Called a nurse to check the person. Stayed with the person.    _____ _____ _____

6. Helped the nurse return the person to bed. Got other staff to help if needed.    _____ _____ _____

**Post-Procedure**

7. Provided for comfort as noted on the inside of the front book cover.    _____ _____ _____

8. Placed the signal light within reach.

9. Raised or lowered the bed rails. Followed the care plan.    _____ _____ _____

10. Completed a safety check of the room as noted on the inside of the front book cover.    _____ _____ _____

11. Reported and recorded the following:
    - How the fall occurred    _____ _____ _____
    - How far the person walked    _____ _____ _____
    - How activity was tolerated before the fall    _____ _____ _____
    - Complaints before the fall    _____ _____ _____
    - How much help the person needed while walking    _____ _____ _____

12. Completed an incident report.    _____ _____ _____

Date of Satisfactory Completion_____   Instructor's Initials_____

Applying Elastic Stockings (NNAAP™)

Name: _____    Date: _____

## Quality of Life

|  |  | S | U | Comments |
|---|---|---|---|---|

- Knocked before entering the person's room.
- Addressed the person by name.
- Introduced yourself by name and title.
- Explained the procedure to the person before beginning and during the procedure.
- Protected the person's rights during the procedure.
- Handled the person gently during the procedure.

## Pre-Procedure

1. Followed "Delegation Guidelines: Elastic Stockings." Reviewed "Promoting Safety and Comfort: Elastic Stockings."
2. Practiced hand hygiene.
3. Obtained elastic stockings in the correct size and length.
4. Identified the person. Checked the ID bracelet against the assignment sheet. Called the person by name.
5. Provided for privacy.
6. Raised the bed for body mechanics. Bed rails were up if used.

## Procedure

7. Lowered the bed rail near you if up.
8. Positioned the person supine.
9. Exposed the legs. Fan-folded top linens toward the thighs.
10. Turned the stocking inside out down to the heel.
11. Slipped the foot of the stocking over the toes, foot, and heel.
12. Grasped the stocking top. Pulled the stocking up the leg. The stocking turned right side out as it was pulled up. The stocking was even and snug.
13. Removed twists, creases, or wrinkles.
14. Repeated steps 10 through 13 for the other leg.

## Post-Procedure

15. Covered the person.
16. Provided for comfort as noted on the inside of the front book cover.
17. Placed the signal light within reach.

*Continued*

| Post-Procedure—cont'd | S | U | Comments |
|---|---|---|---|
| 18. Lowered the bed to its lowest position. | _____ | _____ | _____ |
| 19. Raised or lowered bed rails. Followed the care plan. | _____ | _____ | _____ |
| 20. Unscreened the person. | _____ | _____ | _____ |
| 21. Completed a safety check of the room as noted on the inside of the front book cover. | _____ | _____ | _____ |
| 22. Decontaminated hands. | _____ | _____ | _____ |
| 23. Reported and recorded observations. | _____ | _____ | _____ |

Date of Satisfactory Completion _____      Instructor's Initials_____

## Applying Elastic Bandages

Name: _____     Date: _____

| Quality of Life | S | U | Comments |
|---|---|---|---|

- Knocked before entering the person's room. _____ _____ _____
- Addressed the person by name. _____ _____ _____
- Introduced yourself by name and title. _____ _____ _____
- Explained the procedure to the person before beginning and during the procedure. _____ _____ _____
- Protected the person's rights during the procedure. _____ _____ _____
- Handled the person gently during the procedure. _____ _____ _____

### Pre-Procedure

1. Followed "Delegation Guidelines: Elastic Bandages." Reviewed "Promoting Safety and Comfort: Elastic Bandages." _____ _____ _____
2. Practiced hand hygiene.
3. Collected the following:
   - Elastic bandage as directed by the nurse _____ _____ _____
   - Tape or metal clips (unless the bandage had Velcro) _____ _____ _____
4. Identified the person. Checked the ID bracelet against the assignment sheet. Called the person by name. _____ _____ _____
5. Provided for privacy.
6. Raised the bed for body mechanics. Bed rails were up if used. _____ _____ _____

### Procedure

7. Lowered the bed rail near you if up. _____ _____ _____
8. Helped the person to a comfortable position. Exposed the part to be bandaged. _____ _____ _____
9. Made sure the area was clean and dry. _____ _____ _____
10. Held the bandage so the roll was up. The loose end was on the bottom. _____ _____ _____
11. Applied the bandage to the smallest part of the wrist, foot, ankle, or knee. _____ _____ _____
12. Made two circular turns around the part. _____ _____ _____
13. Made overlapping spiral turns in an upward direction. Each turn overlapped about 2/3 of the previous turn. _____ _____ _____
14. Applied the bandage smoothly with firm, even pressure. It was not tight. _____ _____ _____
15. Ended the bandage with two circular turns. _____ _____ _____
16. Secured the bandage in place with Velcro, tape, or clips. The clips were not under the body part. _____ _____ _____

*Continued*

| Procedure—cont'd | S | U | Comments |
|---|---|---|---|

17. Checked the fingers or toes for coldness or cyanosis. Asked about pain, itching, numbness, or tingling. Removed the bandage if any were noted. Reported observations to the nurse. _____ _____ _____

## Post-Procedure

18. Provided for comfort as noted on the inside of the front book cover. _____ _____ _____
19. Placed the signal light within reach. _____ _____ _____
20. Lowered the bed to its lowest poistion. _____ _____ _____
21. Raised or lowered bed rails. Followed the care plan. _____ _____ _____
22. Unscreened the person. _____ _____ _____
23. Completed a safety check of the room as noted on the inside of the front book cover. _____ _____ _____
24. Decontaminated hands. _____ _____ _____
25. Reported and recorded observations. _____ _____ _____

Date of Satisfactory Completion _____   Instructor's Initials_____

# Applying a Dry Non-Sterile Dressing

Name: _____          Date: _____

| Quality of Life | S | U | Comments |
|---|---|---|---|

- Knocked before entering the person's room.      _____  _____  _____
- Addressed the person by name.      _____  _____  _____
- Introduced yourself by name and title.      _____  _____  _____
- Explained the procedure to the person before beginning and during the procedure.      _____  _____  _____
- Protected the person's rights during the procedure.      _____  _____  _____
- Handled the person gently during the procedure.      _____  _____  _____

## Pre-Procedure

1. Followed "Delegation Guidelines: Applying Dressings." Reviewed "Promoting Safety and Comfort: Applying Dressings."      _____  _____  _____
2. Practiced hand hygiene.
3. Collected needed supplies and equipment:
   - Gloves
   - Personal protective equipment as needed      _____  _____  _____
   - Tape or Montgomery ties
   - Dressings as directed by the nurse
   - Adhesive remover      _____  _____  _____
   - Scissors
   - Plastic bag      _____  _____  _____
   - Bath blanket      _____  _____  _____
4. Identified the person. Checked the ID bracelet against the assignment sheet. Called the person by name.      _____  _____  _____
5. Provided for privacy.      _____  _____  _____
6. Arranged the work area so you would not have to reach over or turn your back on your work area.      _____  _____  _____
7. Raised the bed for body mechanics. Bed rails were up if used.      _____  _____  _____

## Procedure

8. Lowered the bed rail near you if up.      _____  _____  _____
9. Helped the person to a comfortable position.      _____  _____  _____
10. Covered the person with a bath blanket. Fan-folded top linens to the foot of the bed.      _____  _____  _____
11. Exposed the affected body part.      _____  _____  _____
12. Made a cuff on the plastic bag. Placed it within reach.      _____  _____  _____
13. Decontaminated your hands.      _____  _____  _____
14. Put on a gown and mask if needed.      _____  _____  _____
15. Decontaminated hands. Put on the gloves.      _____  _____  _____

*Continued*

| Procedure—cont'd | S | U | Comments |
|---|---|---|---|
| 16. Undid Montgomery ties or removed tape. | _____ | _____ | _____ |
|    a. For Montgomery ties: folded ties away from the wound. | _____ | _____ | _____ |
|    b. For tape: held the skin down. Gently pulled the tape toward the wound. | _____ | _____ | _____ |
| 17. Removed adhesive from the skin if necessary. Wet a 4 × 4 gauze dressing with the adhesive remover. Cleaned away from the wound. | _____ | _____ | _____ |
| 18. Removed gauze dressings. Started with the top dressing. The soiled side was away from the person's sight. Put the dressings in the bag. They did not touch the outside of the bag. | _____ | _____ | _____ |
| 19. Removed the dressing directly over the wound very gently. | _____ | _____ | _____ |
| 20. Observed the wound, drain site, and wound drainage. | _____ | _____ | _____ |
| 21. Removed the gloves and put them into the bag. Decontaminated hands. | _____ | _____ | _____ |
| 22. Put on clean gloves. | _____ | _____ | _____ |
| 23. Opened the dressings. | _____ | _____ | _____ |
| 24. Cut the length of tape needed. | _____ | _____ | _____ |
| 25. Applied dressings as directed by the nurse. | _____ | _____ | _____ |
| 26. Secured the dressings in place. Used tape or Montgomery ties. | _____ | _____ | _____ |
| 27. Removed your gloves and put them in the bag. Decontaminated hands. | _____ | _____ | _____ |

## Post-Procedure

| | S | U | Comments |
|---|---|---|---|
| 28. Provided for comfort as noted on the inside of the front book cover. | _____ | _____ | _____ |
| 29. Placed the signal light within reach. | _____ | _____ | _____ |
| 30. Lowered the bed to its lowest position. | _____ | _____ | _____ |
| 31. Raised or lowered bed rails. Followed the care plan. | _____ | _____ | _____ |
| 32. Discarded supplies into the bag. Tied the bag closed. Discarded the bag according to agency policy. Wore gloves for this step. | _____ | _____ | _____ |
| 33. Cleaned the work surface. Followed the Bloodborne Pathogen Standard. | _____ | _____ | _____ |
| 34. Unscreened the person. | _____ | _____ | _____ |
| 35. Completed a safety check of the room as noted on the inside of the front book cover. | _____ | _____ | _____ |
| 36. Removed the gloves. Decontaminated hands. | _____ | _____ | _____ |
| 37. Reported and recorded observations. | _____ | _____ | _____ |

Date of Satisfactory Completion _____     Instructor's Initials_____

# Applying Heat and Cold Applications

Name: _____     Date: _____

## Quality of Life

|  | S | U | Comments |
|---|---|---|---|

- Knocked before entering the person's room.
- Addressed the person by name.
- Introduced yourself by name and title.
- Explained the procedure to the person before beginning and during the procedure.
- Protected the person's rights during the procedure.
- Handled the person gently during the procedure.

## Pre-Procedure

1. Followed "Delegation Guidelines: Applying Heat and Cold." Reviewed "Promoting Safety and Comfort: Applying Heat and Cold."
2. Practiced hand hygiene.
3. Collected needed equipment.
4. Identified the person. Checked the ID bracelet against the assignment sheet. Called the person by name.
5. Provided for privacy.

## Procedure

6. Prepared the application. Followed agency procedures and the manufacturer's instructions.
7. Placed a dry application in a cover.
8. Placed the application on the affected part. Noted the time.
9. Secured the application in place with ties, tape, or rolled gauze. Did not use pins.
10. Placed the signal light within reach. Unscreened the person.
11. Raised or lowered bed rails. Followed the care plan.
12. Checked the person every 5 minutes. Checked for signs and symptoms of complications. Removed the application if any occurred. Told the nurse at once.
13. Removed the application at the specified time. (If the bed rails were up, lowered the near one for this step.)

## Post-Procedure

14. Provided for comfort as noted on the inside of the front book cover.
15. Placed the signal light within reach.
16. Raised or lowered bed rails. Followed the care plan.

| Post-Procedure—cont'd | S | U | Comments |
|---|---|---|---|
| 17. Unscreened the person. | _____ | _____ | _____ |
| 18. Completed a safety check of the room as noted on the inside of the front book cover. | _____ | _____ | _____ |
| 19. Cleaned the sitz bath with disinfectant solution. Wore utility gloves. | _____ | _____ | _____ |
| 20. Cleaned and returned reusable items to their proper place. Followed agency policy for soiled linen. Wore gloves for this step. | _____ | _____ | _____ |
| 21. Discarded the gloves. Decontaminated hands. | _____ | _____ | _____ |
| 22. Reported and recorded observations. | _____ | _____ | _____ |

Date of Satisfactory Completion _____   Instructor's Initials_____

# Assisting With Coughing and Deep-Breathing Excercises

Name: _____     Date: _____

| Quality of Life | S | U | Comments |
|---|---|---|---|

- Knocked before entering the person's room.          _____  _____  _____
- Addressed the person by name.                       _____  _____  _____
- Introduced yourself by name and title.              _____  _____  _____
- Explained the procedure to the person
  before beginning and during the procedure.          _____  _____  _____
- Protected the person's rights during the procedure. _____  _____  _____
- Handled the person gently during the procedure.     _____  _____  _____

## Pre-Procedure

1. Followed "Delegation Guidelines:
   Coughing and Deep Breathing."                       _____  _____  _____
2. Practiced hand hygiene.                             _____  _____  _____
3. Identified the person. Checked the ID bracelet against
   the assignment sheet. Called the person by name.    _____  _____  _____
4. Provided for privacy.                               _____  _____  _____

## Procedure

5. Helped the person to a comfortable sitting
   position: dangling, semi-Fowler's, or Fowler's.     _____  _____  _____
6. Had the person deep breathe:
   a. Had the person place the hands over the rib cage. _____  _____  _____
   b. Asked the person to exhale. Explained that
      the ribs should move as far down as possible.    _____  _____  _____
   c. Had the person take a deep breath. Reminded the
      person to inhale through the nose.               _____  _____  _____
   d. Asked the person to hold the breath for 3 seconds. _____  _____  _____
   e. Asked the person to exhale slowly through pursed
      lips. The person exhaled until the ribs moved as far
      down as possible.                                _____  _____  _____
   f. Repeated this step 4 more times.                 _____  _____  _____
7. Asked the person to cough:
   a. Had the person interlace the fingers over the incision.
      The person could also hold a pillow or folded towel
      over the incision.                               _____  _____  _____
   b. Had the person take in a deep breath as in step 6. _____  _____  _____
   c. Asked the person to cough strongly twice with
      the mouth open.                                  _____  _____  _____

*Continued*

| Post-Procedure | S | U | Comments |
|---|---|---|---|
| 8. Provided for comfort as noted on the inside of the front book cover. | _____ | _____ | _____ |
| 9. Placed the signal light within reach. | _____ | _____ | _____ |
| 10. Raised or lowered bed rails. Followed the care plan. | _____ | _____ | _____ |
| 11. Unscreened the person. | _____ | _____ | _____ |
| 12. Completed a safety of the room as noted on the inside of the front book cover. | _____ | _____ | _____ |
| 13. Decontaminated hands. | _____ | _____ | _____ |
| 14. Reported and recorded observations. | _____ | _____ | _____ |

Date of Satisfactory Completion _____   Instructor's Initials_____

# Adult CPR—One Rescuer

Name: _____   Date: _____

| Procedure | S | U | Comments |
|---|---|---|---|

**Procedure**  ·  S  ·  U  ·  **Comments**

1. Checked if the person was responding. Tapped or gently shook the person, called the person by name, and shouted "Are you OK?"  _____ _____ _____

2. Called for help. Activated the EMS system or the agency's emergency response system.  _____ _____ _____

3. Positioned the person supine. Logrolled the person so there was no twisting of the spine. The person was on a hard, flat surface. Placed the person's arms alongside the body.  _____ _____ _____

4. Opened the airway. Used the head-tilt/chin-lift method.  _____ _____ _____

5. Checked for breathing. Looked to see if the chest rose and fell. Listened for the escape of air. Felt for the flow of air on your cheek.  _____ _____ _____

6. Gave 2 slow breaths if the person was not breathing or was not breathing adequately. Each breath took 2 seconds. Let the person's lungs deflate between breaths.  _____ _____ _____

7. Checked for a carotid pulse and for breathing, coughing, and moving. This took 5 to 10 seconds. Used your other hand to keep the airway open with the head-tilt/chin-lift method. Started chest compressions if there were no signs of circulation.  _____ _____ _____

8. Gave chest compressions at a rate of 100 per minute. Gave 15 compressions and then 2 slow breaths.  _____ _____ _____

   a. Established a rhythm and counted out loud. (Such as: "1 and, 2 and, 3 and, 4 and, 5 and, 6 and, 7 and, 8 and,9 and, 10 and, 11 and, 12 and, 13 and, 14 and, 15.")  _____ _____ _____

   b. Opened the airway, and gave 2 slow breaths.  _____ _____ _____

   c. Repeated this step until 4 cycles of 15 compressions and 2 breaths were given.  _____ _____ _____

9. Checked for a carotid pulse. Also checked for breathing, coughing, and moving.  _____ _____ _____

10. Continued CPR if the person had no signs of circulation. Began with chest compressions. Continued the cycle of 15 compressions and 2 breaths. Checked for circulation every few minutes.  _____ _____ _____

*Continued*

Procedure—cont'd                                S        U            Comments

11. Did the following if the person had signs of circulation:    _____  _____  _____
    a. Checked for breathing.                   _____  _____  _____
    b. Positioned the person in the recovery    _____  _____  _____
       position if the person was breathing.
    c. Monitored breathing and circulation.     _____  _____  _____
12. Did the following if the person had signs of circulation  _____  _____  _____
    but breathing was absent.
    a. Gave 1 rescue breath every 5 seconds     _____  _____  _____
       (A rate of 10 to 12 breaths per minute).
    b. Monitored circulation.                   _____  _____  _____

Date of Satisfactory Completion _____  Instructor's Initials_____

# Adult CPR—Two Rescuers

Name: _____          Date: _____

| Procedure | S | U | Comments |
|---|---|---|---|

1. Checked if the person was responding.
   Tapped or gently shook the person, called the person
   by name, and shouted "Are you OK?" One rescuer
   activated the EMS system or the agency's emergency
   response system.                                                    _____  _____  _____

2. Opened the airway and checked for breathing.
   Used the head-tilt/chin-lift method.                                _____  _____  _____

3. Gave 2 slow rescue breaths if the person was not
   breathing or if breathing was inadequate. Let the lungs
   deflate between breaths.                                            _____  _____  _____

4. Checked for a pulse using the carotid artery.
   Also checked for breathing, coughing, and moving.                   _____  _____  _____

5. Performed 2-person CPR if there were no signs of
   circulation.

   a. One rescuer gave chest compressions at a rate of
      100 per minute. Counted out loud in a rhythm.
      (Such as: "1 and, 2 and, 3 and, 4 and, 5 and, 6 and,
      7 and, 8 and, 9 and, 10 and, 11 and, 12 and, 13 and,
      14 and, 15.")                                                    _____  _____  _____

   b. The other rescuer gave 2 slow breaths after every
      15 compressions. The rescuer giving chest
      compressions paused for the breaths and continued
      chest compressions after the breaths.                            _____  _____  _____

6. One rescuer did the following after 4 cycles of
   15 compressions and 2 breaths:

   a. Gave 2 slow breaths.                                             _____  _____  _____

   b. Checked for circulation—carotid pulse,
      breathing, coughing, and moving.                                 _____  _____  _____

7. Continued with 15 compressions and 2 slow breaths     _____  _____  _____
   if the person had no signs of circulation. Started with
   chest compressions.

Date of Satisfactory Completion _____          Instructor's Initials_____

# FBAO—The Responsive Adult

Name: _____  Date: _____

| Procedure | S | U | Comments |
|---|---|---|---|
| 1. Asked the person if he or she was choking. | _____ | _____ | _____ |
| 2. Asked if the person could cough or speak. | _____ | _____ | _____ |
| 3. Gave abdominal thrusts. | _____ | _____ | _____ |
|    a. Stood behind the person. | _____ | _____ | _____ |
|    b. Wrapped your arms around the person's waist. | _____ | _____ | _____ |
|    c. Made a fist with one hand. | _____ | _____ | _____ |
|    d. Placed the thumb side of the fist against the abdomen. The fist was in the middle above the navel and below the end of the sternum (breastbone). | _____ | _____ | _____ |
|    e. Grasped your fist with the other hand. | _____ | _____ | _____ |
|    f. Pressed your fist and hand into the person's abdomen with a quick, upward thrust. | _____ | _____ | _____ |
|    g. Repeated thrusts until the object was expelled or the person lost consciousness. | _____ | _____ | _____ |
| 4. Lowered the unresponsive person to the floor or ground. Positioned the person supine. | _____ | _____ | _____ |
| 5. Activated the EMS system or the agency's emergency response system. | _____ | _____ | _____ |
| 6. Did a finger sweep to check for a foreign object. | _____ | _____ | _____ |
|    a. Opened the person's mouth. Used the tongue-jaw lift method. | _____ | _____ | _____ |
|       (1) Grasped the person's tongue and lower jaw with your thumb and fingers. | _____ | _____ | _____ |
|       (2) Lifted the lower jaw upward. | _____ | _____ | _____ |
|    b. Inserted your other index finger into the mouth along the side of the cheek and deep into the throat. The finger was at the base of the tongue. | _____ | _____ | _____ |
|    c. Formed a hook with your index finger. | _____ | _____ | _____ |
|    d. Tried to dislodge and remove the object. Did not push it deeper into the throat. | _____ | _____ | _____ |
|    e. Grasped and removed the object if it was within reach. | _____ | _____ | _____ |
| 7. Opened the airway with the head-tilt/chin-lift method. | _____ | _____ | _____ |
| 8. Gave 1 or 2 rescue breaths. | _____ | _____ | _____ |
| 9. Repositioned the person's head if the chest did not rise. Gave 1 or 2 rescue breaths. | _____ | _____ | _____ |

| Procedure—cont'd | S | U | Comments |
|---|---|---|---|
| 10. Gave up to 5 abdominal thrusts (See procedure "FBAO-The Unresponsive Adult"). | _____ | _____ | _____ |
| 11. Repeated steps 6 through 10 (finger sweeps, rescue breathing, and abdominal thrusts) until rescue breathing was effective. Started CPR if necessary. | _____ | _____ | _____ |

Date of Satisfactory Completion _____ Instructor's Initials_____

# FBAO—The Unresponsive Adult

Name: _____   Date: _____

| Procedure | S | U | Comments |
|---|---|---|---|
| 1. Checked to see if the person was responding. | _____ | _____ | _____ |
| 2. Called for help. Activated the EMS system or the agency's emergency response system. | _____ | _____ | _____ |
| 3. Logrolled the person to the supine position with his or her face up. Arms were at the sides. | _____ | _____ | _____ |
| 4. Opened the airway. Use the head-tilt/chin-lift method. | _____ | _____ | _____ |
| 5. Checked for breathing. | _____ | _____ | _____ |
| 6. Gave 1 or 2 slow rescue breaths. Repositioned the person's head and opened the airway if the chest did not rise. Gave 1 or 2 rescue breaths. | _____ | _____ | _____ |
| 7. Gave 5 abdominal thrusts if you could not ventilate the person. | _____ | _____ | _____ |
| • Straddled the person's thighs. | _____ | _____ | _____ |
| • Placed the heel of one hand against the abdomen. It was in the middle above the navel and below the end of the sternum (breastbone). | _____ | _____ | _____ |
| • Placed your second hand on top of your first hand. | _____ | _____ | _____ |
| • Pressed both hands into the abdomen with a quick, upward thrust. Gave 5 thrusts. | _____ | _____ | _____ |
| 8. Did a finger sweep to check for a foreign object. (See "FBAO—The Responsive Adult") | _____ | _____ | _____ |
| 9. Repeated steps 6 through 8 until rescue breathing was effective. Started CPR if necessary. | _____ | _____ | _____ |

Date of Satisfactory Completion_____   Instructor's Initials_____

## Assisting With Postmortem Care

Name: _____     Date: _____

| Pre-Procedure | S | U | Comments |
|---|---|---|---|

1. Followed "Delegation Guidelines: Postmortem Care." Reviewed "Promoting Safety and Comfort: Postmortem Care."  _____ _____ _____
2. Practiced hand hygiene.  _____ _____ _____
3. Collected the following:
   - Postmortem kit (shroud or body bag, gown, ID tags, gauze squares, safety pins)  _____ _____ _____
   - Bed protectors  _____ _____ _____
   - Wash basin  _____ _____ _____
   - Bath towels and washcloths  _____ _____ _____
   - Denture cup  _____ _____ _____
   - Tape  _____ _____ _____
   - Dressings  _____ _____ _____
   - Gloves  _____ _____ _____
   - Cotton balls  _____ _____ _____
   - Gown  _____ _____ _____
   - Valuables envelope  _____ _____ _____
4. Provided for privacy.  _____ _____ _____
5. Raised the bed for body mechanics.  _____ _____ _____
6. Made sure the bed was flat.  _____ _____ _____

## Procedure

7. Put on the gloves.  _____ _____ _____
8. Positioned the body supine. Arms and legs were straight. A pillow was under the head and shoulders.  _____ _____ _____
9. Closed the eyes. Gently pulled the eyelids over the eyes. Applied moist cotton balls gently over the eyelids if the eyes would not stay closed.  _____ _____ _____
10. Inserted dentures if it was agency policy. If not, put them in a labeled denture cup.  _____ _____ _____
11. Closed the mouth. If necessary, placed a rolled towel under the chin to keep the mouth closed.  _____ _____ _____
12. Followed agency policy about jewelry. Removed all jewelry, except for wedding rings if this was agency policy. Listed the jewelry that you removed. Placed the jewelry and the list in a valuables envelope.  _____ _____ _____

*Continued*

| Procedure—cont'd | S | U | Comments |
|---|---|---|---|

13. Placed a cotton ball over the rings. Taped them in place.  _____ _____ _____

14. Removed drainage containers. Left tubes and catheters in place if there would be an autopsy. Asked the nurse about removing tubes.  _____ _____ _____

15. Bathed soiled areas with plain water. Dried thoroughly.  _____ _____ _____

16. Placed a bed protector under the buttocks.  _____ _____ _____

17. Removed soiled dressings. Replaced them with clean ones.  _____ _____ _____

18. Put a clean gown on the body. Positioned the body as in step 8.  _____ _____ _____

19. Brushed and combed the hair if necessary.  _____ _____ _____

20. Covered the body to the shoulders with a sheet if the family would view the body.  _____ _____ _____

21. Gathered the person's belongings. Put them in a bag labeled with the person's name.  _____ _____ _____

22. Removed supplies, equipment, and linens. Straightened the room. Provided soft lighting.  _____ _____ _____

23. Removed the gloves. Decontaminated hands.  _____ _____ _____

24. Let the family view the body. Provided for privacy. Returned to the room after they left.  _____ _____ _____

25. Decontaminated hands. Put on gloves.  _____ _____ _____

26. Filled out the ID tags. Tied one to the ankle or to the right big toe.  _____ _____ _____

27. Placed the body in the body bag or covered it with a sheet. Or applied the shroud.  _____ _____ _____

    a. Brought the top down over the head.  _____ _____ _____

    b. Folded the bottom up over the feet.  _____ _____ _____

    c. Folded the sides over the body.  _____ _____ _____

    d. Pinned or taped the shroud in place.  _____ _____ _____

28. Attached the second ID tag to the shroud, sheet, or body bag.  _____ _____ _____

29. Left the denture cup with the body.  _____ _____ _____

30. Pulled the privacy curtain around the bed or closed the door.  _____ _____ _____

## Post-Procedure

31. Removed the gloves. Decontaminated hands.  _____ _____ _____

32. Stripped the unit after the body was removed. Wore gloves for this step.  _____ _____ _____

33. Removed the gloves. Decontaminated hands.  _____ _____ _____

34. Reported the following to the nurse:

    • The time the body was taken by the funeral director  _____ _____ _____

    • What was done with jewelry and personal items  _____ _____ _____

    • What was done with dentures  _____ _____ _____

Date of Satisfactory Completion _____     Instructor's Initials_____